Contributions to Psychology and Medicine

Contributions to Psychology and Medicine

The Psychology of Childhood Illness
Christine Eiser

Psychological Aspects of Early Breast Cancer
Colette Ray/Michael Baum

Medical Thinking: The Psychology of Medical Judgment and Decision Making
Steven Schwartz/Timothy Griffin

Women With Cancer: Psychological Perspective
Barbara L. Anderson, Editor

The Somatizing Child: Diagnosis and Treatment of Conversion and Somatization Disorders
Elsa G. Shapiro/Alvin A. Rosenfeld with Norman Cohen and Dorothy Levine

Individual Differences, Stress, and Health Psychology
Michel Pierre Janisse, Editor

The Psychology of the Dentist Patient Relationship
Stephen Bochner

Prospects of Heart Surgery: Psychological Adjustments to Coronary Bypass Grafting
Alan Radley

Neuropsychological and Behavioral Aspects of Diabetes
Clarissa S. Holmes, Editor

Clarissa S. Holmes
Editor

Neuropsychological and Behavioral Aspects of Diabetes

With 12 Illustrations

Springer-Verlag
New York Berlin Heidelberg
London Paris Tokyo Hong Kong

Clarissa S. Holmes
Department of Pediatrics
The University of Iowa Hospitals and Clinics
The University of Iowa
Iowa City, IA 52242
USA

Advisor
J. Richard Eiser
Department of Psychology
Washington Singer Laboratories
University of Exeter
Exeter EX4 4QG
England

Library of Congress Cataloging-in-Publication Data
Neuropsychological and behavioral aspects of diabetes/Clarissa S. Holmes, editor.
p. cm.—(Contributions to psychology and medicine)
Includes index.
ISBN 0-387-97075-4 (alk. paper)
1. Diabetes—Psychological aspects. 2. Clinical neuropsychology.
I. Holmes, Clarissa S. II. Series.
[DNLM: 1. Diabetes Mellitus—psychology. 2. Neuropsychology. WK 810 N494]
RC660.N39 1989
616.4′62′0019—dc20
DNLM/DLC 89-19683

Printed on acid-free paper

Typeset by Caliber Design Planning, Inc.
Printed and bound by R.R. Donnelley & Sons, Harrisonburg, Virginia.
Printed in the United States of America.

9 8 7 6 5 4 3 2 1

ISBN 0-387-97075-4 Springer-Verlag New York Berlin Heidelberg
ISBN 3-540-97075-4 Springer-Verlag Berlin Heidelberg New York

Preface

Behavioral medicine has blossomed as an area of systematic investigation during the past 10–20 years. Throughout its steady growth, there have been increasing interest and specialization in the study of neuropsychological and behavioral aspects of diabetes. This book attempts to capture and report exciting new developments in the study of both insulin-dependent (Type I) and non-insulin-dependent (Type II) diabetes mellitus. Accordingly, it is divided into two major sections.

Physiological aspects of each disease, which differ significantly in pathophysiology and course, are discussed in separate medical overviews that introduce each major section. These overviews are written by Drs. Tsalikian and Zimmerman, leading medical researchers in insulin- and non-insulin-dependent diabetes, respectively. Each section also contains chapters describing neuropsychological and cognitive disease correlates, psychosocial patterns of adjustment, and treatment adherence issues. Psychological aspects of insulin-dependent diabetes have been studied more extensively than non-insulin-dependent diabetes, perhaps because it is more often associated with graver medical complications. Therefore, there is a larger body of research to review and the first section has been divided into chapters on cognitive disease sequelae in populations of children and adults, separately. In his chapter, Dr. Ryan discusses developmental factors related to the unique sensitivity of the brain to metabolic derangement. Dr. Holmes reviews studies of adults with diabetes and the cognitive correlates of both acute and chronic blood glucose disruption. Developmental disease issues are further covered in Dr. Delamater's chapter of children's adaptation to disease following initial diagnosis, and Dr. Johnson's review of adherence and health issues in children. Familial adaptation of pediatric and adult patients is discussed in Dr. Anderson's chapter.

Because of the relatively fragile metabolic balance of patients with Type I diabetes, these patients are particularly vulnerable to the effects of eating disorders. Further, since individuals with insulin-dependent diabetes must conscientiously monitor, calculate, and manage their food intake, such undue attention may place them at increased risk for eating disorders. This evidence is reviewed by Dr. Marcus in her chapter describing eating problems. Dr. Gonder-Frederick and her colleagues discuss the ability of patients to perceive, and ultimately to treat, variations in blood glucose levels. This issue is important, given the lability of blood glucose fluctuation in Type I diabetes, and the risk of severe hypoglycemia.

Non-insulin-dependent diabetes more frequently occurs in obese adults than does the insulin-dependent type; accordingly, different disease management issues are present. The effect of stress interacts systematically with metabolic control in Type II diabetes, and the physiological framework, and experimental findings, of this work are described by Dr. Surwit in his chapter. Strategies for weight loss and their relative success are reviewed by Dr. Wing, for both the adult population as a whole, and those with non-insulin-dependent diabetes. Dr. Perlmuter and colleagues describe studies of cognitive functioning and its relation to both disease and motivational variables.

Dr. Geringer's chapter on affective disorders points out some of the hormonal similarities between Type I and II diabetes. Both environmental and, most interestingly, physiological evidence is reviewed that may relate to elevated rates of depression with these diseases. Studies of affective disorders in diabetic populations frequently compare the status of patients with both types of disease; therefore, depression in these two groups is reviewed within the same chapter.

It is the hope of the editor that collection of this information into one source will aid both researchers and practitioners in the evaluation of relevant disease factors that may require further study or clinical monitoring and intervention.

June, 1989

Acknowledgments

The editor wishes to express her appreciation to Dr. Suzanne Bennett Johnson and Dr. Lawrence Perlmuter for their assistance in identifying potential contributors to the book. Kathy Funk was instrumental in her typing assistance and in her help with coordinating various aspects of the project. Finally, the editor wishes to thank her family, Bill and Ashley Cooper, for the inspiration and fortitude that they have provided for her.

Contents

Contributors

BARBARA J. ANDERSON, PH.D.
Joslin Clinic, Boston, MA 02215, USA

DANIEL J. COX, PH.D.
Department of Psychiatry, University of Virginia School of Medicine, Charlottesville, VA 22901, USA

ALAN M. DELAMATER, PH.D.
Department of Psychology, Wayne State University, Detroit, MI 48202, USA

LEONARD H. EPSTEIN, PH.D.
University of Pittsburgh School of Medicine, Pittsburgh, PA 15213, USA

MARK N. FEINGLOS, M.D.
Division of Endocrinology, Department of Medicine, Duke University Medical Center, Durham, NC 27710, USA

EDITH S. GERINGER, M.D.
Department of Psychiatry, Massachusetts General Hospital, Boston, MA 02108, USA

STEVEN H. GOLDFINGER, PH.D.
VA Outpatient Clinic, Boston, MA 02108, USA

LINDA A. GONDER-FREDERICK, PH.D.
University of Virginia, Charlottesville, VA 22901, USA

CLARISSA S. HOLMES, PH.D.
Departments of Psychology and Pediatrics, Tulane University, New Orleans, LA 70118, USA

SUZANNE BENNETT JOHNSON, PH.D.
Department of Psychiatry, J. Hillis Miller Health Center, University of Florida, Gainesville, FL 32610, USA

MARSHA D. MARCUS, PH.D.
Western Psychiatric Institute and Clinic, University of Pittsburgh School of Medicine, Pittsburgh, PA 15213, USA

DAVID M. NATHAN, M.D.
Harvard Medical School, Boston, MA 02108, USA

LAWRENCE PERLMUTER, PH.D.
Memory and Learning Clinic, VA Outpatient Clinic, Boston, MA 02108, USA

SUZANNE L. ROSS, PH.D.
Division of Medical Psychology, Department of Psychiatry, Duke University Medical Center, Durham, NC 27710, USA

CHRISTOPHER M. RYAN, PH.D.
Western Psychiatric Institute and Clinic, University of Pittsburgh School of Medicine, Pittsburgh, PA 15213, USA

ANNE R. SHORE, B.A.
Memory and Learning Clinic, VA Outpatient Clinic, Boston MA, 02108, USA

RICHARD S. SURWIT, PH.D.
Division of Medical Psychology, Department of Psychiatry, Duke University Medical Center, Durham, NC 27710, USA

EVA TSALIKIAN, M.D.
Division of Pediatric Endocrinology, Department of Pediatrics, University of Iowa Hospitals and Clinics, Iowa City, IA 52242, USA

RENA R. WING, PH.D.
Western Psychiatric Institute and Clinics, University of Pittsburgh School of Medicine, Pittsburgh, PA 15213, USA

BRUCE R. ZIMMERMAN, M.D.
Department of Endocrinology, Mayo Clinic, Rochester, MN 55905, USA

Section I

Insulin-Dependent Diabetes

1

Insulin-Dependent (Type I) Diabetes Mellitus: Medical Overview

Eva Tsalikian

Insulin-dependent diabetes mellitus (IDDM) or Type I diabetes is a syndrome of impaired energy homeostasis caused by inadequate insulin supply from the beta cells of the pancreatic islets in order to meet insulin requirements by peripheral tissues. This imbalance in the supply and demand for insulin results in abnormal carbohydrate, fat, and protein metabolism. This syndrome can present at any age but it is commonly first diagnosed during childhood and adolescence. Only a very small percentage of young individuals diagnosed with diabetes have non-insulin-dependent or Type II diabetes, whereas in the adult population IDDM has a very low incidence in comparison with non-insulin-dependent diabetes mellitus (NIDDM). The two syndromes are distinctly different in their etiology and pathophysiology and should not be confused. The old nomenclature of juvenile-onset diabetes for IDDM and maturity-onset diabetes for NIDDM is not considered accurate and is not used any longer.

Etiology—Epidemiology

At the time of presentation of IDDM a large number of insulin-secreting cells of the pancreatic islets is already destroyed from a process that is now widely believed to be of autoimmune etiology (Eisenbarth, 1986; Gorsuch, Spencer, Lister, et al. 1981). The timing and course of this destructive process is not clearly understood and therefore the exact causative factors are not yet identified. Genetic factors that control the body's immune responses, age, seasonal variation, or chemicals have all been implicated in the etiology of diabetes although no one single factor has been yet identified as capable of causing IDDM. Epidemiologic studies on the prevalence, incidence, geographic distribution, and variation with age and sex have attempted to elucidate the factors affecting the onset of IDDM. In recent years research in the etiology and epidemiology of IDDM has immensely contributed to our understanding of the disease.

Approximately 1 in 500 children less than 18 years of age in the United States will contract diabetes (LaPorte, Fishbein, Drash et al., 1981). This incidence is primarily observed in white children. Black children are affected less frequently. Geographical distribution in the few countries where studies have been completed indicates wide variation with highest incidence in Finland and Norway and lowest in Japan (WHO Study Group, 1985). The age of onset is also variable with a peak in the frequency of new onset observed during the early pubertal years (LaPorte et al., 1981). The peak seems to be at an earlier age for females than males as it would be expected considering the differential time of the growth spurt and onset of puberty for males and females. Recent studies indicate that there may be a slightly higher incidence of IDDM in boys than in girls younger than 15 years of age (Dahlquist, Blom, Holmgren et al., 1985).

As is true for several diseases with autoimmune etiology, IDDM is closely associated with the major histocompatibility genes located on the short arm of chromosome 6. More than 90% of children with IDDM are HLA DR3 and/or HLA DR4 positive (Cahill & McDevitt, 1981) but these antigens still appear to be insufficient genetic factors for the development of IDDM. It has been hypothesized that since these antigens are important in regulating the immune response, their presence results in specific susceptibility in the individuals endowed with them. This susceptibility under the right circumstances, i.e., insults from viruses, chemicals, etc., will result in the initiation of the destructive process against the beta cell, mediated by cellular or humoral immunologic mechanisms (Scott, Nerup, & Lernmark, 1985).

Presentation—Management

Destruction of the pancreatic beta cell results in inadequate insulin supply. Insulin is the main hormone necessary for glucose and energy homeostasis. Glucose is provided to the body by the carbohydrate content of diet. Only a portion of dietary glucose intake is introduced into the circulation for utilization by peripheral tissues for energy. The rest is stored into the liver as glycogen and released as needed. Insulin regulates the fine balance between glucose supply by the liver and uptake by peripheral tissues except for the brain. In IDDM low serum insulin concentrations allow glycogen breakdown and release of glucose by the liver while peripheral glucose uptake is inhibited resulting in hyperglycemia. Hyperglycemia leads to glycosuria which, in turn, causes excessive urine excretion resulting in polyuria and polydipsia. Because of the excessive loss of water and the inadequate energy supply to the tissues, weight loss is also manifested. Polyuria, polydipsia, and weight loss are the most common presenting symptoms. Furthermore, inadequate insulin supply results in excessive fat breakdown and accumulation in the circulation of the end products of this process, the ketone bodies, and eventual excretion in the urine (ketonuria). High plasma glucose and ketone body concentrations if not treated promptly leads to diabetic ketoacidosis, a severe condition manifested by vomiting, dehydration, Kussmaul respiration, and finally coma.

Presentation of IDDM is not different in children and adults but treatment and management of the disease may vary in the two age groups. In this chapter emphasis will be mostly on the management of diabetes in children. At the time of original diagnosis, signs and symptoms usually have been present from a few days to a few weeks.

Treatment of children with diabetes is first directed toward normalization of the metabolic disturbances observed at presentation. Careful rehydration and insulin administration are used in the first 24–48 hours following diagnosis. Subsequently, treatment is directed toward achievement of long-term glucose and overall metabolic control for maintenance of symptom-free growth and development in these children and for prevention of diabetes complications. In order to achieve this goal insulin administration, dietary management, and physical fitness are all very closely related functions that need to be incorporated in the everyday management of diabetes with equally weighted importance and intensity. In recent years an attempt has been made to use immunosuppressive agents in the treatment of children with newly diagnosed diabetes. Although cyclosporin therapy is frequently successful in eliminating insulin requirements (Bougneres, Carel, Castano et al., 1988), the beneficial effect is only present with continuous treatment. Prolonged treatment with cyclosporin has both short- and long-term side effects (Myers, Ross, Newton et al., 1984) and therefore is not recommended for treatment at this time until further studies are completed. To this day, insulin administration remains the mainstay of treatment.

Several regimens and modes of insulin administration have been at times popular. The most common method is the use of two subcutaneous injections of a mixture of short- and intermediate-acting insulin given in the morning before breakfast and before supper in the evening. Approximately two thirds of the total daily dose is given in the morning and one third in the evening. The doses depend on the size and pubertal stage of the child and the time since diagnosis. Shortly after diagnosis a period of decreased insulin dose requirement is associated with regaining some residual function from the cell of the pancreas commonly called the "honeymoon period." This period lasts from a few weeks to several months and it is more prolonged in newly diagnosed adolescents. The mechanism contributing to this phenomenon is not well understood. There are no cases of sustained total reversal and regaining of full function of the pancreatic beta cells. Pubertal and postpubertal children and adolescents require slightly higher doses of insulin per kilogram body weight. Insulin doses are adjusted individually until metabolic control is achieved.

In children with diabetes, dietary needs in terms of caloric intake and composition are the same as in all other healthy children who do not have diabetes. Because of the fixed dose and time of insulin administration, meal timing and caloric intake has to be consistent on a daily basis (Brink, 1988). A common meal plan consists of three meals at usual times and three snacks at midmorning, midafternoon, and before bedtime. Contribution of calories in the diet is recommended as 55% of total from carbohydrate, 30% from fat, and 15% from protein. Higher-fiber-containing foods should be regularly included as long as they are compatible with the child's taste and eating habits. In devising a meal plan for a growing child the specific needs should be addressed, including variable intake according to activity level as well as allowing "extras" such as sweets on special occasions so that the child does not feel restricted and excluded from peer social activities.

Physical exercise in a child with diabetes should be encouraged and at no time restricted. Correct management of glucose control, taking into consideration the variable times of physical activity each day, can allow for uneventful participation to all types of activities including competitive sports for the older child and adolescent. Exercise is commonly believed to cause hypoglycemia because of the rapid utilization of substrates and is usually recommended as a way to improve metabolic control. Although activity and exercise are very important factors for maintenance of a well-balanced program of metabolic control, exercise may cause hyperglycemia mostly when the child is already in poor control when exercise starts. Therefore correction of poor metabolic control is recommended prior to intense activity. One of the problems encountered during intense activity is the rapid absorption of insulin from the site of injection (Zimman, Murray, Vranic et al., 1977). This rapid absorption may result in hypoglycemia. It is recommended that insulin is not given to limbs that will be exercised shortly following an injection.

In the last 10–15 years good glucose control has been achieved much easier and more accurately because of the introduction of home blood glucose monitoring. Children and adolescents and their families are able to assess blood glucose control at home by obtaining capillary blood several times a day ("Symposium on Home Glucose Monitoring," 1980). A commonly used schedule calls for children to assess their capillary blood glucose three or four times a day, record the readings, and consult with the record daily so that appropriate insulin dose adjustments are made as necessary. Urinary glucose monitoring is not deemed necessary if the above schedule of capillary blood glucose is followed. Ketonuria is monitored only with concomitant pronounced hyperglycemia. Overall long-term glucose control can be monitored with glycosylated hemoglobin measurements at regular intervals (Gabbay, Hasty, Breslow et al., 1977).

Glycosylated hemoglobin comprises a percentage of total hemoglobin A proportional to the blood glucose concentration during the 2–3 months prior to the measurement (Nathan, Singer, Hurxthal, & Goodson, 1984). Hemoglobin A is a short-lived protein (life span 2–3 months) the structure of which can be altered by nonenzymatic attachment of the glucose molecule on the amino terminus of this protein. The product of this alteration of the HgA molecule is the HgA_1 or glycosylated hemoglobin. Separation of glycosylated hemoglobin or HgA_1 from total hemoglobin is done by chromatrographic techniques. HgA_1 is comprised of three different peaks $HgA_1(a + b + c)$, the peak most accurately reflecting hyperglycemia is HgA_{1c} and it is measured most commonly. The normal range for HgA_{1c} concentration is lower than total glycosylated HgA or HgA_1 (Garlick, Mazer, Higgins, & Bunn, 1983).

Although HgA_{1c} has been widely used for monitoring of long-term glycemia, there are shortcomings to this method, one of which is the possible effect of the blood glucose concentration at the time of measurement on the level of glycosylated hemoglobin (Goldstein, Peth, England, Hess, & Da Costa, 1980).

In children and mostly in adolescents it is difficult to maintain the levels of HgA_{1c} at normal range reflecting the difficulty in maintaining euglycemia in these patients (Goldstein, Walker, Rawlins et al., 1980). The goal of treatment should be to strive to maintain HgA_{1c} and therefore glucose and overall metabolic control as close to the normal range as possible. This goal should not interfere with the child's normal physical and psychological development.

Hypoglycemia

Optimal metabolic control with the goal to achieve euglycemia most of the times of day and night is complicated occasionally by frequent hypoglycemia. Hypoglycemia is usually the result of excess insulin, inadequate caloric intake, and/or untimely excess activity, each alone or in some combination. Hypoglycemia is manifested by symptoms of hunger, shakiness, lightheadedness, unconsciousness, seizures, and coma, depending on severity. Symptoms and signs of hypoglycemia depend also on age. The ability of the child and parents to recognize and respond to the first signs of hypoglycemia will many times determine the extent of symptoms. When recognized, early hypoglycemia is easily treated with rapidly absorbed glucose by mouth such as sugar added in orange juice. If symptoms have progressed and the child is unable to swallow, an injection of glucagon rapidly reverses hypoglycemic symptoms (Aman & Wranne, 1988).

Physiologically hypoglycemia stimulates counterregulatory hormones such as glucagon, growth hormone, and epinephrine. These hormones increase glucose release by the liver and decrease peripheral uptake of glucose by tissues resulting in reversal of hypoglycemia. Prolonged duration of IDDM may cause a delayed response of these hormones (Bolli et al., 1983). Furthermore, symptoms may vary in the very young or even in the older child which may prevent prompt recognition of hypoglycemia. Both of these reasons may result in untreated prolonged hypoglycemia. This unrecognized prolonged hypoglycemia will be a further stimulus for counterregulatory hormone release with the end result being excessive hyperglycemia. Commonly, this phenomenon has been observed in the early morning when hyperglycemia following nocturnal hypoglycemia is called the Somogyi phenomenon.

Except for the Somogyi phenomenon, early morning hyperglycemia, a rather common phenomenon complicating metabolic control, can be caused by lack of adequate insulin in the early morning hours or a physiologic phenomenon called the Dawn phenomenon. This latter hyperglycemic phenomenon is probably present as well in nondiabetic individuals and is believed to be due to the physiologic nocturnal surge of growth hormone (Bolli & Gerich, 1984). Treatment of early morning hyperglycemia should be instituted according to the perceived cause for the hyperglycemia. A middle of the night capillary blood glucose check can provide information on the existence of hypoglycemia prior to hyperglycemia and direct to the appropriate insulin adjustment.

Complications of IDDM

The major cause for morbidity and mortality in patients with IDDM is from the long-term microvascular and macrovascular complications of diabetes and peripheral neuropathy. The macrovascular complications result in an increased incidence of heart disease and cerebrovascular episodes in individuals with IDDM as well as peripheral vascular occlusion resulting in limb amputations. The microvascular changes affect primarily the eyes and kidneys. Diabetic retinopathy and nephropathy lead to blindness and renal failure. Diabetes is the most common cause of blindness in the United States and kidney transplants for renal failure due to diabetes are performed most commonly than for any other cause. Diabetic retinopathy and nephropathy has an incidence of up to 30–40% following 20 years of duration of the disease (Krolewski et al., 1986). These complications are never present prior to at least 5–10 years of duration and according to most of the studies they are not present prior to puberty in children regardless of duration (Burger, Hovener, Dusterhus, Hartman, & Weber, 1986). The pathophysiology of the microangiopathic complications of diabetes is not clearly understood. Recent studies have demonstrated alterations of the structure and function of tissue proteins by nonenzymatic glycosylation (Brownlee, Vlassara, & Cerami, 1984) that most probably result in the microangiopathic changes present in diabetes. These mechanisms imply a direct role of hyperglycemia on the pathogenesis of diabetes complications. Likewise for the neuropathic complications of diabetes, recent studies have shown that abnormal myoinositol metabolism due to hyperglycemia (Greene, Lattimer, Ulbrecht, & Carroll, 1985) is the etiologic mechanism for this common complication of diabetes. The question whether good metabolic control is related to the presentation and incidence of diabetes complications is a very important one and remains unanswered. A prospective national study is underway to address this question (The DCCT Research Group, 1987). Furthermore, the effect of specific genetic predisposition on the incidence of these complications remains a question that has been addressed but without satisfactory answers at this time. Existing evidence presently dictates trying to achieve as good metabolic control as possible with the therapeutic measures presently available.

The future for patients with IDDM holds a multitude of avenues for hope for more effective treatment either by new agents directed against the primary etiologic insult or by pancreas or islet transplantation. Furthermore it is reasonable to believe that prevention of diabetes is not such a distant and unreachable goal anymore and that the work of multiple investigators in the field (Maclaren, 1988) will yield success for definitive prevention and cure.

References

Aman, J., & Wranne, L. (1988). Hypoglycaemia of childhood diabetes. II. Effect of subcutaneous or intramuscular injection of different doses of glucagon. *Acta Paediatrica Scandinavica 77*, 548–553.

Bolli, G., De Feo, P., Compagnucci, P., Cartechini, M., Angeletti, G., Santeusanio, F., Brunetti, P., & Gerich, J. (1983). Abnormal glucose counterregulation in insulin-dependent diabetes mellitus: Interaction of anti-insulin antibodies and impaired glucagon and epinephrine secretion. *Diabetes 32*, 134–141.

Bolli, G., & Gerich, J. (1984). The dawn phenomenon—a common occurrence in both non-insulin dependent and insulin-dependent diabetes mellitus. *New England Journal of Medicine 310*, 746–750.

Bougneres, P.F., Carel, J.C., Castano, L., et al. (1988). Factors associated with early remission of Type I diabetes in children treated with cyclosporine. *New England Journal of Medicine 318*, 663–670.

Brink, S.J. (1988). Pediatric, adolescent, and young-adult nutrition issues in IDDM. *Diabetes Care 11*, 192–200.

Brownlee, M., Vlassara, H., & Cerami, A. (1984). Nonenzymatic glycosylation and the pathogenesis of diabetic complications. *Annals of Internal Medicine 101*, 527–537.

Burger, W., Hovener, G., Dusterhus, R., Hartmann, R., & Weber, B. Prevalance and development of retinopathy in children and adolescents with type I (insulin-dependent) diabetes mellitus. A longitudinal study. *Diabetologia 29*, 17–22.

Cahill, G.F., & McDevitt, H.O. (1981). Insulin-dependent diabetes mellitus: The initial lesion. *New England Journal of Medicine 304*, 1454–1465.

Dahlquist, G., Blom, L., Holmgren, G., et al. (1985). The epidemiology of diabetes in Swedish children 0–14 year—A six-year prospective study. *Diabetologia 28*, 802–808.

Eisenbarth, G.S. (1986) Type I diabetes mellitus: A chronic autoimmune disease. *New England Journal of Medicine 314*, 1360–1368.

Gabbay, K.H., Hasty, K., Breslow, J.L., et al. (1977). Glycosylated hemoglobin and long-term blood glucose control in diabetes mellitus. *Journal of Clinical Endocrinology and Metabolism 44*, 859.

Garlick, R.L., Mazer, J.S., Higgins, P.J., & Bunn, H.F. (1983). Characterization of glycosylated hemoglobins. *Journal of Clinical Investigation 71*, 1062–1072.

Goldstein, D.E., Peth, S.B., England, J.D., Hess, R.L., & Da Costa, J. Effects of acute changes in blood glucose on HbA_{1c}. *Diabetes 29*, 623–628.

Goldstein, D.E., Walker, B., Rawlings, S.S., et al. (1980). Hemoglobin Alc levels in children and adolescents with diabetes mellitus. *Diabetes Care 3*, 503.

Gorsuch, A.N., Spencer, K.M., Lister, J., et al. (1981). The natural history of type I (insulin-dependent) diabetes mellitus: Evidence for a long prediabetic period. *Lancet 2*, 1363–1365.

Greene, D.A., Lattimer, S., Ulbrecht, J., & Carroll, P. (1985). Glucose-induced alterations in nerve metabolism: Current perspective on the pathogenesis of diabetic neuropathy and future directions for research and therapy. *Diabetes Care 8*, 290–299.

Krolewski, A.S., Warram, J.H., Rand, L.I., Christlieb, A.R., Busick, E.J., & Kahn, C.R. (1986). Risk of proliferative diabetic retinopathy in juvenile-onsent type I diabetes: A 40-year follow-up study. *Diabetes Care 9*, 443–452.

LaPorte, R.E., Fishbein, H.A., Drash, A.L., et al. (1981). The Pittsburgh insulin-dependent diabetes mellius (IDDM) registry: The incidence of insulin-dependent diabetes mellitus in Allegheny County Pennsylvania (1965–1976). *Diabetes 30*, 279–284.

Maclaren, N.K. (1988). How, when, and why to predict IDDM. *Diabetes 37*, 1591–1594.

Myers, B.D., Ross, J., Newton, L., et al. (1984). Cyclosporine-associated chronic nephropathy. *New England Journal of Medicine 11*, 699–705.

Nathan, D.M., Singer, D.E., Hurxthal, K., & Goodson, J.D. (1984). The clinical information value of the glycosylated hemoglobin assay. *New England Journal of Medicine 310*, 341–346.

Scott, J., Nerup, J., & Lernmark, A. (1985). Immunologic factors in diabetes mellitus. In, W.F. Rosse (Ed.), *Clinical immunology update* (pp. 53–85) New York: Elsevier.

Symposium on home glucose monitoring. (1980). *Diabetes Care 3*, 57.

The DCCT Research Group. (1987). Diabetes control and complications trial (DCCT): Results of feasibility study. *Diabetes Care 10*, 1–19.

WHO Study Group (1985). *Diabetes mellitus*. WHO Technical Reports Series 727. World Health Organization: Geneva.

Zimman, G., Murray, F.T., Vranic, M., et al. (1977). Glucoregulation during moderate exercise in insulin treated diabetics. *Journal of Clinical Endocrinology and Metabolism 45*, 641.

2

Adaptation of Children to Newly Diagnosed Diabetes

Alan M. Delamater

The most common metabolic disease of childhood is insulin-dependent or Type I diabetes mellitus. The disease usually is diagnosed between infancy and 35 years of age. Two peaks of incidence have been noted in children, at about 5–6 and 11–13 years of age (Drash, 1979). The onset of symptoms is acute and includes polyuria, polyphagia, polydipsia, weakness, weight loss, and fatigue. These symptoms are due to the inability of the individual to metabolize glucose and the subsequent utilization of fat as a source of alternative energy. With severe insulin deficiency, fatty acids are converted to ketones and reach high levels in the blood and urine. Unless this condition is treated, diabetic ketoacidosis occurs, resulting in loss of consciousness, coma, and death.

When a child is diagnosed, it is both a medical crisis and a crisis of adaptation for the child and family. Within a brief period of time, usually a few weeks, the child's health deteriorates, diabetes is diagnosed, and the child is hospitalized. Generally, the child's physical condition is quickly stabilized in the hospital with IV fluids and insulin. During the first few days after diagnosis, patients and families must learn a complex set of skills necessary for daily diabetes management. Typically, diabetes education occurs in several massed learning sessions during the approximately 5 days of hospitalization at diagnosis. After discharge from the hospital, outpatient follow-up care is provided at regular intervals.

When they are sent home, the child and family are faced with the prospect of daily management of a disease which has no cure and could quickly become life-threatening. Assuming such responsibility can be very stressful to many families (Hamburg & Inoff, 1983). Successful adaptation to diabetes involves a reorganization of the family itself, since the regimen affects essential aspects of daily life, including planning and modification of eating and exercise, as well as daily administration of insulin and monitoring of glucose levels. Roles and responsibilities must be clarified, expectations communicated, and specific behaviors monitored and reinforced. In addition, the family begins to form and develop a new set of relationships with the health-care team members, with whom they will be in regular contact and upon whom they will rely.

Children with diabetes will eventually have an absolute insulin deficiency. However, during the first 24 months after diagnosis, their pancreas may produce some insulin (Ludvigsson & Heding, 1976). This period is often referred to as the "honeymoon" period, since metabolic control is easier to achieve. Residual pancreatic beta-cell activity is determined by measurement of C-peptide. Studies have indicated that stimulated C-peptide, as determined by radio-immunoassay techniques, is inversely correlated with duration of diabetes (Ludvigsson & Heding, 1976; Madsbad, Faber, & Binder, 1978) and is associated with better metabolic control (Beischer et al., 1978; Madsbad, McNair, & Faber, 1980). In a study by Dahlquist and colleagues (Dahlquist et al., 1982) of 131 children, C-peptide correlated with glycosylated hemoglobin A1 (a long-term measure of antecedent blood glucose control) better than age, duration, insulin dose, or number of insulin injections per day. Since residual beta-cell activity continues to some extent throughout the first 24 months after diagnosis of diabetes (Ludvigsson & Heding, 1976), it is crucial to measure C-peptide during this period in order to partial out its effects on metabolic control so that the impact of other variables may be more clearly ascertained.

The adaptation process has not been studied well until fairly recently. Clinical observations have suggested that the diagnosis poses a considerable stress to the child and family (Geist, 1979; Tarnow & Tomlinson, 1978; Wishner & O'Brien, 1978) and that reactions to diagnosis may predict later ways of coping with disease management (Tietz & Vidmar, 1972). The purpose of this chapter is to review recent empirical research which has focused on the adaptation of newly diagnosed children and families. This research has considered the psychosocial adaptation of children and parents in longitudinal studies, age at onset in relation to psychosocial adjustment and cognitive abilities, and treatment outcome studies. The chapter will conclude with a discussion of methodological issues and future research.

Psychosocial Adaptation

Child Variables

Ahnsjo, Humble, Larsson, Settergren-Carlsson, and Sterky (1981) reported a longitudinal study of psychosocial adjustment of newly diagnosed children. Sixty-four diabetic children aged 4–17-years-old were compared with 30 matched controls on various measures of psychosocial functioning within 5 months of diagnosis and 9 years postdiagnosis. No differences were observed between the groups at either point in time. These authors concluded that the onset of diabetes does not impact adversely on psychosocial adjustment. However, several methodological difficulties limit this conclusion, including the use of non-blind raters and nonstandardized measures.

A recent study by Kovacs and colleagues (Kovacs, Feinberg, Paulauskas et al., 1985) employed more reliable methods for documenting the psychological status of children during the first year of diabetes. Seventy-four children (representing 76% of those contacted for participation) between the ages of 8 and 13 were evaluated 2–3 weeks after discharge from the hospital and several additional times during the first year. There was a normal amount of life stress and preexisting psychological problems in the year prior to diagnosis of diabetes. Results indicated that soon after diagnosis 36% of the children exhibited reactions that met criteria for psychiatric disorder, the most frequent of which was adjustment disorder with depression. However, 50% of these children had recovered by 3 months, and 93% had recovered by 9 months postdiagnosis. Marital distress and low socioeconomic status were more likely among those children who had psychiatric disorder. Kovacs et al. concluded that the majority of children coped well with the new life demands that diabetes imposes. The 36% prevalence of psychiatric disorder suggests that, while serious psychological distress at diagnosis is not the norm, it is also not necessarily pathologic, given the good recovery expected by 9 months post-diagnosis. For the 64% of children who did not experience significant distress, initial normative responses included depressed mood, anxiety, social withdrawal, and feelings of friendlessness. These psychological reactions were fairly transient.

In another report based on the same subjects, Kovacs, Brent, Steinberg, Paulauskas, and Reid (1986) investigated children's self-reports of psychological adjustment and coping strategies during the first year. Soon after diagnosis, self-ratings on standardized measures of depression, anxiety, and self-esteem indicated few emotional symptoms and positive self-esteem. Emotional symptoms decreased over the year, while feelings of self-esteem increased. Disease-related coping strategies were measured with a semistructured interview. Common behavioral strategies included information seeking and regimen-related behaviors, while common cognitive strategies included wishful thinking, thoughts of forbidden foods, and feelings of shock, bewilderment, and resentment. Coping strategies were unrelated to psychological variables.

Jacobson and colleagues (Jacobson et al., 1986) also studied the psychological adjustment of newly diagnosed children. In their study, 64 children between the ages of 9 and 15 years (representing 76% of those asked to participate) were compared with 68 control children (representing 54% of those asked to participate) who had experienced a recent acute medical problem (such as fractures, infections, appendicitis). Psychological variables examined included standardized self-report measures of self-esteem, locus of control, behavior problems, and diabetes adjustment. The evaluation took place at an average duration of 5 months for both groups, although the range was quite variable: 42% of diabetics were studied within the first 3 months and 28% studied between 6 and 12 months of diagnosis; 18% of the control patients were studied within 3 months of their illness, while 37% were evaluated between 6 and 12 months after their illness.

Results indicated no differences between the groups on measures of locus of control, behavior problems, or general self-esteem; the only difference between the groups was that diabetics reported decreased school-related competence. Although the authors suggest that the diagnosis of diabetes does not lead to psychological disruption, it is difficult to conclude anything about the impact of diagnosis in this study since prediagnosis measures were not obtained. In addition, because subjects were studied at variable intervals from the time of diagnosis, disruption in psychological functioning may have been obscured when group means were considered in the analyses. However, the findings do support the view that psychological adaptation in the first year of diabetes appears normal using standardized self-report measures.

It is interesting to note in this study that general measures of psychological functioning correlated significantly with a disease-specific measure of adjustment (i.e., the Diabetes Adjustment Scale). Better adjustment to having diabetes was associated with high self-esteem and self-competence, and less behavioral symptoms; worse adjustment to diabetes was associated with external locus of control. Jacboson et al. (1986) suggest that early adaptation to diabetes is related to overall personality development and coping patterns.

Family Variables

These same two sets of investigators have also examined family functioning with respect to the diagnosis of diabetes in children. While Jacobson and colleagues have studied the family environment and interactions as related to child functioning and in comparison with a control group, Kovacs and colleagues have studied the psychological responses of parents to the diagnosis of their child.

Hauser, Jacobson, Wertlieb, Brink, and Wentworth (1985) found that families of newly diagnosed diabetic children reported significantly more organization and recreational activities as compared with a control group of families with a child who experienced medical treatment for a recent acute problem. The authors suggest that families tend to pull together after the diagnosis as a coping response. This observation contrasts somewhat, but is not incompatible with the earlier clinical observations that diagnosis is stressful to family members (Krosnick, 1970; Wishner & O'Brien, 1978).

In testing the assumption that family factors are important mediators of the psychological adaptation of children to diagnosis, Wertlieb, Hauser, & Jacobson (1986) compared 46 newly diagnosed children with 29 acute illness control children on mother-rated measures of behavior problems (using the Child Behavior Checklist) and child-rated measures of family environment (using the Family Environment Scale). Evaluations were conducted at various points during the first year. There were no differences in either behavior problems or family environment, with both groups in the normative range. However, in correlating behavior problems with family environment, a different pattern emerged for the groups. For diabetics, problems increased with family conflict and decreased with organization and control, while for the comparison group, problems increased with organization and control and decreased with cohesion. The authors suggest that newly diagnosed families must deal with issues of control, limits, and rules somewhat differently than in nondiabetic families where a family's emphasis on control is related to behavioral problems in young adolescents.

In another report by these investigators (Hauser et al., 1986), direct observations were used to determine the effects of diagnosis on family interactions. Fifty-six diabetic families and 49 controls with recent acute illness participated. Subjects were apparently studied about 5–7 months after diagnosis. Results showed more enabling speech (i.e., focusing, problem-solving, and active understanding) in the patients and mothers, and more constraining (i.e., indifference, judgmental, devaluing) interactions among fathers of diabetics, compared with control families. The authors suggest that these patterns reflect the influence of the child's diabetes on family interactions, corresponding to the emotional tone of the family's reaction to the diagnosis. In other words, the enabling interactions reflect the hopefulness, optimism, and support felt by the family members, and the constraining interactions reflect the distress experienced by the family as the implications of the life-long condition are realized. Since mothers are typically more involved in the care-giving role in the family, the enabling pattern is more evident in the mother–child interaction, while negative affect is presumably more easily expressed by fathers. These suggestions would be more easily supported with both prediagnosis and postdiagnosis measures of family interaction so that the impact of diagnosis could be determined.

The psychological responses of parents to the diagnosis of their children were investigated in a longitudinal study by Kovacs, Finkelstein, et al., (1985). Both mothers and fathers of 74, 8- to 13-year-old children were studied. These were primarily intact, middle-class families. The initial assessment occurred 2–3 weeks after discharge from the hospital at diagnosis, with additional assessments 6–7 months and 1 year postdiagnosis. Standardized self-report measures of depression (the Beck Depression Inventory) and psychiatric symptoms (the SCL-90) were utilized, as well as clinician ratings of depression and anxiety (Hamilton Rating Scale) and clinical interviews to determine parental concerns and involvement in the regimen.

Results indicated that shortly after diagnosis, there was little evidence of major emotional distress. The average levels of depression, anxiety, and overall distress were subclinical; however, a greater proportion of mothers were considered depressed than would be expected in the general population. In general, mothers were more symptomatic than fathers. Symptoms were unrelated to child age and sex, but were associated with degree of maternal concern and worry. Over time, emotional symptoms decreased, with the significant decline occurring by 6 months postdiagnosis. No changes were observed during the first year in marital status, marital harmony, or physical health and medication use by parents. The authors concluded that most parents deal very well with the diagnosis of their child, and that emotional responses are similar to a mourning process, with initial distress and recovery after a few months.

Regimen Adherence and Metabolic Control

Psychosocial factors have also been studied as predictors of regimen adherence and metabolic control in newly diagnosed children, although there are only a few studies in the literature. Jacobson et al. (1987) investigated psychological predictors of regimen adherence in a sample of 57, 9- to 15-year-old patients during the first 18 months of diabetes. Ratings of adherence were made by the health care providers at clinic visits every few months. Ratings were made on 4-point scales for each of several regimen components. Reliability studies indicated adequate reliability for ratings of diet, metabolic monitoring, and insulin use, and poor reliability for ratings of exercise. A composite index was devised based on the three reliable regimen adherence ratings. It is possible, however, that adherence ratings were biased by knowledge of metabolic control.

Adherence was studied over time, comparing the first and second 9-month periods. In addition, psychological data obtained during the first year were used as predictors of adherence. Results indicated a significant decline in adherence during the second 9-month period. Preadolescents were more adherent than adolescents. Correlations of psychosocial variables with the composite index revealed that better adherence was associated with increased self-esteem and social functioning, fewer behavior problems, internal locus of control, and better diabetes adjustment. Regression analysis indicated that 55% of the variance in adherence during the first 9 months could be accounted for by child age, self-esteem, and social functioning. A similar analysis of the second 9-month adherence composite revealed that age, diabetes adjustment, and social functioning accounted for 57% of the variance in adherence.

Shouval, Ber, and Galatzer (1982) reported a positive correlation between a highly organized family environment and better regimen adherence in newly diagnosed children. In addition, these investigators reported that independence, cohesiveness, and expressiveness (as measured by the Family Environment Scale) were associated with better metabolic control in the sample. Measures of family functioning obtained at diagnosis were used to predict metabolic control 1 year later by Baker and colleagues (Baker, Rosman, Sargent, Nogueira, & Stanley, 1982) in a study of 25 children. High levels of family supportiveness and competence and clear parental communication were associated with improved metabolic control in the children. These investigators similarly reported in a prospective study of 43 newly diagnosed children that positive family interactions at diagnosis were associated with improved metabolic control 3 years later (Sargent, Rosman, Baker, Nogueira, & Stanley, 1985). The findings reported in these three studies are difficult to interpret, however, because of the absence of data concerning residual pancreatic activity (i.e., C-peptide) which may affect the metabolic control data (i.e., glycosylated hemoglobin A1).

Hamman and colleagues (1985) examined predictors of acute complications in newly diagnosed children. In a retrospective design, these investigators found that children classified as having a "severe" illness at diabetes onset (based on serum pH and bicarbonate), or with parents of lower socioeconomic status, or those aged 10–14, had significantly greater subsequent ketoacidosis episodes and diabetes-related hospitalizations. Similarly, Fishbein, Faich, and Ellis (1982) reported higher subsequent diabetes-related hospitalization rates for newly diagnosed children of low socioeconomic status.

Effects of Age at Diabetes Onset

Psychosocial Functioning

Two studies have investigated the effects of age at diagnosis on psychosocial functioning. Ryan and Morrow (1986) studied self-esteem (as measured by the Piers–Harris Scale) in 125 adolescents as a function of gender and early (<5 years old) versus late (greater than or equal to

5 years) onset. A significant interaction was obtained which revealed that early onset females had poorer self-esteem than early onset males. The effect was limited to the physical appearance and anxiety subscales of the self-esteem measure. The self-esteem scores were unaffected by degree of metabolic control (as measured by hemoglobin A1) or illness duration. The authors suggest that boys and girls may have different strategies for coping with diabetes in terms of their self-feelings. Early diabetes onset in girls may interfere with the development of a positive body image, possibly due to delayed sexual maturity and culturally heightened sensitivity to physical appearance, while early onset boys may utilize more denial.

Rovet, Ehrlich, and Hoppe (1987) studied a variety of measures of psychosocial adjustment in diabetic preadolescents as a function of age at onset and gender. Twenty-seven early onset (less than or equal to 3 years old at diagnosis), 24 late onset (≥ 4 years old), and 30 sibling controls were studied. Dependent variables included measures of behavior problems and social competence, self-concept, temperament, and school performance. Results indicated that late onset boys had more internalizing behavioral problems than early onset boys or girls. There was also some evidence that early onset girls had more difficulty at school, both in terms of academic and social adjustment. Effects of onset on self-concept were not observed. These findings are limited, however, due to the 55% participation rate in the early onset group, the relatively small sample sizes in the subgroups, and the large number of statistical comparisons.

Cognitive Functioning

An early observation by Ack, Miller, and Wil (1961) suggested that children who developed diabetes prior to age 5 had significantly lower IQ's than nondiabetic siblings. Although only 38 siblings pairs were studied, this finding has inspired more recent research.

Ryan, Vega, and Drash (1985) examined cognitive functioning in 46 early onset (<5 years old at diagnosis) and 79 late onset adolescents who were randomly selected from a large outpatient sample. All subjects were diabetic for at least 3 years at the time of the testing. A nondiabetic control group was also evaluated. The evaluation protocol included standardized measures of intelligence, memory, academic achievement, and neuropsychological functioning. Factor analysis was used to reduce the data to five factors. Multivariate analysis revealed that the early onset group had significantly poorer cognitive performance on all factors, particularly for visual-spatial functioning.

In a recent study by Rovet, Ehrlich, and Hoppe (1988), 27 children with early onset (<4 years), 24 with late onset (>4 years), and 30 siblings controls were compared on a variety of cognitive and school performance measures. Results indicated that children with early onset had significantly lower visuospatial, but not verbal, performance. Girls with early onset were especially affected. In addition, early onset children were more likely to have school problems and increased frequency of hypoglycemic reactions. Regression analyses indicated that age at onset, diabetes duration and history of hypoglycemic reactions were significant predictors of spatial ability, but accounted for only 14% of the variance.

Studies by Anderson et al. (1984) and Holmes & Richman (1985) have provided additional data indicating that children and adolescents who develop diabetes early in their life may be at risk for later neurocognitive deficits. Based on the available data, it appears that visuospatial deficits may be secondary to history of frequent hypoglycemic reactions (Ryan, Longstreet, & Morrow, 1985). However, verbal skills deficits may be attributed to more frequent school absences in children with early onset (Ryan et al., 1985). These mechanisms await confirmation in prospective studies.

Treatment Studies

Few treatment studies have been conducted with newly diagnosed children. Using a retrospective design, Galatzer, Amir, Gil, Karp, and Laron (1982) compared a psychosocially oriented crisis intervention program given at one hospital to routine clinic care provided at several other hospitals. The intervention program was administered by interdisciplinary staff in the period just after diagnosis. Subjects were 223 patients, aged from 7 to 24 years, with a mean of 15 years, who had been in follow-up periods ranging from 3 to 15 years. Results indicated that patients who received the crisis intervention program were rated as significantly better adjusted with respect to regimen adherence, family relationships, and sociability. Within each group, patients of higher socioeconomic status were rated as better adjusted. These findings are qualified, however, by several methodological limitations, including the retrospective design with variable follow-up intervals, lack of randomization, poor specification of treatment procedures, and use of global, subjective ratings of adjustment.

Nerup and Larsen (1983), in a randomized prospective study, investigated the effects of a home-based intervention for newly diagnosed patients. Although some children and adolescents were included, most of the patients studied were adults. Patients were randomized to standard outpatient care or to an intervention program consisting of five home follow-up visits by a nurse during the first year after diagnosis.

Compared with the control group of patients who did not receive the follow-up visits, patients in the home-based follow-up program had better metabolic control, as evidenced by lower glycosylated hemoglobin values and decreased hospital admissions for ketoacidosis. Residual pancreatic activity, however, was not considered, making the metabolic outcomes inconclusive.

Delamater, Bubb et al., (1988) studied the effects on metabolic control of a family-based self-management program with newly diagnosed children. Thirty-six children (representing 90% of patients meeting study criteria) ranging from 3 to 16 years of age participated in the study. All patients were hospitalized at diagnosis and received standard in-hospital diabetes education and standard outpatient procedures, involving regular outpatient contact with the health care team. Patients were stratified by age, sex, and risk status (based on socioeconomic status and illness severity) and randomized to either the self-management program, a supportive counseling program, or to standard outpatient procedures. The groups were well matched with respect to age, sex, socioeconomic status, and illness severity at diagnosis.

Patients randomized to the self-management training group participated in seven follow-up sessions held in the 4 months following discharge from the hospital. These were individual sessions with the patient and parent(s) which focused on increasing parental contingent praise for appropriate regimen adherence, utilization of self-monitoring of blood glucose, and development of problem-solving strategies. The goal of the treatment was to help patients and their families to integrate data from glucose monitoring in order to guide decisions concerning diabetes self-management. Additional contact for review and reinforcement of self-management strategies occurred at 6 and 12 months postdiagnosis. Patients randomized to the supportive counseling group were seen for seven follow-up sessions during the 4 months after diagnosis at the same schedule as the experimental patients. This group served as an attention-placebo to control for the effects of therapist contact in the self-management patients.

The primary comparison of the study was between the patients receiving self-management training and those in standard care. The follow-up period in the study was 2 years. The glycosylated hemoglobin A1 values at 2 years were subjected to analysis of covariance, with initial hemoglobin A1 and 2-year stimulated C-peptide as covariates. Results indicated that the self-management patients had significantly lower hemoglobin A1 than did patients in the standard group. Though not significant, experimental patients also had lower hemoglobin A1 than patients who received supportive counseling. Patients in the self-management group maintained lower hemoglobin A1 than patients in the other groups throughout the follow-up period.

Methodological Issues and Future Research

The question of how children adapt to newly diagnosed diabetes can only be answered in prospective, longitudinal research designs. Issues related to this involve consideration of control groups, premorbid status and age at onset, and specification of outcome variables and timing of assessment. Ultimately, the utility of such research will be demonstrated when predictors of adjustment can be clearly identified, so that preventive intervention programs can be implemented with high-risk patients and families.

It is evident in the current review that few investigators have conducted prospective, longitudinal studies of newly diagnosed children. Some of these have been concerned with psychosocial adaptation (Ahnsjo et al., 1981; Jacobson et al., 1986; Kovacs, Feinberg et al., 1985), while only one was a controlled treatment outcome study (Delamater, Bubb et al., 1988). The studies of psychosocial adaptation have compared diabetic children to healthy controls (Ahnsjo et al., 1981), acuately ill controls (Jacobson et al., 1986), and to normative data using standardized measures (Kovacs, Feinberg et al., 1985). The results have consistently shown the majority of patients to do quite well after the initial period of adjustment. However, the impact of diagnosis has not been conclusively shown, since premorbid measures of functioning were obtained in only one study (Kovacs, Feinberg et al., 1985). Prospective studies of genetically high-risk children (of diabetic parents) would be helpful in this regard. Short of such studies, it would at least be informative to have retrospective evaluation of prediagnosis levels of functioning and coping abilities. Furthermore, it is currently not known whether the impact of diagnosis is unique to diabetes or to chronic disease in general. To answer this question requires a study incorporating an appropriate control group. From a methodological point of view, a prospective study with premorbid measures comparing diabetic children with children with another chronic illness, e.g., renal disease, would be necessary in order to separate the effects of diabetes from chronic illness in general.

Timing of assessment of psychosocial functioning is another important consideration. As Kovacs, Feinberg et al. (1985) have shown, a significant minority of children do experience psychological distress in their initial adaptation, but these effects resolve within 6–9 months. Therefore, the studies by Ahnsjo et al. (1981) and Jacobson et al. (1986), in which variable time intervals after diagnosis were used in the initial assessment, probably obscured the effects of adaptation in particular individuals when group comparisons were made. One could argue that these issues are not all that significant, however, since most patients appear in the normative range on standardized measures of psychosocial functioning. However, this conclusion would appear premature until more extended follow-up is conducted of patients experiencing significant distress in the initial period after diagnosis. It may be that clinically significant initial distress is predictive of later difficulties in adaptation to diabetes. Future research should examine the relationship of initial coping efforts and psychosocial adjustment to later psychosocial functioning, regimen adherence, and metabolic control.

One is always concerned with the composition of the study groups in terms of their representativeness of the population. Both the studies by Kovacs and colleagues and Jacobson and colleagues had participation rates of 76%. It remains to be shown whether nonparticipants differed in significant ways from participants. In addition, the 55% participation rate of the control group in the Jacobson studies cast doubt on the validity of that comparison group. Another pertinent issue here is the socioeconomic status of the patients. This is especially important since it appears that this variable is predictive of adjustment problems in terms of psychosocial adaptation (Galatzer et al., 1982; Kovacs, Feinberg et al., 1985) and metabolic control (Hamman et al., 1985). It should be noted that the available studies have been conducted with white, primarily middle and upper class patients. Further research should address the question of adaptation in lower socioeconomic and minority groups.

As indicated in the literature review, age at onset appears to be a significant factor in terms of psychosocial and cognitive functioning. The effects of this variable must at this point be considered preliminary, however, due to the cross-sectional designs employed in these studies. It cannot be assumed that patients evaluated at different points in the course of diabetes are sampled from similar populations. Changes in functioning due to a chronic disease such as diabetes can only be determined from longitudinal research designs in which the same patients are studied on multiple occasions.

Another methodological issue concerns blood glucose levels at the time of assessment in studies of cognitive functioning in diabetic patients. Cognitive performance of diabetic individuals has been shown to be affected by blood glucose levels at the time of the assessment (Holmes, Hayford, Gonzalez, & Weydert, 1983; Holmes, Koepke, Thompson, Gyves, & Weydert, 1984). The studies described in this review have not considered this variable, thus limiting the reliability of the findings. Future research on the effects of age at diabetes onset must therefore control for this potential confound.

The effects of diagnosis of diabetes on psychosocial adaptation of children clearly depends on the developmental stage of the children. The available research has studied children in the 8- to 16-year-old range, without looking specifically at younger versus older children. Although there is clinical discussion of the impact of diagnosis on children at various developmental levels (e.g., Hamburg & Inoff, 1983), there has not to this date been systematic study of developmental effects in this population, particularly of children diagnosed prior to age 6 or older than 16. It would be especially important to study the differential impact of diagnosis on preschool, school-aged, and adolescent patients, since the understanding of disease process depends upon cognitive developmental level (Burbach & Peterson, 1986). The implications of diabetes management would also be expected to impact differentially on children at various ages because of the different developmental issues involved. This interaction between particular disease-related behaviors and the working at and resolution of specific developmental tasks (such as autonomy, peer group identity, etc.) have only just begun to be addressed. One recent example of research in this area has shown associations between cognitive maturity and self-management behaviors in adolescents (Ingersoll, Orr, Herrold, & Golden, 1986).

Psychosocial factors have been shown to differentiate diabetic youth in good versus poor metabolic control, particularly family factors such as conflict, cohesion, communication patterns regarding roles and responsibilities, and reinforcement of regimen-related behavior (Anderson & Auslander, 1980; Delamater, 1986; Johnson, 1988). Studies with newly diagnosed children have begun to consider the role of such factors as predictors of later adaptation; however, more work in this area is needed. Studies evaluating adaptation in terms of metabolic control must include measures of residual pancreatic beta-cell activity (i.e., C-peptide) in order to clearly delineate relationships between psychosocial factors and metabolic control.

Alternatively, studies which investigate the impact of diagnosis on family factors such as marital satisfaction, divorce rates, parent–child relationships, and effects on siblings are also needed. There have been equivocal findings regarding marital satisfaction and divorce rates (Anderson & Auslander, 1980) due to methodological limitations of early studies. While Kovacs, Finkelstein et al. (1985) found no effects on marital stability during the first year, further research on this question during more extended follow-up is needed. There is a paucity of work on the effects of diabetes on sibling functioning.

A final issue concerns research on the effects of initial education and treatment of newly diagnosed children. Although diabetes education is routinely provided at diagnosis, little is known about the effects of such programs. This education is obviously a critical component of the initial management of diabetes, yet it is typically provided during a time of great stress—not an optimal time for learning and retaining all that is required for effective diabetes management. Controlled studies of the effects of diabetes education programs with newly diagnosed have not been conducted. Studies with established adult patients generally show the education program to have no impact on regimen adherence and metabolic control (Bloomgarden et al., 1987). The importance of follow-up education and training is dramatized by findings of poor recall of self-care recommendations (Page, Verstraete, Robb, & Etzwiler, 1981), and lack of diabetes knowledge (Johnson et al., 1982) and skill with dietary (Delamater, Smith, Kurtz, & White, 1988) and glucose monitoring (Delamater et al., 1989) components of the regimen. The only prospective, controlled treatment-outcome study to date with newly diagnosed children indicates that follow-up education and training in behavioral self-management strategies leads to improved metabolic control which is evident 2 years after diagnosis (Delamater, Bubb et al., 1988). The so-called "honeymoon" period would appear to be an optimal time for prevention-based intervention, rather than a time for patients and families to develop inappropriate self-care behaviors which may set them up for later problems. More work in this area is needed.

Summary

It is clear that the diagnosis of diabetes poses a considerable challenge to young patients and their families. Results of recent prospective studies of psychosocial adaptation in newly diagnosed children indicate that about one third of patients experience clinically significant psychological distress in the first few months, but symptoms subside within 9 months for the majority of children. Overall, it can be concluded that most young patients adapt well to life with diabetes. Their psychosocial adaptation appears to be related to personality factors (e.g., self-esteem), family environment, marital distress, and socioeconomic status. Similarly, most parents deal well with the diagnosis of their child. Although there is little evidence of major psychological distress, emotional responses of parents are similar to a mourning process, with initial distress and recovery after a few months.

Age at diabetes onset has been studied in relation to cognitive and psychosocial functioning. Results of cross-sectional studies indicate that onset of diabetes prior to age 5 may be associated with later cognitive deficits. The mechanisms of this effect remain to be demonstrated in prospective studies, but it appears at this point that visual-spatial deficits may be related to history of hypoglycemic reactions whereas verbal deficits may be attributed to school absences. The data on psychosocial functioning are less clear, but suggest that early onset for girls is associated with poorer self-esteem and greater difficulties at school, while later onset for boys is associated with more behavior problems.

There are relatively few studies of predictors of later adaptation to diabetes in terms of psychosocial functioning, regimen adherence, and metabolic control. The available results suggest that child variables such as age, self-esteem, social functioning, and diabetes adjustment may predict later regimen adherence, whereas family factors such as organization, cohesiveness, and supportiveness are associated with better subsequent metabolic control. Severity of illness at diagnosis, as well as lower socioeconomic status, has been associated with subsequent metabolic control problems in young patients. Such findings suggest that intervention programs with high-risk children and families during the months following diagnosis may prevent later adaptation problems. There is evidence from one treatment-outcome study with newly diagnosed children that family-based self-management training provided soon after diagnosis leads to improved metabolic control which is maintained 2 years postdiagnosis.

Research concerning adaptation to diabetes requires prospective, longitudinal studies evaluating multiple outcome variables. At the present time there are few such studies in the literature, and those which have been conducted have primarily studied white 8- to 16-year-old children of middle or upper socioeconomic status. Future research should consider the adaptation of minority children and those of lower socioeconomic status, as well as very young children and those aged 16 or more at diagnosis. Particular attention should be focused on attainment of normal developmental tasks, rather than measuring only psychopathology in determining psychosocial adaptation. In addition, research should examine the relationship of initial coping efforts to later psychosocial and disease-related outcomes. More studies of the effects of initial education and intervention programs with newly diagnosed are also needed.

References

Ack, M., Miller, I., & Weil, W.B. (1961). Intelligence in children with diabetes mellitus. *Pediatrics, 28*, 764–770.

Ahnsjo, S., Humble, K., Larsson, Y., Settergren-Carlsson, G., & Sterky, G. (1981). Personality changes and social adjustment during the first three years of diabetes in children. *Acta Paediatrica Scandinavica, 70*, 321–327.

Anderson, B., & Auslander, W. (1980). Research on diabetes management and the family: A critique. *Diabetes Care, 3*, 696–702.

Anderson, B., Hagen, J., Barclay, C., Goldstein, G., Kandt, R., & Dacon, G. (1984). Cognitive and school performance in diabetic children. *Diabetes, 33* (Suppl. 1), 21A.

Baker, L., Rosman, B., Sargent, J., Nogueira, J., & Stanley, C.A. (1982). Family factors predict glycosylated hemoglobin (HbA_1) in juvenile diabetes: A prospective study. *Diabetes, 31* (Suppl. 2), 15a.

Beischer, W., Kerner, W., Raptis, S., Keller, L., Beischer, B., & Pfeiffer, E.F. (1978). Insulin therapy in relation to circulating C-peptide levels. *Diabetes* (Supplement 1), *27*, 235–240.

Bloomgarden, Z.T., Karmally, W., Metzger, M.J., Brothers, M., Nechemias, C.,

Bookman, J., Faierman, D., Ginsberg-Fellner, F., Rayfield, E., & Brown, W.V. (1987). Randomized, controlled trial of diabetes patient education: Improved knowledge without improved metabolic status. *Diabetes Care, 10*, 263–272.

Burbach, D.J., & Peterson, L. (1986). Children's concepts of physical illness: A review and critique of the cognitive-developmental literature. *Health Psychology, 5*, 307–325.

Dahlquist, G., Blom, L., Bolme, P., Hagerfeldt, L., Lindgren, F., Persson, D., Thalme, B., Theorell, M., & Westin, S. (1982). Metabolic control in 131 juvenile-onset diabetic patients as measured by HbA_{1c}: Relation to age, duration, C-peptide, insulin dose, and one or two insulin injections. *Diabetes Care, 5*, 399–406.

Delamater, A.M. (1986). Psychological aspects of diabetes mellitus in children. In B.B. Lahey & A.E. Kazdin (Eds.). *Advances in clinical child psychology* (Vol. 9). New York: Plenum.

Delamater, A.M., Bubb, J., Smith, J.A., Davis, S.G., White, N.H., & Santiago, J.V. (1988). Self-management training with newly diagnosed diabetic children: 2-year follow-up. *Diabetes*, 37 (Suppl. 1), 55A.

Delamater, A.M., Davis, S.G., Bubb, J., Santiago, J.V., Smith, J.A., & White, N.H. (1989). Self-monitoring of blood glucose by adolescents with diabetes: Technical skills and utilization of data. *The Diabetes Educator, 15*, 56–61.

Delamater, A.M., Smith, J.A., Kurtz, S.M., & White, N.H. (1988). Dietary skills and adherence in children with insulin-dependent diabetes mellitus. *The Diabetes Educator, 14*, 33–36.

Drash, A.L. (1979). The child with diabetes. In B. Hamburg, L. Lipsett, G. Inoff, & A. Drash (Eds.). *Behavioral and psychosocial issues in diabetes* (pp. 33–42). U.S. Department of Health and Human Service (NIH Publication No. 80-1993).

Fishbein, H.A., Faich, G.A., & Ellis, S.E. (1982). Incidence and hospitalization patterns of insulin-dependent diabetes mellitus. *Diabetes Care, 5*, 630–633.

Galatzer, A., Amir, S., Gil, R., Karp, M., & Laron, Z. (1982). Crisis intervention program in newly diagnosed diabetic children. *Diabetes Care, 5*, 414–419.

Geist, R.A. (1979). Onset of chronic illness in children and adolescents. *American Journal of Orthopsychiatry, 49*, 4–23.

Hamburg, B.A. & Inoff, G.E. (1983). Coping with predictable cases of diabetes. *Diabetes Care, 6*, 409–416.

Hamman, R.F., Cook, M., Keefer, S., et al. (1985). Medical care patterns at the onset of insulin-dependent diabetes mellitus: Association with severity and subsequent complications. *Diabetes Care, 8* (Suppl. 1), 94–100.

Hauser, S.T., Jacobson, A.M., Wertlieb, D., Brink, S., & Wentworth, S. (1985). The contribution of family environment to perceived competence and illness adjustment in diabetic and acutely ill adolescents. *Family Relations, 34*, 99–108.

Hauser, S.T., Jacobson, A.M., Wertlieb, D., Weiss-Perry, B., Follansbee, D., Wolfsdorf, J., Herskowitz, R.D., Houlihan, J., & Rajapark, D. (1986). Children with recently diagnosed diabetes: Interactions with their families. *Health Psychology, 5*, 273–296.

Holmes, C.S., Hayford, J.T., Gonzales, J.L., & Weydert, J.A. (1983). A survey of cognitive functioning at different glucose levels in diabetic persons. *Diabetes Care, 6*, 180–185.

Holmes, C.S., Koepke, K.M., Thompson, R.G., Gyves, P.W., & Weydert, J.A. (1984). Verbal Fluency and naming performance in Type 1 diabetes at different blood glucose concentrations. *Diabetes Care, 7*, 454–459.

Holmes, C.S., & Richman, L.C. (1985). Cognitive profiles of children with insulin-dependent diabetes mellitus. *Developmental and Behavioral Pediatrics, 6*, 323–331.

Ingersoll, G.M., Orr, D.P., Herrold, A.J., & Golden, M.P. (1986). Cognitive maturity and self-management among adolescents with insulin-dependent diabetes mellitus. *Journal of Pediatrics, 108*, 620–623.

Jacobson, A.M., Hauser, S.T., Wertlieb, D., Wolfsdorf, J., Orleans, J., & Viegra, M. (1986). Psychological adjustment of children with recently diagnosed diabetes mellitus. *Diabetes Care, 9*, 323–329.

Jacobson, A.M., Hauser, S.T., Wolfsdorf, J., Houlihan, J., Milley, J., Herskowitz, R.D., Wertlieb, D., & Watt, E. (1987). Psychologic predictors of compliance in children with recent onset of diabetes mellitus. *Journal of Pediatrics, 110*, 805–811.

Johnson, S.B. (1988). Diabetes mellitus in childhood. In D.K. Routh (Ed.). *Handbook of pediatric psychology*. New York: Guilford.

Johnson, S.B., Pollak, T., Silverstein, J.H., Rosenblum, A.L., Spillar, R., McCallum, M., & Harkavy, J. (1982). Cognitive and behavioral knowledge about insulin-dependent diabetes among children and parents. *Pediatrics, 69*, 708–713.

Kovacs, M., Brent, D., Steinberg, T.F., Paulauskas, S., & Reid, J. (1986). Children's self-reports of psychologic adjustment and coping strategies during the first year of insulin dependent diabetes mellitus. *Diabetes Care, 9*, 472–479.

Kovacs, M., Feinberg, T.L., Paulauskas, S., Finkelstein, R., Pollock, M., & Crouse-Novak, M. (1985). Initial coping responses and psychosocial characteristics of children with insulin dependent diabetes mellitus. *Journal of Pediatrics, 106*, 827–834.

Kovacs, M., Finkelstein, R., Feinberg, T.L., Crouse-Novak, M., Paulauskas, S., & Pollock, M. (1985). Initial psychologic responses of parents to the diagnosis of insulin dependent diabetes mellitus in their children. *Diabetes Care, 8*, 568–575.

Krosnick, A. (1970). Psychiatric apsects of diabetes. In M. Ellenberg, & H. Rifkin (Eds.). *Diabetes mellitus: Theory and Practice*. New York: McGraw-Hill.

Ludvigsson, J., & Heding, L.G. (1976). C-peptide in children with juvenile diabetes. *Diabetologia, 12*, 627–630.

Madsbad, S., Faber, O.K., & Binder, C. (1978). Prevalence of residual beta cell function in insulin dependent diabetics in relation to age at onset and duration of diabetes. *Diabetes, 27* (Supplement 1), 262–264.

Madsbad, S., McNair, P., & Faber, O.K. (1980). Beta-cell function and metabolic control in insulin-treated diabetics. *Acta Endocrinology, 93*, 196–200.

Nerup, V.A., & Larsen, D.F. (1983). Home education and instruction of newly diagnosed IDDM patients. Unpublished manuscript. Stano Memorial Hospital, Gentofte, Denmark.

Page, P., Verstraete, D.G., Robb, J.R., & Etzwiler, D.D. (1981). Patient recall of self-care recommendations in diabetes. *Diabetes Care, 4*, 96–98.

Rovet, J.F., Ehrlich, R., & Hoppe, M. (1987). Behavior problems in children with diabetes as a function of sex and age of onset of disease. *Journal of Child Psychology and Psychiatry, 28*, 477–491.

Rovet, J.F., Ehrlich, R., & Hoppe, M. (1988). Specific intellectual deficits in children with early onset diabetes mellitus. *Child Development, 59*, 226–234.

Ryan, C.M., Longstreet, C., & Morrow, L.A. (1985). The effects of diabetes mellitus on the school attendance and school achievement of adolescents. *Child: Care, Health, and Development, 11*, 229–240.

Ryan, C.M., & Morrow, L.A. (1986). Self-esteem in diabetic adolescents: Relationship between age at onset and gender. *Journal of Consulting and Clinical Psychology, 54*, 730–731.

Ryan, C.M., Vega, A., & Drash, A. (1985). Cognitive deficits in adolescents who developed diabetes early in life. *Pediatrics, 75*, 921–927.

Sargent, J., Rosman, B., Baker, L., Nogueira, J., & Stanley, C. (1985). Family interaction and diabetic control: A prospective study. *Diabetes, 34* (Suppl. 1), 77A.

Shouval, R., Ber, R., & Galatzer, A. (1982). Family social climate and the length status and social adaptation of diabetic youth. In Z. Laron (Ed.). *Psychological aspects of diabetes in children and adolescents*. Basel: Karger.

Tarnow, J., & Tomlinson, N. (1978). Juvenile diabetes: Impact on the child and family. *Psychosomatics, 19*, 487–491.

Tietz, W., & Vidmar, J.T. (1972). The impact of coping styles on the control of juvenile diabetes. *Psychiatry in Medicine, 3*, 67–74.

Wertlieb, D., Hauser, S.T., & Jacobson, A.M. (1986). Adaptation to diabetes: Behavior symptoms and family context. *Journal of Pediatric Psychology, 11*, 463–479.

Wishner, W.J., & O'Brien, M.D. (1978). Diabetes and the family. *Medical Clinics of North America, 62*, 849–856.

3

Adherence Behaviors and Health Status in Childhood Diabetes

Suzanne Bennett Johnson

Defining adherence to the diabetes regimen is difficult for several reasons. First, there is the vast array of regimen behaviors required. Insulin injections must be given at regular times and appropriately timed in relationship to meals. Dietary proscriptions are numerous; small meals must be taken frequently and certain types of foods, those high in concentrated sweets and fats, are to be minimized. Regular exercise is considered beneficial as it improves insulin utilization and lowers blood glucose, but it must be carefully coordinated with food intake so as to avoid hypoglycemia. Since current treatment methods only approximate normal pancreatic function, wide swings in blood glucose can and do occur. For this reason, patients are encouraged to test their blood glucose two or more times a day. These data are then utilized by the physician and/or patient to make insulin dose, dietary, or other changes to the patient's daily regimen. Consequently, defining adherence in childhood diabetes means defining numerous regimen behaviors.

This process is further complicated by well-documented knowledge, skill, and provider/patient communication deficits in this population. Patients may believe and report that they are highly compliant but, due to deficits in knowledge or skill, they inadvertently behave in very noncompliant ways. Studies of children injecting insulin or testing glucose have reported significant procedural errors in a substantial proportion of the children observed (Epstein, Coburn, Becker, Drash, & Siminerio, 1980; Johnson, et al., 1982). Yet, these children believed that they were performing in a highly compliant manner. While physicians are usually responsible for patients' diabetes regimen prescriptions, there are often large discrepancies between what providers believe they have told their patients and what the patients actually recall (Hulka,

Kupper, Cassel, Mayo, 1975; Page, Verstraete, Robb, & Etzwiler, 1981). When such discrepancies occur, patients may inadvertently behave in ways that differ significantly from their doctors' orders.

For many aspects of the diabetes regimen, the provider may give no or an unclear prescription. For example, although excercise is considered beneficial, not all patients are told to engage in regular exercise. Or, if exercise is mentioned, a very general prescription may be given (e.g., "get some exercise"). In such cases, it is extremely difficult to define adherence since a provider prescription is nonexistent or unclear. For this reason, Glasgow, Wilson, and McCaul (1985) have recommended that the term "levels of diabetes self-care behaviors" be utilized when there is no clear provider prescription available; they suggest that the term "adherence" or "compliance" be reserved for those relatively rare diabetes management behaviors for which there exists a documented provider prescription. Glasgow et al.'s point is well taken: defining adherence requires some sense of an ideal standard, clearly documented by the physician or by the investigator.

Adherence and Health Status: Conceptual Issues

Because insulin-dependent diabetes mellitus (IDDM) is a chronic illness with multiple regimen behaviors, it is the patient who manages this disease on a daily basis. The physician serves as a consultant, making management prescriptions and suggestions, rather than providing direct daily care. The physician is dependent upon the patient to operationalize medical advice. Since the goal of treatment is to maintain blood glucose levels as close to normal as possible, the patient's cooperation must be obtained if this goal is to be attained. The serious long-term complications of diabetes (i.e., blindness, renal disease, heart disease, leg amputations) are thought to be delayed, diminished, or even prevented by maintenance of blood glucose in or near the normal range. Consequently, there is increasing interest in improving patient adherence behaviors since they are seen as so central to the successful management of this disease.

While adherence and diabetes control are presumably linked, there are few empirical tests of this assumption. In fact, there exists a conceptual confounding of terms in which compliance and diabetes control are often used interchangeably, as if they were referring to the same construct or process. Many health providers simply assume that their well-controlled patients are compliant and their poorly controlled patients are noncompliant. The interchangeable use of these terms is often so ingrained that the provider and patient may be unaware of this confounding or its implications. Such confounding may be of little practical import if adherence behaviors were the sole determinants of diabetes control. In fact, this is not the case. At the most basic level, diabetes control is determined by the adequacy of the treatment regimen. Prescribed insulin doses that are too high or too low will negatively impact upon the child. To be sure, an adequate treatment regimen will be rendered ineffective by patient failure to comply. At the same time, even perfect compliance will not make an inadequate treatment prescription effective. Great care must be taken to select the appropriate insulin dose, frequency and timing of injections, dietary intake, and so on. Further, an adequate treatment regimen may become inadequate as a consequence of biological (e.g., increasing disease duration, puberty, illness), environmental (e.g., increased stress), or life-style (e.g., increased or decreased exercise) changes. Selecting an appropriate insulin dose and regimen prescription is not a static event; the health care provider must remain sensitive to the changing needs of the patient.

When compliance and diabetes control are treated as interchangeable constructs, determinants of diabetes control, other than compliance, may be ignored and remain unexplored. The patient may be subtly (or not so subtly) blamed for his or her condition. And, adherence/health status linkages remain untested.

Assessing Adherence

The paucity of empirical research linking adherence behaviors to diabetes control is a product of a conceptual confounding of terms but is also the result of problems associated with efforts to measure adherence. A variety of approaches have been utilized: health status indicators, physician ratings, self-reports, behavioral observations, and permanent products.

Health Status Indicators

Since compliance and control are frequently treated as interchangeable terms, utilizing a measure of metabolic status to index compliance should come as no surprise. Indeed, this approach is used more often than not. In a recent survey of U.S. pediatric diabetologists, over 89% reported using glycosylated hemoglobin levels (the most widely accepted measure of diabetes control) to assess compliance (Clarke, Snyder, & Nowacek, 1985). These providers did not assess adherence behaviors directly. Rather, they inferred them from this single indicator of the patient's metabolic status. Obviously, studies that utilize health status indicators to measure adherence can never adequately address the relationship between adherence to the diabetes regimen and diabetes control.

Physician Ratings

Physician or health care provider ratings of a patient's compliance to a treatment regimen is another common assessment strategy. Unfortunately, reliability and validity data are rarely provided. Early studies found physicians' estimates of patients' adherence to be extremely poor, although none of these studies were conducted with chronically ill childhood populations (Caron & Roth, 1968; Charney et al., 1967; Davis, 1968). A more recent study of physician estimates of diabetes adolescents' adherence yielded more favorable results (Bobrow, AvRuskin, & Siller, 1985). In general, however, there is little psychometric data addressing the adequacy of physician or health care provider ratings of adherence. More importantly, physician ratings risk confounding compliance with diabetes control. Physicians are very much aware of their patients' health status. Knowledge of the patient's metabolic status could very well influence a physician's rating of the patient's adherence; once again, compliance and diabetes control are conceptually confounded. Studies utilizing this assessment strategy could easily produce a spurious relationship between patient adherence and diabetes control, reflecting physician beliefs about adherence/control relationships rather than a valid link between the two.

Self-Reports

Most health care providers rely on the patient's or parent's report when assessing adherence behaviors. Unfortunately, what patients say they do may bear little resemblance to actual behavior, and may be markedly influenced by what the patient believes the doctor wants to hear. Although there is some evidence that patient reports of noncompliance may be accurate (Epstein & Cluss, 1982), reports of highly compliant behavior remain suspect. Some investigators utilize composite scores based on patient adherence ratings to specific components of the diabetes regimen (e.g., Hanson, Henggeler, & Burghen, 1987b). Psychometric evidence supporting the reliability or validity of these self-ratings is rarely provided. Composite scores are also problematic because they are based on a unidimensional conceptualization of compliance; the level of adherence is presumed to be consistent across the wide variety of adherence behaviors demanded by the treatment regimen. There is increasing evidence that adherence in IDDM is a multidimensional, rather than a unidimensional, construct (Glasgow, McCaul, & Schafer, 1987; Johnson, Silverstein, Rosenbloom, Carter, & Cunningham, 1986; Schafer, Glasgow, McCaul, & Dreher, 1983). If so, composite scores may not adequately reflect this underlying complexity. We will return to this point later.

Self-recording of diabetes adherence behaviors on a daily basis is a more labor-intensive approach, in which the patient or parent keeps a written record of the patient's diabetes-relevant activities. Glasgow and his colleagues have used this approach in conjunction with other methods (Glasgow et al., 1987; Schafer, McCaul, & Glasgow, 1986). In our own work, we have found daily written records provide reliable estimates of adherence behaviors, if patients and families keep complete records. Unfortunately, in our particular patient sample, only half of the youngsters and their families kept complete records, severely limiting the practical utility of this approach.

We have had some success using 24-hr recall interviews as a method of assessing diabetes regimen adherence. This particular self-report method will be described in more detail in the next section of this chapter.

Behavioral Observations

Behavioral observation of targeted adherence behaviors has been successfully used in a number of studies (e.g., Epstein et al., 1981). Lowe and Lutzker (1979), for example, had a mother observe her diabetic daughter's foot care, urine testing, and dietary behaviors. Reliability, intermittently assessed by the child's older sister and by the experimenters, ranged from 81 to 100% agreement. While good-quality observational data can be obtained on an individual case basis, the large number of regimen behaviors required of diabetic youngsters and the labor-intensive nature of behavioral observation procedures make this an impractical general screening strategy for most patients. The approach remains useful for selected children and families who have one or two easily identified problem behaviors, and who are sufficiently motivated to closely monitor and record the behaviors targeted for change.

Permanent Products

Counting permanent products associated with adherence behaviors is an interesting, but rarely used, adherence assessment technique. This approach is ineffective as a general assessment strategy because adherence behaviors are not always reliably associated with a permanent product that can be easily observed and measured. However, in some cases, permanent products can be creatively employed to corroborate self-reports or other types of adherence data. Gross (1983), for example, asked four 10- to 12-year-old diabetic boys to monitor their urine glucose four times per day. Since urine testing requires the use of test tablets, the boys' reports of the number of urine tests conducted could be verified by a weekly count of urine test tablets; the number of test tablets depleted on a weekly basis should have agreed with the boys' reports of the number of tests conducted. Indeed, in this particular study, there was an 80% agreement between the boys' reports of testing frequency and the number of tests estimated by a weekly count of test tablets.

The recent development of meters for home blood-glucose monitoring with large memory capacities offers a number of permanent products useful to patients, providers, and investigators interested in this particular aspect of diabetes care. These meters store in memory the date and time, as well as the result of a blood glucose test. The provider and patient can access this stored data to help make treatment decisions. The interested investigator can also use the stored data to assess glucose-testing adherence or to evaluate the accuracy of patients' self-reports of glucose-testing behavior.

Assessing Daily Diabetes Management by 24-Hour Recall Interview

The 24-hr recall interview has long been a standard dietary assessment technique and is considered the best of the available self-report methods (Marquis, Ware, & Relles, 1979). We expanded the interview to include all diabetes-relevant behaviors to test its viability as a general adherence assessment strategy. Also unlike the usual dietary assessment procedure in which one interview is conducted with a single informant, we conduct at least three interviews to ensure a more representative sample of daily diabetes management behavior. Instead of using a single informant, we conduct interviews with both the youngster and his or her mother. Each is interviewed separately about the youngster's behavior during the preceding 24 hr. The previous day's events are recalled in temporal sequence beginning with the child's awakening in the morning and ending with retiring to bed. To encourage honest reporting, all interviews are conducted by trained nonmedical personnel who are not associated with the clinic staff. Obtaining adherence data from both mother and child permits estimates of parent/child agreement which bear on the reliability and validity of the procedure. Combining data obtained from both informants also helps reduce memory errors associated with any recall procedure.

Thirteen different adherence behaviors are quantified from the 24-hr recall data: four injection, three exercise, five dietary measures, and a glucose testing frequency measure. Each is constructed so that a range of scores is possible, with higher scores indicating relative noncompliance and scores close to zero indicating relative compliance. A brief description of the 13 adherence measures is provided in Table 3.1. The reader is referred to a previous paper for further details concerning their definition and quantification (Johnson et al., 1986).

Table 3.1. A Brief Description of 13 Adherence Measures Quantified from 24-Hour Recall Interview Data

Injection Behaviors

Injection Regularity: The degree to which injections are given at the same time every day.

Injection Interval: The degree to which the time between injections approaches ideal.

Injection–Meal Timing: The degree to which injections are given 30–60 min. before eating.

Regularity of Injection–Meal Timing: The degree to which the time between injection and eating is consistent across days.

Exercise Behaviors

Exercise Frequency: How often a youngster exercises on a daily basis.

Exercise Duration: How long a youngster exercises on any exercise occasion.

Exercise Type: The strenuousness of the youngster's exercise.

Dietary Behaviors

% Calories: Carbohydrate: Percentage of total calories consumed consisting of carbohydrates in relationship to the 60% ideal recommended by the American Diabetes Association (Nuttal & Brunzall, 1979).

% Calories: Fat: Percentage of total calories consumed consisting of fats in relationship to the 25% ideal recommended by the American Diabetes Association (Nuttal & Brunzall, 1979).

Calories Consumed: The youngster's ideal total number of daily calories (based on age, sex, and height) subtracted from the youngster's reported daily calorie consumption.

Concentrated Sweets: The average number of concentrated sweet exchange units eaten on a daily basis (40 calories of any concentrated sweet equals one concentrated sweet exchange unit).

Eating Frequency: How often a youngster eats on a daily basis.

Glucose Testing Behavior

Testing Frequency: How often a youngster conducts a glucose test on a daily basis.

Note: For additional details concerning the definition and quantification of the 13 adherence measures, see Johnson et al. (1986).

Estimates of parent/child agreement provide important psychometric information relevant to the reliability and validity of this procedure. Although perfect agreement cannot be expected since parents do not observe all of their children's activities, statistically significant correlations between child and parent reports have been documented in three separate samples (Freund, Johnson, Silverstein, & Thomas, 1989; Johnson et al., 1986; Spevack, Johnson, & Riley, 1988, see Table 3.2); most are in the moderate to high range. The correlations depicted in Table 3.2 were based on data obtained from three 24-hr recall inter-

Table 3.2. Parent/Child Agreement for 13 Diabetes Management Behaviors

Adherence Measures	Johnson et al. (1986) ($n=168$) r ($p<$)	Freund et al. (1989) ($n=78$) r ($p<$)	Spevack et al. (1988) ($n=64$) r ($p<$)
Injection Behaviors			
Injection regularity	.61 (.0001)	.62 (.0001)	.65 (.0001)
Injection interval	.77 (.0001)	.74 (.0001)	.75 (.0001)
Injection–meal timing	.67 (.0001)	.64 (.0001)	.54 (.0001)
Regularity of injection–meal timing	.42 (.0001)	.33 (.005)	.09 (ns)
Exercise Behaviors			
Exercise frequency	.62 (.0001)	.75 (.0001)	.68 (.0001)
Exercise duration	.59 (.0001)	.72 (.0001)	.29 (.02)
Exercise type	.54 (.0001)	.76 (.0001)	.64 (.0001)
Dietary Behaviors			
Eating frequency	.45 (.0001)	.65 (.0001)	.72 (.0001)
Calories consumed	.77 (.0001)	.72 (.0001)	.73 (.0001)
% Calories: carbohydrate	.64 (.0001)	.76 (.0001)	.72 (.0001)
% Carlories: fat	.64 (.0001)	.75 (.0001)	.78 (.0001)
Concentrated sweets	.62 (.0001)	.67 (.0001)	.63 (.0001)
Glucose Testing Behavior			
Testing frequency	.78 (.0001)	.94 (.0001)	.90 (.0001)

Note: ns: nonsignificant.

views conducted with each parent and with each child. The Freund et al. (1989) study provided additional data relevant to interview frequency effects on estimates of parent/child agreement. These data are provided in Table 3.3. For 8 of the 13 adherence measures, parent/child agreement was significantly enhanced when 9, as compared to 3, interviews were used to quantify the adherence measures. Since parent/child agreement was respectable for most measures based on three interviews, the increased reliability obtained with the use of nine interviews must be weighed against the additional costs of conducting more than three interviews.

In the Freund et al. (1989) investigation, nine interviews were conducted with the parent and with the child over a 3-month interval. This permitted an examination of the stability of adherence behaviors over the course of the investigation. Adherence measures quantified using the first three interviews collected during the first month of the study could be compared to the same measures quantified using interviews conducted during the second and third months of this investigation. The relevant correlations are provided in Table 3.4. All correlations

Table 3.3. Interview Frequency Effects on Parent/Child Agreement

Adherence Measures	3 Interviews r ($p<$)	9 Interviews r ($p<$)
Injection Behaviors		
* Injection regularity	.62 (.0001)	.81 (.0001)
Injection interval	.74 (.0001)	.72 (.0001)
* Injection–meal timing	.64 (.0001)	.85 (.0001)
* Regularity of injection–meal timing	.33 (.005)	.59 (.0001)
Exercise Behaviors		
Exercise frequency	.75 (.0001)	.76 (.0001)
* Exercise duration	.72 (.0001)	.90 (.0001)
Exercise type	.76 (.0001)	.76 (.0001)
Dietary Behaviors		
* Eating frequency	.65 (.0001)	.81 (.0001)
Calories consumed	.72 (.0001)	.77 (.0001)
* % Calories: carbohydrate	.76 (.0001)	.88 (.0001)
* % Carlories: fat	.75 (.0001)	.88 (.0001)
* Concentrated sweets	.67 (.0001)	.82 (.0001)
Glucose Testing Behavior		
Testing frequency	.94 (.0001)	.94 (.0001)

Source: Freund et al., (1989).
* Correlations significantly different.

were statistically significant, with one exception, suggesting that diabetes regimen behaviors are quite stable over intervals as long as 3 months. There did appear to be some differences in the degree of stability exhibited by the different regimen behaviors. Glucose testing and dietary behaviors appeared to be the most stable, followed by exercise and injection behaviors. These data are consistent with that previously reported by Glasgow et al. (1987) who monitored adherence behaviors of adolescent and adult IDDM patients over 2-month and 6-month test–retest intervals. Although their method of assessing adherence varies from ours, the pattern of results obtained is quite similar. Glasgow et al. (1987) found glucose testing behaviors to be the most stable, followed by dietary, insulin injection, and exercise behaviors. These authors' test–retest reliability estimates for the 6-month interval were generally lower than for the 2-month interval, suggesting that while adherence behaviors may be quite stable over 2 or 3 months, significant variation may occur over longer intervals.

While the available parent/child agreement and test–retest data sup-

Table 3.4. Stability of Adherence Behaviors over 3 months

Adherence Measures	Months 1 & 2 ($n = 66–74$) r ($p <$)	Months 2 & 3 ($n = 65–72$) r ($p <$)	Months 1 & 3 ($n = 64–72$) r ($p <$)
Injection Behaviors			
Injection regularity	.24 (.04)	.35 (.004)	.06 (ns)
Injection interval	.49 (.0001)	.43 (.0003)	.38 (.001)
Injection–meal timing	.71 (.0001)	.58 (.0001)	.65 (.0001)
Regularity of injection–meal timing	.30 (.01)	.31 (.009)	.24 (.05)
Exercise Behaviors			
Exercise frequency	.40 (.0005)	.63 (.0001)	.47 (.0001)
Exercise duration	.42 (.0002)	.51 (.0001)	.74 (.0001)
Type of exercise	.39 (.0006)	.48 (.0001)	.37 (.001)
Dietary Behaviors			
Eating frequency	.74 (.0001)	.77 (.0001)	.63 (.0001)
Calories consumed	.74 (.0001)	.72 (.0001)	.67 (.0001)
% Calories: carbohydrate	.61 (.0001)	.45 (.0001)	.58 (.0001)
% Carlories: fat	.63 (.0001)	.51 (.0001)	.60 (.0001)
Concentrated sweets	.53 (.0001)	.51 (.0001)	.53 (.0001)
Glucose Testing Behavior			
Testing frequency	.76 (.0001)	.75 (.0001)	.72 (.0001)

Source: Freund et al., (1989).
Note: ns: nonsignificant.

port the reliability of this method, they do not address the underestimation bias, due to errors of memory, that is frequently associated with recall data. Reynolds, Johnson, and Silverstein (in press) attempted to address this issue by comparing 24-hr recall interview data, obtained from 7- to 12-year-old children attending a diabetes summer camp, with actual observations of their behavior. There were only minor child/observer differences with regard to insulin injection and glucose testing behaviors. However, underestimation was a significant problem for most of the dietary behaviors and for one of the exercise measures (see Table 3.5). The youngsters underestimated both the frequency of eating and the amount of food consumed. They also underestimated the strenuousness of their exercise. In this study, only relatively young children were interviewed and no parent report data were collected. Interviewing both parent and child and combining data from both respondents should help minimize the underestimation bias associated with single informant data.

In summary, the 24-hr recall interview, when conducted with multi-

Table 3.5. Observer Versus Child Report of Diabetes Management Behaviors

Adherence Measures	Mean Child Report	Mean Observer Report
Injection Behaviors		
* AM injection time	7:28	7:41
PM injection time	17:43	17:48
Exercise Behaviors		
Exercise frequency	3.0	3.6
* Exercise duration (minutes)	47.2	45.7
* Exercise type (KCAL per min)	0.0784	0.0961
Dietary Behaviors		
Breakfast time	8:04	8:08
Dinner time	18:10	18:12
* Eating frequency	3.7	4.9
* Calories consumed	2336	2979
% Calories: carbohydrate	36.4	35.4
* Grams: carbohydrate	209	262
* % Calories: fat	47.4	50.0
* Grams: fat	125	166
* Concentrated sweets (exchange units)	2.2	3.4
Glucose Testing Behaviors		
Testing frequency	1.9	2.1
Test results (ranked data)	8.9	8.9

Source: Reynolds, Johnson, and Silverstein (in press).
* Observer/child reports significantly different.

ple informants on multiple occasions, appears to provide the investigator with a reliable method of assessing a wide range of diabetes adherence behaviors.

Adherence in Childhood Diabetes: Developmental Issues

Since our focus is childhood diabetes, no discussion of adherence in this population would be complete without some consideration of developmental issues. Age-related differences have been found in both the reliability of adherence data reported by children and in the actual level of adherence behaviors they exhibit.

Using the 24-hr recall approach, children as young as 6 years have

Table 3.6. Parent/Child Agreement for 6 to 9- and 10 to 12-Year-Olds for 13 Diabetes Adherence Behaviors

	Johnson et al. (1986)		Freund et al. (1989)	
	6–9 Yrs $n=26–31$	10–12 yrs $n=65–70$	6–9 yrs $n=8–12$	10–12 yrs $n=21–22$
Adherence Measures	r ($p<$)	r ($p<$)	r ($p<$)	r ($p<$)
Injection Behaviors				
Injection regularity	.46 (.02)	.68 (.0001)	.16 (ns)	.82 (.0001)
Injection interval	.36 (.05)	.71 (.0001)	.31 (ns)	.64 (.002)
Injection–meal timing	.53 (.002)	.54 (.0001)	.18 (ns)	.61 (.0003)
Regularity of injection meal timing	−.23 (.002)	.50 (.0001)	.18 (ns)	.20 (ns)
Exercise Behaviors				
Exercise frequency	.62 (.0001)	.72 (.0001)	.90 (.0001)	.49 (.02)
Exercise duration	.03 (ns)	.96 (.0001)	.20 (ns)	.38 (.08)
Exercise type	.74 (.0001)	.99 (.0001)	.86 (.0004)	.53 (.01)
Dietary Behaviors				
Eating frequency	.67 (.0001)	.47 (.0001)	.83 (.0008)	.68 (.0006)
Calories consumed	.79 (.0001)	.80 (.0001)	.51 (ns)	.52 (.02)
% Calories: carbohydrate	.44 (.01)	.63 (.0001)	.90 (.0001)	.74 (.0002)
% Calories: fat	.50 (.005)	.63 (.0001)	.87 (.0002)	.72 (.0004)
Concentrated sweets	.47 (.007)	.71 (.0001)	.80 (.002)	.83 (.0001)
Glucose Testing Behavior				
Testing frequency	.81 (.0001)	.73 (.0001)	.92 (.0001)	.97 (.0001)

Note: ns: nonsignificant.

been interviewed. Compared to their older counterparts (e.g., 10–12-year-olds), younger children (6–9 years) show poorer parent/child agreement on adherence measures involving time (i.e., all four injection measures and the exercise duration measure). Relevant data from two separate studies are provided in Table 3.6. On simple frequency measures (e.g., eating, exercise, and testing frequency) and on more qualitative measures (e.g., type of exercise and type of foods consumed), young children demonstrate agreement with their parents that is comparable to the parent/child agreement exhibited by older youngsters. It is not surprising that 6–9-year-olds have problems reliably reporting behaviors involving time since these require more complex mathematical concepts. However, data provided by Freund et al. (1989) suggest that, with practice, children as young as 6 years may become reliable reporters of all adherence behaviors, including those involving time. As was mentioned previously, parents and children in this study were interviewed on nine occasions across 3 months. This permitted an assessment of possible change in parent/child agreement across time. While parent/child agreement exhibited marked stability for most adherence measures in all age groups, the youngest children studied showed substantial improvement in parent/child agreement for the injection measures, all of which require an accurate report of the timing of injections and/or the timing of meals. As is depicted in Table 3.7, parent/child agreement for the 6–9-year-olds markedly improved between interviews 1–3 and interviews 4–6. By interviews 4–6, these young children were exhibiting parent/child agreement comparable to the 10–12-year-olds studied. Further, this improvement in parent/child agreement was maintained throughout the rest of the investigation. In summary, the available data suggest that youngsters as young as 6 years of age are reliable reporters concerning most adherence behaviors. Very young children do have some problems accurately reporting behaviors involving time. However, these problems appear to be overcome with practice.

Developmental differences also emerge when the actual level of adherence behaviors of different aged children are examined. In general, adolescents are less adherent than their younger counterparts. Rele-

Table 3.7. Parent/Child Agreement With Practice for 6 to 9- and 10 to 12-Year-Olds for the Injection Adherence Measures

	Age Group	
Adherence Measures	6–9 yrs. n=8–12 *r* (*p*<)	10–12 yrs. n=19–22 *r* (*p*<)
Injection regularity		
Interviews 1–3	.16 (ns)	.82 (.0001)
Interviews 4–6	.88 (.002)	.50 (.02)
Interviews 7–9	.74 (.02)	.81 (.0001)
Injection interval		
Interviews 1–3	.31 (ns)	.64 (.002)
Interviews 4–6	.89 (.003)	.87 (.0001)
Interviews 7–9	.76 (.02)	.89 (.0001)
Injection–meal timing		
Interviews 1–3	.18 (ns)	.61 (.003)
Interviews 4–6	.68 (.02)	.71 (.0004)
Interviews 7–9	.62 (.06)	.96 (.0001)
Regularity of injection–meal timing		
Interviews 1–3	−.16 (ns)	.20 (ns)
Interviews 4–6	.67 (.07)	.49 (.03)
Interviews 7–9	.53 (ns)	.51 (.04)

Source: Freund et al. (1989).
Note: ns: nonsignificant.

vant data from two different studies are presented in Table 3.8. The cross-study consistency of significant age-related effects is noteworthy. In both studies, adolescents, when compared to younger patients, took their injections less regularly, exercised less frequently, ate less frequently, ate too few carbohydrates, ate too many fats, and glucose tested less often. Although the clinical literature has often remarked upon the disruptive influence of adolescence on adequate diabetes care (e.g., Tattersall & Lowe, 1981), there have been few empirical tests of this assertion. The data presented in Table 3.8 suggest that the concerns frequently expressed by clinicians are quite justified; adolescents do appear to be remarkably nonadherent with the demands of their daily diabetes regimen. Intervention programs need to be designed that specifically address the special needs and problems presented by this population.

Adherence in Childhood Diabetes: A Unitary or Multidimensional Concept?

Physicians often describe patients as "compliant" or "noncompliant" as if adherence was a unitary trait or characteristic of the patient. Researchers have also treated adherence as a unitary construct, utilizing a clinician's rating, a composite score of patient self-ratings, or even a laboratory assay of metabolic status, as a single index of adherence. There is increasing evidence that diabetes adherence behaviors are not strongly correlated with one another and that a multidimensional conceptualization of diabetes adherence is more accurate. We approached this problem by subjecting 13 diabetes adherence behaviors, quantified from 24-hr recall data collected from a sample of 168 IDDM children and adolescents, to a principle component factor analysis (Johnson et al., 1986). If diabetes adherence is a unitary construct, a single factor should have emerged. Instead, a five-factor solution resulted, accounting for over 70% of the variance. The five factors were rotated to simple structure using the varimax procedure to ease interpretation; the factors and their loadings are presented in Table 3.9. All three exercise measures loaded on the first factor and all four injection measures loaded on Factor 2. Dietary behaviors did not load on a single factor. The type of food consumed (Factor 3) was unrelated to the frequency of eating (Factor 4) and the amount of calories consumed (Factor 5). Glucose testing frequency was related to eating frequency (Factor 4); children who were careful to eat frequently also tested frequently. The amount of calories consumed was related to concentrated sweet consumption; children who ate excess calories also ate excess sweets (Factor 5). Confirmatory factor analysis was applied to the adherence data collected from a second sample of 162 IDDM children and adolescents

Table 3.8. Age-Related Differences in Diabetes Adherence Behaviors (Johnson et al., 1986; 1989)

Adherence Measures* (N)	Age Group: 6–9 yrs. Study 1 (31–32)	6–9 yrs. Study 2 (12)	10–12 yrs. Study 1 (67–71)	10–12 yrs. Study 2 (21–22)	13–15 yrs. Study 1 (38–42)	13–15 yrs. Study2 (26–28)	16–19 yrs. Study 1 (21–23)	16–19 yrs. Study 2 (16)
Injection Behaviors								
Injection regularity (min)[a,b]	29.4	41.4	36.0	37.7	52.2	43.0	64.8	59.9
Injection interval (min)[a]	38.4	56.1	48.0	53.2	72.0	54.1	99.6	83.4
Injection–meal timing (min before meal)[a]	25.8	17.0	18.6	24.8	9.6	13.9	1.8	23.5
Regularity of injection–meal timing (min)	23.5	28.2	18.8	18.6	23.9	23.1	42.6	33.1
Exercise Behaviors								
Exercise frequency (per day)[a,b]	1.9	2.1	2.0	1.9	1.7	1.7	1.3	1.3
Exercise duration (min)	20.6	20.3	23.0	15.8	19.4	17.8	20.2	17.9
Exercise type (kcal/min)	.029	.028	.032	.025	.026	.024	.021	.019
Dietary Behaviors								
Eating frequency (per day)[a,b]	5.4	5.3	5.3	5.3	5.2	4.8	4.8	4.5
Calories consumed (above or below ideal)[b]	9	533	44	538	−60	162	−233	−220
% Calories: carbohydrates[a,b]	40.6	37.5	37.2	35.6	36.1	34.2	34.8	31.4
% Calories: fat[a,b]	44.4	46.6	47.2	49.0	48.4	49.8	50.0	53.0
Concentrated sweets (per day)	1.6	1.5	1.7	2.3	2.6	2.1	2.2	1.5
Glucose Testing Behavior								
Testing frequency (per day)[a,b]	2.1	1.9	1.9	1.7	1.5	1.5	.9	.8

Study 1: Johnson et al. (1986).
Study 2: Johnson et al. (1989).
[a]Age-related significant differences for Study 1, $p<.05$.
[b]Age-related significant differences for Study 2, $p<.05$.
*Presented are interpretations of the adherence measures using familiar measurement scales.

Table 3.9. Factor Analysis of Adherence Measures: Factor Loadings

Adherence Measure	Factor 1: Exercise	Factor 2: Injection	Factor 3: Diet Type	Factor 4: Testing/Eating Frequency	Factor 5: Diet Amount
Injection regularity	−.071	.736	.054	.018	−.077
Injection interval	.095	.852	.176	.005	.102
Injection–meal timing	.041	.724	.038	−.068	.003
Regularity of injection–meal timing	.007	.522	−.022	.361	.190
Calories consumed	−.090	.079	.262	−.408	.696
Percentage of calories from fat	.006	.124	.965	.090	.070
Percentage of calories from carbohydrates	.010	.108	.971	.028	−.008
Concentrated sweets	−.011	.024	−.088	.216	.845
Eating frequency	−.048	−.075	.250	.740	−.116
Exercise duration	.959	.007	−.017	−.005	−.042
Exercise type	.941	−.086	.040	.028	−.007
Exercise frequency	.667	.109	−.010	.151	−.022
Glucose testing frequency	.239	.116	−.082	.656	.121
Percentage of variance accounted for	18.0	16.4	15.8	10.5	9.9

Note: High factor loadings are underscored, indicating the adherence measures belonging to each factor.

From Johnson, Silverstein, Rosenbloom, Carter, Cunningham, "Assessing Daily Management in Childhood Diabetes," *Health Psychology*, 5(6), 1986. Reprinted with permission.

(Johnson, Tomar, Cunningham, & Henretta, in press). The first four factors were confirmed. Calories consumed and concentrated sweets, which comprised Factor 5 in the initial exploratory factor analysis, exhibited a similar relationship to one another in both samples but their relationships to the other adherence measures differed between samples. These data suggest that calories consumed and concentrated sweets are probably best treated as separate, single indicator constructs.

Our factor analytic work and earlier correlational research reported by Glasgow and his colleagues (Glasgow et al., 1987; Schafer et al., 1983) support a multidimensional conceptualization of adherence. How the youngster and family manage childhood diabetes cannot be characterized by a unitary trait. Since different regimen behaviors are likely to be unrelated to one another, attempts to measure adherence using single indicator assessment methods will not adequately capture its complexity; assessment methods that focus on the multiple components of diabetes management are more appropriate.

Adherence/Health Status Relationships in Childhood Diabetes: Summary of Current Knowledge Base

While adherence to the diabetes regimen is presumably linked to health status, there have been few empirical tests of this assumption. Early work by Williams, Watkins, and their colleagues noted numerous adherence problems in a sample of diabetic adults they interviewed and observed at home. However, the level of the patients' adherence appeared to be unrelated to the patients' diabetes control (Watkins, Williams, Martin, Hogan, & Anderson, 1967; Williams, Martin, Hogan, Watkins, & Ellis, 1967). Investigators have since taken greater care to separate diabetic populations by disease type (i.e., insulin-dependent versus non-insulin-dependent). Nevertheless, researchers have failed to document consistent, clinically significant relationships between compliance and diabetes control in IDDM samples. Using self-report data yielding a single adherence composite score, several researchers have reported low but statistically significant correlations between adherence and diabetes control (Brownlee-Duffeck, Peterson, Simonds, Goldstein, Kilo, & Hoette, 1987; Hanson, Henggeler, & Burghen, 1987a). However, others using similar measures of adherence and diabetes control have failed to find significant relationships (Cox, Taylor, Nowacek, Holley-Wilcox, & Pohl, 1984; Hanson, Henggeler, & Burghen, 1987b; Simonds, Goldstein, Walker, & Rawlings, 1981). Kaplan, Chadwick, and Schimmel's (1985) report is noteworthy because of its high reported correlation between 19 IDDM adolescents' self-reported adherence behavior and their level of glycosylated hemoglobin, the single most well-accepted measure of diabetes control ($r = -.78$). The authors report a similar significant correlation between the adolescents' glycosylated hemoglobin levels and their scores on a Lie Scale, raising questions as to the validity of the adolescents' self-reported adherence data. Further, there is increasing evidence that adherence behaviors in diabetes are relatively independent of one another (Glasgow et al., 1987; Johnson et al., 1986; Schafer, et al., 1983; Webb et al., 1984). Consequently, global ratings or composite scores of adherence may not adequately reflect the complexity of diabetes regimen behaviors.

Some investigators have studied particular diabetes adherence behaviors, such as dietary practices or blood glucose monitoring, and have attempted to link these specific behaviors to diabetes control. Again, inconsistent findings have emerged. Webb et al. (1984) reported that dietary compliance appeared to be related to diabetes control in a sample of IDDM adults. However, two intervention studies that improved patients' dietary adherence failed to produce concomitant changes in their diabetes control (Webb et al., 1984; Webb, Dobson, Tupling et al., 1982). Christensen, Terry, Wyatt, Pichert, and Lorenz (1983) reported that dietary compliance appeared to be associated with better diabetes control, but their statistical tests of this relationship only approached significance. Kaar, Akerblom, Huttunen, Knip, and Sakkinen (1984) reported that a nurse's rating of children's dietary compliance was related to the youngster's diabetes control. However, this study can be criticized for measurement dependence; the nurses who made the dietary compliance ratings also knew the patient's current diabetes control status which may have spuriously inflated the relationship between the two. An interesting study by Wing and her colleagues (Wing, Nowalk, Marcus, Koeske, & Finegold, 1986) did not assess daily dietary practices, but did find that unusual dietary behaviors, most notably bulemic behaviors, were associated with poorer diabetes control in IDDM adolescents.

Home glucose monitoring is the other specific regimen behavior that has attracted considerable empirical attention. Once again, highly compliant glucose testing behavior has not always been linked to good diabetes control. Gonder-Frederick, Julian, Cox, Clarke, and Carter (1988) reported that adult patients' self-reports of home blood glucose monitoring were linked to diabetes control but Wilson and Endres (1986) were unable to document such a relationship in a sample of IDDM adolescents. Some early intervention studies that used behavior therapy to improve patient adherence with glucose testing found concomitant changes in the patient's diabetes control (Carney, Schechter, & Davis, 1983; Schafer, Glasgow, & McCaul, 1982), but others did not (Epstein et al., 1981). More recent studies that have successfully increased the frequency and accuracy of home blood glucose monitoring in IDDM patients were unable to document subsequent improvements in diabetes control (Daneman, Siminerio, Transue, Betschart, Drash, & Becker, 1985; Mazze, Pasmantier, Murphy, & Shamoon, 1985).

Glasgow and his colleagues have published the most comprehensive studies of adherence/diabetes control relationships in IDDM populations. They treat insulin injection, dietary, exercise, and glucose testing behaviors as separate aspects of the diabetes regimen, instead of using a single compliance rating or composite score. Their early work documented some relationship between dietary, insulin injection, and glucose testing behaviors and diabetes control in a small sample IDDM adolescents (Schafer et al., 1983) but their subsequent studies, conducted with larger samples and with greater methodological sophistication, failed to find any consistent relationship between patients' regimen behaviors and their diabetes control (Glasgow et al., 1987; Schafer et al., 1986).

Studies that have attempted to link adherence behaviors to health status in IDDM have varied in methodological rigor. Some studies have used global measures of adherence that may be insensitive to the complexities of the diabetes regimen. Most use self-report measures of adherence that are uncorroborated by another family member. None have repeatedly assessed multiple adherence behaviors across time to ensure that the temporal interval during which adherence is assessed is congruent with the temporal interval indexed by the diabetes control measure. In view of the inconsistencies found in the literature to date, future studies must approach this area with increased scientific expertise.

Methodological Issues and Guidelines for Future Research

Certainly, failure to take insulin injections on a daily basis will have dire consequences for the child. However, failure to take insulin injections appears to be a relatively rare phenomenon. In our own work, we originally quantified 14 adherence behaviors from 24-hr recall interview data. The 14th measure was the percent of insulin injections prescribed that were actually taken. We found the percentage to be so high and the variability so low that we were forced to drop it as an adherence measure. Glasgow et al. (1987) have reported failure to take insulin injections to be a rare event in their study samples as well. When a physician or a psychologist is faced with a child whose failure to take injections has been well documented, each should be aware of the pathology this failure represents both from a medical and a psychological point of view; these children are not only physically ill but their failure to take insulin represents a significant deviation from the behavior exhibited by most youngsters with this disease. Clearly, failure to take insulin injections explains very little of the variance in health status in this population because it is such a rare event. Yet beyond this single basic adherence behavior, there is little evidence that the myriad of other adherence behaviors requested of the child have any notable impact on diabetes control. Nevertheless, it is probably premature to accept the null hypothesis that adherence behaviors are unrelated to health status outcomes in this disease. We must continue to address this issue with more sophisticated research. This last section will outline ways in which we can improve upon past research in future attempts to delineate adherence/health status relationships in childhood diabetes.

The first three guidelines have been mentioned in earlier sections of this chapter. First, it is critical that adherence and diabetes control be treated and measured as independent constructs. Earlier studies have sometimes indexed adherence by measures of diabetes control. However, more subtle confounding can and does occur. Whenever physician or health provider ratings of adherence are used, possible confounding between adherence and diabetes control can occur. Although the provider ratings may appear to be independent of the diabetes control indices, the provider's knowledge of the patient's diabetes control could influence the provider's ratings of adherence. It is most difficult to obtain provider adherence ratings that are "blind" to the patient's health status as this is inimical to the physician's central role; without knowledge of the patient's current metabolic status, the physician cannot make appropriate recommendations for improved care. For all of these reasons it is probably best to avoid health provider ratings of patient adherence.

The multivariate nature of diabetes adherence behaviors has also been discussed in a previous section of this chapter. Since adherence behaviors are not highly related to one another, investigators interested in the broad spectrum of diabetes adherence behaviors should avoid adherence composite scores or other single indicator measures of adherence. There is increasing evidence that the multiple components of the diabetes regimen can be reliably measured using the 24-hr recall interview with parent and child. Alternatively, the researcher could choose to focus on one component of the regimen, such as blood glucose testing, thereby reducing the measurement demands of the study.

Since our focus is children, it is not surprising that developmental issues have and will continue to emerge. Compared to older children and adolescents, there is evidence that 6–9-year-olds provide less reliable data when interviewed about adherence behaviors involving time. However, it also appears that with a short period of practice, these young children quickly learn to become highly reliable reporters about all adherence behaviors, including those involving time. While adolescents appear to be able to provide reliable data concerning their diabetes adherence behaviors, their actual level adherence is markedly poorer than that exhibited by their younger counterparts. The adolescent developmental period is also associated with a marked deterioration in diabetes control. For years, adolescents' poorer diabetes control was presumed to be "caused" by their poorer adherence. But, studies of adolescents, like studies of IDDM patients in general, have failed to document consistent, clinically significant associations between adherence behaviors and diabetes control. Clearly, explanatory variables other than, and in addition to, adherence behaviors must be considered. We will return to this issue later.

The remaining guidelines have not been mentioned in previous sections of this chapter and relate to both research design and variable selection.

Most, if not all, previous studies can be faulted for their failure to ensure temporal congruity between their adherence and health status measures. For example, glycosylated hemoglobin, the most widely accepted index of diabetes control, represents the average of the patient's blood glucose over the preceding 2–3 months (Ziel & Davidson, 1987). To test whether adherence behaviors are related to glycosylated hemoglobin, adherence behaviors should be monitored for 2–3 months preceding the blood draw for the glycosylated hemoglobin assay.

Earlier studies have used cross-sectional designs in which a single measure of diabetes control, such as glycosylated hemoglobin, is related to one or more adherence measures. This is analogous to assessing the relationship between calorie consumption and weight; by measuring both at the same point in time, the relationship between the two will be underestimated by fat people who are dieting to lose weight and very thin people who are consuming excess calories in an attempt to gain weight. A better approach would be to use a longitudinal design in which weight is measured at study entry, calories consumed are monitored for a specified interval, and then weight is remeasured at study end. Similarly, longitudinal designs that permit some statistical control of diabetes control at study entry, with adherence behaviors monitored during an interval temporally congruent with the same diabetes control measure collected at study end, may offer a more sensitive test of adherence/health status relationships.

Glycosylated hemoglobin is a standard index of diabetes control used by most clinicians and investigators. The inability of many researchers to predict glycosylated hemoglobin using behavioral measures raises questions as to its use as the sole dependent measure in studies that attempt to link adherence behaviors to diabetes control. As mentioned previously, glycosylated hemoglobin provides an index of the patient's average blood glucose during the preceding 2–3 months. As such, it is relatively insensitive to blood glucose variability. Most clinicians would agree that one goal of treatment is reduced variability in blood glucose, in addition to a general lowering of blood glucose levels to the near-normal range. The results of a glycosylated hemoglobin assay may offer information about the second goal but will provide little insight into the first. Patients may differ considerably in terms of blood glucose variability while their average blood glucose levels may be the same. Such patients may exhibit very similar glycosylated hemoglobin levels, leading to the false conclusion that they are responding to diabetes in the same way. It is possible that adherence behaviors influence blood glucose variability more than mean blood glucose levels. This is simply an hypothesis that awaits empirical verification. However, testing this hypothesis may prove difficult since blood glucose variability data would require multiple glucose tests at varying times across days. Such data would be difficult to acquire on an outpatient basis since the patient would have to provide it. The availability of memory meters that record the time, date, and results of all blood glucose tests may prove helpful in this regard. Nevertheless, the investigator remains dependent upon the patient to conduct all of the necessary tests. Our data suggest that few patients are highly adherent glucose testers. This would limit such studies to the subsample of patients who would willingly conduct the multiple glucose tests requested by the researcher. Nevertheless, such studies could provide some initial insights as to the relative influence of adherence behaviors on blood glucose variability as compared to mean blood glucose.

Also noteworthy is the fact that past research has focused exclusively on glucose metabolism, utilizing blood glucose, urine glucose, or glycosylated hemoglobin measures. To our knowledge, there have been no published reports of adherence/lipid metabolism relationships in this population. This is an interesting oversight in view of the fact that triglyceride and cholesterol levels are often elevated in poorly controlled diabetes youngsters (Glasgow, August, & Hung, 1981; Lopes-Virella, Wohlthmann, Loadholt, & Buse, 1981; Peterson, Koenig, Jones, Saudek, & Cerami, 1977; Sosenko, Breslow, Miettinen, & Gabbay, 1980). Further, children with diabetes are most likely to die of athersclerotic heart disease in adulthood (Barrett-Conner & Orchard, 1985). Future studies should assess both glucose and lipid metabolism in order to determine whether adherence behaviors have differential effects on these two different aspects of metabolism in diabetes patients.

In order to obtain reasonable sample sizes, many earlier studies attempted to link adherence to health status in very heterogeneous groups of patients. Recent studies have taken greater care to distinguish between the insulin-dependent and the non-insulin-dependent forms of diabetes. While homogeneous in terms of diabetes type, most samples remained heterogeneous in terms of patient age, disease duration, pubertal status, the ability of the patient to produce some insulin of his/her own, insulin dose, and so on. This heterogeneity may be introducing so much variability that adherence/health status relationships are very difficult to detect. Since it is impossible to study completely homogeneous patient groups, the investigator should give some thought as to which variables should be the focus of efforts to restrict patient samples.

In our own work with IDDM children and adolescents, we have been repeatedly impressed with the predictive power of patient age and disease duration on diabetes control. Since patient age and disease duration per se explain nothing, we have considered possible mechanisms underlying these associations. Two biological factors seem particularly worthy of future study. Disease duration is associated with patients' ability to produce insulin on their own; this ability diminishes with increasing disease duration (Travis, Brouhard, & Schreiner, 1987). It is quite possible that adherence behaviors will have differential effects on those children who continue to produce some endogenous insulin, compared to those who no longer retain this ability. In future research, C-peptide assays could be performed in order to identify which children are endogenous insulin producing (Schade, Santiago, Skyler, & Rizza, 1983).

In childhood populations, increasing age is associated with pubertal development. There is recent evidence that insulin resistance increases in nondiabetic as well as diabetic youngsters during the adolescent period (Amiel, Sherwin, Simonson, Lauritano, & Tamborlane, 1986). While the causal mechanisms underlying this increased insulin resistance is unknown, hormonal factors associated with puberty are strongly suspected. Adolescent IDDM populations are most interesting because of the deterioration in diabetes control and in regimen adherence associated with this developmental period. Yet, the available literature has failed to document a consistent, clinically significant association between adolescents' adherence behaviors and their diabetes control. Perhaps hormonal factors associated with puberty are sufficiently powerful to obscure or diminish the influence of adherence behaviors on IDDM adolescents' metabolic status. Future studies can better address this issue by including assessments of pubertal status, in addition to measures of adherence behaviors, and indices of diabetes control.

The appropriateness of the insulin dose prescribed presents additional problems for the investigator studying adherence/health status relationships. In any given sample, some children are probably underinsulinized, others are overinsulinized, and still others are on an appropriate insulin dose. Insulin dose is yet one more variable responsible for increased hereogeneity in any study sample. However, issues surrounding the appropriateness of insulin dose prescriptions present significant theoretical problems as well. Adherence should impact upon health status only when the medical treatment prescribed is effective. Even perfect adherence cannot make an inappropriate treatment regimen effective. In cases of faulty regimen prescriptions, highly adherent behaviors may have no impact upon patient health status or could even prove harmful. Theoretically, in any given sample of IDDM youngsters, adherence behaviors should exhibit expected relationships to health status only in youngsters prescribed an appropriate insulin dose. For those who are underinsulinized or overinsulinized, very different adherence/health status relationships may emerge. Unfortunately, there are no readily available, objective criteria as to the appropriateness of any insulin dose. Units of insulin per kilogram is a crude index sometimes used by clinicians and investigators. However, it is unsatisfactory because insulin needs can vary greatly between patients. Glycosylated hemoglobin assay is also used as an index of the appropriateness of the child's insulin dose. This too is unsatisfactory because variables other than insulin dose (i.e., adherence behaviors) are presumed to effect glycosylated hemoglobin levels. Daily blood glucose tests are a third method of determining an appropriate insulin dose. Daily determinations of blood glucose level and variability are entirely dependent upon patient cooperation and, once again, are presumed to be effected by factors (i.e., adherence behaviors) other than, or in addition to, insulin dose. In future research, greater attention needs to be given to the identification of each child's "ideal" insulin dose. Laboratory assays relevant to this issue (e.g., assays of exogoneous insulin availability and utilization, insulin antibodies, and other indices of insulin resistance) may become less costly and more reliable. In the meantime, health care providers need to be reminded that a high glycosylated hemoglobin level is an indication that something is wrong but not what is wrong. The problem could lie with the patient's behavior or with the provider's prescription. In most cases, a great deal of additional information will need to be collected to make an educated determination as to how best to proceed. Psychologists working with patients to improve their adherence behaviors should coordinate their efforts with those of the patient's physician. In cases where improved adherence results in no discernible change in diabetes control, the physician should be encouraged to review the appropriateness of the patient's prescribed insulin dose.

Most studies that attempt to link adherence behaviors to diabetes control have used between-subjects designs. Group designs presume that adherence behaviors affect diabetes control in much the same way across subjects. It is quite possible that the same adherence behaviors have very different effects on the metabolic status of different individuals. If so, group designs would be insensitive to true, but highly individualized, adherence/diabetes control relationships. When group designs fail to detect significant associations between adherence and diabetes control, within-subject designs may be able to elucidate these relationships more clearly. There is some precedent for this approach within the available IDDM literature (Cox, Gonder-Frederick, Pohl, & Pennebaker, 1983; Freund, Johnson, Rosenbloom, Alexander, & Hansen, 1986; Pennebaker, et al., 1981). These studies, which focused on symptom–blood glucose relationships in IDDM populations, failed to find any significant association between patient symptomotology and episodes of hypoglycemia or hyperglycemia when a group design was used. When the data were reanalyzed using a within-subjects approach, multiple significant associations emerged. In other words, most patients exhibited one or more symptoms that were consistently associated with hypoglycemia or hyperglycemia. But, the pattern of these symptom/glycemic relationships differed across patients. While these studies did not address possible associations between adherence behaviors and diabetes control, they nicely demonstrate the very discrepant findings that may emerge when between-subjects versus within-subject designs are used.

Since adherence behaviors are presumed to be causally linked to health status in IDDM populations, the failure of the available literature to clearly and consistently document such a relationship is disturbing to clinicians and researchers alike. However, our efforts to date are not without merit. We have developed better measures of adherence, we have developed better conceptualizations of the phenomena we seek to study, and we have developed clearer guidelines that should improve research on this important topic in the future.

Acknowledgment. Supported by grants #R01 HD13820 and K04 HD00686 from the National Institute of Child Health and Human Development.

References

Amiel, S.A., Sherwin, R.S., Simonson, D.C., Lauritano, A.A., & Tamborlane, W.V. (1986). Impaired insulin action in puberty: A contributing factor to poor glycemic control in adolescents with diabetes. *The New England Journal of Medicine, 315*, 215–219.

Barrett-Connor, E., & Orchard, T. (1985). Diabetes and heart disease. In National Diabetes Data Group (Eds.). *Diabetes in America* (pp. XVI: 1–41) (NIH Publication No. 85-1468). Washington, D.C.: U.S. Department of Health and Human Services/Public Health Service.

Bobrow, E.S., AvRuskin, T.W., & Siller, J. (1985). Mother-daughter interaction and adherence to diabetes regimens. *Diabetes Care, 8*, 146–151.

Brownlee-Duffeck, M. Peterson, L., Simonds, J.F., Goldstein, D., Kilo, C., & Hoette, S. (1987). The role of health beliefs in the regimen adherence and metabolic control of adolescents and adults with diabetes mellitus. *Journal of Consulting and Clinical Psychology, 55*, 139–144.

Carney, R.M., Schecter, K., & Davis, T. (1983). Improving adherence to blood glucose testing in insulin-dependent diabetic children. *Behavior Therapy, 14*, 247–254.

Caron, H.S., & Roth, H.P. (1968). Patients' cooperation with a medical regimen: Difficulties in identifying the noncooperator. *The Journal of the American Medical Association, 203*, 120–124.

Charney, E., Bynum, R., Eldredge, D., Frank, D., MacWhinney, J.B., McNabb, N., Scheiner, A., Sumpter, E.A., & Iker, H. (1967). How well do patients take oral penicillin? A collaborative study in private practice. *Pediatrics, 40*, 188–195.

Christensen, N.K., Terry, R.D., Wyatt, S., Pichert, J.W., & Lorenz, R.A. (1983). Quantitative assessment of dietary adherence in patients with insulin-dependent diabetes mellitus. *Diabetes Care, 6*, 245–250.

Clarke, W.L., Snyder, A.L., & Nowacek, G. (1985). Outpatient pediatric diabetes-I. Current practices. *Journal of Chronic Diseases, 38*, 85–90.

Cox, D.J., Gonder-Frederick, L., Pohl, S., & Pennebaker, J.W. (1983). Reliability of symptom–blood glucose relationships among insulin-dependent adult diabetics. *Psychosomatic Medicine, 45*, 357–360.

Cox, D.J., Taylor, A.G., Nowacek, G., Holley-Wilcox, P., & Pohl, S.L. (1984). The relationship between psychological stress and insulin-dependent diabetic blood glucose control: Preliminary investigations. *Health Psychology, 3*, 63–75.

Daneman, D., Siminerio, L., Transue, D., Betschart, J., Drash, A., & Becker, D. (1985). The role of self-monitoring of blood glucose in the routine management of children with insulin-dependent diabetes mellitus. *Diabetes Care, 8*, 1–4.

Davis, M.S. (1968). Physiologic, psychological and demographic factors in patient compliance with doctors' orders. *Medical Care, 6*, 115–122.

Epstein, L.H., Beck, S., Figueroa, J., Farkas, G., Kazdin, A.E., Daneman, D., & Becker, D. (1981). The effects of targeting improvements in urine glucose on metabolic control in children with insulin dependent diabetes. *Journal of Applied Behavior Analysis, 14*, 365–375.

Epstein, L.H., & Cluss, P.A. (1982). A behavioral medicine perspective on adherence to long-term medical regimens. *Journal of Consulting and Clinical Psychology, 50*, 950–971.

Epstein, L.H., Coburn, P.C., Becker, D., Drash, A., & Siminerio, L. (1980). Measurement and modification of the accuracy of determinations of urine glucose concentration. Diabetes Care, 3, 535–536.

Freund, A., Johnson, S.B., Rosenbloom, A., Alexander, B., & Hansen, C.A. (1986). Subjective symptoms, blood glucose estimation, and blood glucose concentrations in adolescents with diabetes. *Diabetes Care, 9*, 236–243.

Freund, A., Johnson, S.B., Silverstein, J., & Thomas, J. (1989). Assessing daily management of childhood diabetes using 24-hr. recall interviews: Reliability and stability. Unpublished manuscript, University of Florida.

Glasgow, A.M., August, G.P., & Hung, W. (1981). Relationship between control and serum lipids in juvenile-onset diabetes. *Diabetes Care, 4*, 76–80.

Glasgow, R.E., McCaul, K.D., & Schafer, L.C. (1987). Self-care behaviors and glycemic control in type I diabetes. *Journal of Chronic Disease, 40*, 399–417.

Glasgow, R.E., Wilson, W., & McCaul, K.D. (1985). Regimen adherence: A problematic construct in diabetes research. *Diabetes Care, 8*, 300–301.

Gonder-Frederick, L.A., Julian, D.M., Cox, D.J., Clarke, W.L., & Carter, W.R. (1988). Self-measurement of blood glucose: Accuracy of self-reported data and adherence to recommended regimen. *Diabetes Care, 11*, 579–585.

Gross, A.M. (1983). Self-management training and medication compliance in children with diabetes. *Child and Family Behavior Therapy, 4*, 47–55.

Hanson, C.L., Henggeler, S.W., & Burghen, G.A. (1987a). Race and sex differences in metabolic control of adolescents with IDDM: A function of psychosocial variables? *Diabetes Care, 10*, 313–318.

Hanson, C.L., Henggeler, S.W., & Burghen, G.A. (1987b). Model of associations between psychosocial variables and health-outcome measures of adolescents with IDDM. *Diabetes Care, 10*, 752–758.

Hulka, B.S., Kupper, L.L., Cassel, J.C., & Mayo, F. (1975). Doctor-patient communication and outcomes among diabetic patients. *Journal of Community Health, 1*, 15– 27.

Johnson, S.B., Freund, A., Silverstein, J., Hansen, C., & Malone, J., (1989). Adherence/health status relationships in childhood diabetes. Unpublished manuscript, University of Florida.

Johnson, S.B., Pollak, T., Silverstein, J.H., Rosenbloom, A.L., Spillar, R., McCallum, M., & Harkavy, J. (1982). Cognitive and behavioral knowledge about insulin dependent diabetes among children and parents. *Pediatrics, 69*, 708–713.

Johnson, S.B., Silverstein, J., Rosenbloom, A., Carter, R., & Cunningham, W. (1986). Assessing daily management in childhood diabetes. *Health Psychology, 5*, 545–564.

Johnson, S.B., Tomer, A., Cunningham, W.R., & Henretta, J. (in press). Adherence in childhood diabetes: Results of a confirmatory factor analysis. *Health Psychology*.

Kaplan, R.M., Chadwick, M.W., & Schimmel, L.E. (1985). Social learning intervention to promote metabolic control in type I diabetes mellitus: Pilot experiment results. *Diabetes Care, 8*, 107–206.

Kaar, M.-L., Akerblom, H.K., Huttunen, N.-P., Knip, M., & Sakkinen, K. (1984). Metabolic control in children and adolescents with insulin-dependent diabetes mellitus. *Acta Paediatrica Scandinavica, 73*, 102–108.

Lopes-Virella, M.F., Wohlthmann, H.J., Loadholt, C.B., & Buse, M.G. (1981). Plasma lipids and lipoproteins in young insulin-dependent diabetic patients: Relationship with control. *Diabetologia, 21*, 216–223.

Lowe, K., & Lutzker, J.R. (1979). Increasing compliance to a medical regimen with a juvenile diabetic. *Behavior Therapy, 10*, 57–64.

Marquis, K.H., Ware, J.E., Jr., & Relles, D.A. (1979). *Measures of diabetic patient knowledge, attitudes and behavior regarding self-care: Summary Report.* Atlanta, GA: Center for Disease Control (NTIS No. PB83-134528).

Mazze, R.S., Pasmantier, R., Murphy, J., & Shamoon, H. (1985). Self-monitoring of capillary blood glucose: Changing the performance of individuals with diabetes. *Diabetes Care, 8*, 207–213.

Page, P., Verstraete, D.G., Robb, J.R., & Etzwiler, D.D. (1981). Patient recall of self-care recommendations in diabetes. *Diabetes Care, 4*, 96–98.

Pennebaker, J.W., Cox, D.J., Gonder-Frederick, L., Wunsch, M.G., Evans, W.C., & Pohl, S. (1981). Physical symptoms related to blood glucose in insulin-dependent diabetics. *Psychosomatic Medicine, 43*, 489–500.

Peterson, C.M., Koenig, R.J., Jones, R.L., Saudek, C.D., & Cerami, A. (1977). Correlation of serum triglyceride levels and hemoglobin concentrations in diabetes mellitus. *Diabetes, 26*, 507–509.

Reynolds, L., Johnson, S.B., and Silverstein, J. (in press). Assessing daily diabetes management by 24-hr. recall interview: The validity of children's reports. *Journal of Pediatric Psychology*.

Schade, D.S., Santiago, J.V., Skyler, J.S., & Rizza, R.A. (1983). *Intensive insulin therapy*. Amsterdam: Excerpta Medica.

Schafer, L.C., Glasgow, R.E., & McCaul, K.D. (1982). Increasing the adherence of diabetic adolescents. *Journal of Behavioral Medicine, 5*, 353–362.

Schafer, L.C., Glasgow, R.E., McCaul, K.D., & Dreher, M. (1983). Adherence to IDDM regimens: Relationship to psychosocial variables and metabolic control. *Diabetes Care, 6*, 493–498.

Schafer, L.C., McCaul, K.D., & Glasgow, R.E. (1986). Supportive and nonsupportive family behaviors: Relationships to adherence and metabolic control in persons with Type I diabetes. *Diabetes Care, 9*, 179–185.

Simonds, J., Goldstein, D., Walker, B., & Rawlings, S. (1981). The relationship between psychological factors and blood glucose regulation in insulin-dependent diabetic adolescents. *Diabetes Care, 4*, 610–615.

Sosenko, J.M., Breslow, J.L., Miettinen, O.S., & Gabbay, K.H. (1980). Hyperglycemia and plasma lipid levels: A prospective study of young insulin-dependent diabetic patients. *New England Journal of Medicine, 302*, 650–654.

Spevack, M. Johnson, S.B., & Riley, W. (1988). The effect of diabetes summer camp on adherence behaviors and glycemic control. Presented at the Florida Conference on Child Health Psychiology, Gainesville, Florida.

Tattersall, R.B., & Lowe, J. (1981). Diabetes in adolescence. *Diabetologia, 20*, 517–523.

Travis, L.B., Brouhard, B.H., & Schreiner, B. (1987). *Diabetes mellitus in children and adolescents*. Philadelphia: W.B. Saunders Co.

Watkins, J.D., Williams, F., Martin, D.A., Hogan, M.D., & Anderson, E. (1967). A study of diabetic patients at home. *American Journal of Public Health, 57*, 452–459.

Webb, K.L., Dobson, A.J., Tupling, H.E., Harris, G.W., O'Connell, D.L., Atkinson, J., Sulway, M.J., & Leeder, S.R. (1982). Evaluation of a diabetes education programme. *Australian/New Zealand Journal of Medicine, 12*, 153–160.

Webb, K.L., Dobson, A.J., O'Connell, D.L., Tupling, H.E., Harris, G.W., Moxon, J.A., Sulway, M.J., & Leeder, S.R. (1984). Dietary compliance among insulin-dependent diabetics. *Journal of Chronic Disease, 37*, 633–643.

Williams, T.F., Martin, D.A., Hogan, M.D., Watkins, J.D., & Ellis, E.V. (1967). The clinical picture of diabetic control, studied in four settings. *American Journal of Public Health, 57*, 441–451.

Wilson, D.P., & Endres, R.K. (1986). Compliance with blood glucose monitoring in children with Type I diabetes mellitus. *The Journal of Pediatrics, 108*, 1022–1024.

Wing, R., Nowalk, M., Marcus, M., Koeske, R., & Finegold, D. (1986). Subclinical eating disorders and glycemic control in adolescents with Type I diabetes. *Diabetes Care, 9*, 162–167.

Ziel, R.H., & Davidson, M.B. (1987). The role of glucosylated serum albumin in monitoring glycemic control in stable insulin-requiring diabetic out-patients. *Journal of Clinical Endocrinology and Metabolism, 64*, 269–273.

4

Neuropsychological Consequences and Correlates of Diabetes in Childhood

Christopher M. Ryan

Introduction

There is now no doubt that a link exists between diabetes mellitus and the development of "neuropsychological" or "neurobehavioral" or "cognitive" disturbances. That is not to say that diabetes is *invariably* associated with cognitive dysfunction. It is not. Indeed, *as a group*, diabetic patients are not all that dissimilar from nondiabetic individuals—at least from a neuropsychological perspective. Nevertheless, studies conducted during this decade have demonstrated that cognitive dysfunction does appear in certain diabetic children and adults. Sometimes this dysfunction is manifested as a series of clinically significant deficits that are so serious that they disrupt the ability of the individual to function effectively in the world. More commonly, this dysfunction is much more subtle. In fact, it is probably more accurate to consider this so-called neuropsychological dysfunction as a *decrement* in mental efficiency rather than as an intellectual *deficit*.

Conceptualizing the disease of diabetes as having both biomedical and psychosocial components, I shall draw on a series of recent studies of neuropsychological functioning in children and adolescents, and attempt to delineate the link between juvenile-onset diabetes and decrements in information-processing efficiency. My goal is not only to describe the nature and extent of neuropsychological disturbances associated with diabetes in childhood, but to more accurately attribute these disturbances to specific disease parameters. To that end, I shall begin with a brief discussion of the theoretical reasons for predicting the existence of neuropsychological dysfunction in diabetic youngsters. I shall then summarize the early studies (and the methodological problems inherent in those studies), and follow with a more detailed discussion of the neuropsychological studies conducted on children during the past 10 years. In response to Fritsch and Hitzig's (1870) admonition that "the method creates the results," I shall focus on methodological issues (both problems and innovations) whenever possible.

The Relationship Between Diabetes, Brain Dysfunction, and Psychosocial Disorders

If one believes that performance on neuropsychological tests can serve as an index of the integrity of the brain, one would *expect* to find significant neuropsychological impairments in diabetic patients. It is well known that the central nervous system (CNS) may be affected directly or indirectly by the biomedical complications of diabetes mellitus as well as by the physiological changes produced by insulin treatment of that disorder.

Considered as complications of diabetes are those biomedical disorders that are manifested as changes within the peripheral nervous system, the small blood vessels, and the blood-brain barrier (for comprehensive review see Mooradian, 1988). Retinopathy and peripheral neuropathy are two of the earliest, most common complications; renal disease and cardiovascular disturbances tend to develop somewhat later in life. These complications appear to be a function of chronic, high blood glucose levels (hyperglycemia), and are positively correlated with the duration of disease. Although few studies of humans have provided direct evidence of neuropathologic changes *within* the brain that are secondary to diabetes-related cerebrovascular changes (but see Reske-Nielsen, Lundbaek, & Rafaelsen, 1965), animal research has provided indirect evidence for a relationship between diabetes and the development of brain abnormalities at the vascular, biochemical, and neuroendocrine level (e.g., Bestetti & Rossi, 1982; Luse, Gerritsen, & Dulin, 1970; Mukai, Hori, & Pomeroy, 1980). Most impressive are the recent animal studies suggesting that the integrity of the blood-brain barrier may be altered in such a way that the normal delivery of nutrients to the brain is blocked, and the normal transport of toxic substances out of the brain is disrupted (Junker, Jaggi, Bestetti, & Rossi, 1985).

On the other hand, the use of exogenous insulin injections to treat diabetes can also have an adverse effect on the brain. Too much insulin, or a normal dose of insulin in an individual who has increased their level of exercise and/or reduced their intake of carbohydrates, will eventuate in a reduction of ambient blood glucose levels (hypoglycemia). Because cerebral metabolism requires consistent, very high levels of glucose for normal functioning, a decline in blood glucose levels to approximately 60 mg/dl or less will usually trigger a series of autonomic changes (e.g., sweating, weakness, irritability) as well as a series of neuroglycopenic changes, best characterized as a transient reduction in overall mental efficiency. At very low blood glucose levels, permanent severe brain damage may be produced, and seizures or coma may occur. While hypoglycemia may occur in the diabetic patient at any age, very young diabetics seem to have an increased risk of hypoglycemia (Ternand, Go, Gerich, & Haymond, 1982).

If one believes that performance on neuropsychological tests can be influenced by psychosocial or psychiatric factors, one would also expect to find significant neuropsychological impairments in diabetic patients. A very extensive literature has examined the possibility that juvenile-onset diabetes may interfere with normal psychosocial functioning, and disrupt a child's performance in the classroom. Early cross-sectional studies supported that view with data indicating that youngsters with diabetes of several years duration had a higher incidence of behavior problems (Katz, 1957), significantly more psychiatric pathology as well as a greater degree of anxiety, dysphoria, and dependency (Swift, Seidman, & Stein, 1967), lower self-esteem and more depression (Sullivan, 1978), and evidence of more psychopathology within the family (Gath, Smith & Baum, 1980; Stein, & Charles, 1971; Sterky, 1963).

Those conclusions must be tempered by results from several more recent studies that have found little evidence of significant psychopathology. When diabetic youngsters were compared with demographically similar healthy children or with children having other chronic diseases, few between-group differences were seen on measures of depression, anxiety, and perceived quality of life (e.g., Kellerman, Zeltzer, Ellenberg, Dash, & Rigler, 1980; Ryan, Leahy, Morrow, & George, in press; Tavormina, Kastner, Slater, & Watt, 1976). Although a prospective study of newly diagnosed diabetic children has demonstrated that 36% of these youngsters met DSM-III criteria for a psychiatric disorder shortly after diagnosis, this disorder was transient: within 9 months of initial diagnosis of IDDM, 93% of the children had recovered psychiatrically (Kovacs et al., 1985). The lack of a consensus between different investigators may be a consequence of variations in methodology—particularly in subject sampling strategies. Clearly, the effect of diabetes on psychosocial functioning in children remains controversial at the present time. Nevertheless, most clinicians would argue that regardless of the empirical data, many of their pediatric diabetic patients seem to manifest serious behavioral and psychiatric problems.

There are several reasons why ascertaining the presence or absence of psychosocial/psychiatric problems in this patient population is extremely important for the neuropsychologist. The first of these has to do with the sensitivity and specificity of neuropsychological tests in detecting brain dysfunction. Although the overall sensitivity of neuropsychological measures to serious brain dysfunction is high, the specificity of these measures to structural brain damage is low. That is, individuals may perform poorly on standard clinical neuropsychological tasks for a variety of reasons that are unrelated, or only indirectly related, to a brain lesion. Depressed individuals tend to perform in the "impaired" and "borderline impaired" range on a wide variety of tasks (for review, see Miller, 1975). Those tasks most likely to be affected in depression are the very same measures that are most sensitive to the effects of a cortical or subcortical lesion—tasks assessing concentration and memory skills (Weingartner, Cohen, Murphy, Martello, & Gerdt, 1981). Anxious individuals may also manifest impairments on certain neuropsychological tests for essentially the same reason: their high level of psychological distress interferes with their ability to concentrate and expend the mental effort to carry out certain cognitive operations (Cummings, 1985).

Poor performance on certain neuropsychological tests may also be noted in individuals who have impoverished, or incomplete, educational or cultural experiences. This is particularly the case on measures of "crystallized intelligence," where an individual is asked to recall or otherwise manipulate information that is typically acquired in a particular environment, or at a particular developmental stage. One can correctly answer a question like "Where is Mexico?" only because of certain cultural or educational experiences. Studies of both children (Amante, VanHouten, Grieve, Bader, & Margules, 1977) and adults (Heaton, Grant, & Matthews, 1986; Ryan, Morrow, Bromet, & Parkinson, 1987) have repeatedly demonstrated the influence of educational and cultural or experiential factors on neuropsychological test performance.

From this brief review, one would predict that neuropsychological deficits would be quite prominent in diabetic patients. The biomedical complications of diabetes and the use of insulin to treat diabetes may, independently, disrupt the structural and functional integrity of the brain and in that way interfere with performance on standard clinical neuropsychological measures. That is, learning, memory, problem-solving ability, and speed and dexterity should all be impaired to a certain extent in diabetic patients because these cognitive processes are most susceptible to any type of diffuse cortical dysfunction. The high degree of psychosocial disruption frequently found in diabetic children and their families is an additional reason why one would expect to see prominent neuropsychological deficits in the diabetic youngster. Again, such deficits should be most apparent on measures of learning, memory, and speed and dexterity, but, in addition, one might expect to see performance decrements on measures of crystallized intelligence (e.g., Verbal IQ scores, academic achievement tests) if the psychosocial disorder is associated with behavioral problems in the classroom or otherwise interferes with the normal process of cognitive development.

Early Studies of Cognitive Functioning in Diabetic Children

Although early investigators did not specifically articulate the hypothesis that juvenile-onset diabetes may be associated with widespread cognitive impairment, between 1935 and 1965 there was certainly a great deal of interest in the intellectual capacity of diabetic children, as indexed by their performance on standardized measures of intelligence. In virtually all instances, the Stanford–Binet Intelligence Test was administered to diabetic youngsters, and their scores compared with the normative data. For example, Grishaw, West, and Smith (1939) studied a group of diabetic patients drawn from their private practice and administered the Stanford–Binet to a subset of 62 randomly selected children, all of whom had been diagnosed before the age of 16 years. They concluded that diabetic youngsters are "well in advance of the normal distribution . . ." (p. 799), having found that 42% of their subjects had IQs above 110 (as compared with 10.5% from Terman's normative sample), and only 10.5% had IQs below 90 (as compared with 19.4% from the normative group). Additional support for the view that diabetic children are brighter than nondiabetics comes from Joslin's (1935) study of 169 diabetic youngsters treated at a specialty clinic in Boston. He and his associates found that twice as many tested above 110 as tested below 90.

Unfortunately, these conclusions have not been supported by other investigators. Shirley and Greer (1940) concluded that diabetic youngsters, as a group, were somewhat *less* intelligent than nondiabetics. In their investigations they evaluated 155 diabetic youngsters who were referred to a university psychiatry clinic. Almost all of these children came from families that were either indigent or were drawn from the lower economic classes. Unlike Joslin or Grishaw and associates, the Stanford–Binet IQ scores of these children tended to somewhat lower than Terman's normative sample. Only 21% fell in the "superior" or "very superior" range, whereas 22% fell in the "dull normal" range and 12% fell in the "mentally retarded" range. On the other hand, both McGavin and associates (1940) and Brown (1938) reported a distribution of IQ scores that did not differ from that of the normal population.

Because of the high degree of variability in results from study to study, these early descriptive reports provide no useful information about the cognitive capacity of diabetic children. They do, however, illustrate a methodological problem which continues to plague investigators studying clinical samples: the possibility of sampling bias. It is likely that those children drawn from a private practice (e.g., Grishaw et al., 1940) or from a diabetes specialty clinic (e.g., Joslin, 1935) during the Depression will have come from more affluent, better educated families. Because scores on cognitive tests are associated with social class level (e.g., Amante et al., 1977), it is not at all surprising to find these middle- and upper-class children performing better than the normative sample on the Stanford–Binet. For that same reason, it is not surprising to find that those youngsters drawn from an indigent population and specifically *referred* to a psychiatric clinic (because of clinically significant behavioral and psychiatric disturbances?) would tend to perform below normal on intelligence tests (Shirley & Greer, 1940). While this would be less of a concern if the diabetic patients were being compared with a control group composed of demographically similar nondiabetics, in most instances such comparisons were not made. Rather, the IQ distributions of the diabetic subjects were compared with the published normative IQ distributions which were based on a representative sample of the U.S. population.

The two studies that found essentially normal intelligence in diabetic youngsters (Brown, 1938; McGavin et al., 1940) were those that ascertained the socioeconomic status of each subject's family and demonstrated that their samples were truly representative of either the state or U.S. population. Indeed, Brown (1938) went a step further and included a comparison group comprised of healthy siblings, in an effort to more closely control for socioeconomic differences between diabetic and nondiabetic subjects. Although some have recently argued that the siblings of children with a chronic disease may not always be an ideal "normal" group because they may also manifest mild cognitive or behavioral problems (e.g., Breslau, Weitzman, & Messenger, 1981), the inclusion of a sib control group probably remains the most efficient means of ensuring that the "normal" comparison group is demographically similar to the targeted patient group.

Virtually all of these early studies were purely descriptive *group* studies that made no effort to examine the relationship between IQ scores and diabetes-related variables (e.g., degree of metabolic control, duration of disease, age at diagnosis, presence of specific biomedical complications, etc.). The one exception to that generalization is a study conducted by Ack, Miller, and Weil (1961). In their investigation, they evaluated 38 diabetic children who were drawn from a broad socioeconomic spectrum and ranged in age from 3 to 18.5 years. They administered the Stanford–Binet to both diabetic children and their siblings, but rather than comparing the two groups of subjects, they compared each diabetic with his or her sib and calculated the mean difference in IQ scores between each of the 38 pairs of subjects. Contrary to expectation, they did not find an obvious relationship between duration of diabetes and these IQ difference scores. On the other hand, a significant effect of age at onset was found: those youngsters who developed diabetes before 5 years of age earned IQ scores that were significantly lower than their nondiabetic sib (10-point difference on average), whereas those who developed diabetes after that age performed as well as their sibling (less than a 1-point difference).

Ack and associates provided both a psychosocial and neurological justification for using an age at onset of 5 years to subdivide their diabetic sample. They suggested that very young diabetic children were more likely than older diabetic children to experience a significant degree of psychosocial distress, in part because these younger children have relatively limited personality resources to cope with the disturbing events associated with diabetes (hospitalization; frequent injections and monitoring of blood and urine). They also argued that the first 5 years of life are the period of greatest growth and change within the central nervous system (CNS), and for that reason, a serious biochemical insult during that interval is more likely to have a long-lasting adverse effect. Some support for that latter possibility was found when they examined the relationship between the IQ scores and the number of metabolic crises. Though there was no association between IQ and the number of hypoglycemic seizures and/or episodes of ketoacidosis in the later onset diabetic group, there appeared to be a trend in the early onset group: the greater the number of serious metabolic disturbances (either as a consequence of excessively low or high blood glucose levels), the lower the child's IQ, relative to their sibling. Unfortunately, these trends failed to reach statistical significance, perhaps because of the small number of subjects, as well as the difficulty in accurately quantifying the number of metabolic crises.

These early studies provided no compelling evidence that juvenile-onset diabetes significantly disrupts cognitive functioning and for that reason, interest in examining the relationship between diabetes and neuropsychological performance dropped off. This decision may have been premature, in large part because of the serious methodological problems associated with these studies. In addition to the sampling problems detailed above, two other methodological deficiencies deserve mention.

First, the level of statistical analysis was, at best, primitive. Most authors merely presented the proportion of diabetic patients falling in the "average," "above average," and "below average" range (e.g., Brown, 1938; Grishaw et al., 1939; McGavin et al., 1940). The one exception to that is the study by Ack et al. (1961) who used both parametric and nonparametric techniques to compare diabetic and nondiabetic subjects.

Second, the types of measures employed to assess cognitive status are relatively insensitive to cognitive, or neuropsychological, *dys*function. In nearly all instances, investigators relied on the Stanford–Binet Intelligence Test and computed only a single, global measure of competence —the IQ score. No effort was made to examine possible patterns of strengths and weaknesses on individual subtests, nor was any effort made to examine relatively circumscribed cognitive processes, like learning, memory, problem-solving, and motor coordination. This is a rather puzzling omission because several very early papers (e.g., Dashiell, 1930; Miles & Root, 1922) used a variety of measures (e.g., mental arithmetic; memory span; speed and dexterity) and found that diabetic patients experience dramatic deterioration on these more specific types of tasks.

Juvenile-Onset Diabetes and Neuropsychological Functioning: The Age at Onset Effect

A resurgence of interest in the possible relationship between diabetes and neuropsychological dysfunction in children has occurred during the past 10 years. At least four reasons for this change come to mind. First, several groups of European investigators have recorded electroencephalograms (EEGs) from diabetic and nondiabetic children and concluded that diabetic youngsters have an elevated risk of brain abnormalities (Eeg-Olofsson & Petersen, 1966; Gilhaus, Daweke, Lülsdorf, Sachsse, & Sachsse, 1973; Haumont, Dorchy, & Pelc, 1979). Of particular note is the finding of Gilhaus and associates that those children who developed diabetes early in life seem to be much more likely to manifest abnormalities than those with a somewhat later onset. Second, several studies of diabetic *adults* suggested that these individuals may indeed be at risk for cognitive deficits. Evidence of clinically significant impairment was found on measures of learning efficiency (Bale, 1973), on tasks requiring rapid responding and focused attention (Meuter, Thomas, Grüneklee, Gries, & Lohmann, 1980), and on complex problem-solving tests (Rennick, Wilder, Sargent, & Ashley, 1968). Third, there has been a renewed interest in the psychological well-being of diabetic patients, particularly children. This interest led to a national conference on that topic held in 1979 (Hamburg, Lipsett, Inoff, & Drash, 1980) which articulated strategies for new research on psychological aspects of diabetes mellitus. Finally, the growth and formalization of the specialized field of neuropsychology has provided both a range of assessment instruments and an appreciation for the value of such procedures.

Age at Onset and Widespread Cognitive Dysfunction in Adolescents

It is within this context that we initiated a series of studies in 1980 on diabetic adolescents. Because so little was known about the nature and extent of neuropsychological dysfunction in these individuals, we took an inductive, rather than a deductive, approach and administered a comprehensive battery of tests that would allow us to determine the neuropsychological *correlates* of juvenile-onset diabetes. Although the initial plan was to rely on measures drawn primarily from the Halstead–Reitan Neuropsychological Battery (e.g., Vega, 1980), that approach was later discarded because of the general insensitivity of the Halstead–Reitan measures to relatively circumscribed, subtle impairment—particularly in children. Substituted in its place was a battery that would allow us to take a "process approach" to assessment (Milberg, Hebben, & Kaplan, 1986), and examine discrete cognitive processes, like learning, memory, attention, mental flexibility, and visuospatial processes. Our goal was to take an epidemiologic approach and administer these measures to a large, randomly selected sample of children drawn from the Allegheny County Diabetes Registry (Drash et al., 1983). We restricted our evaluation to adolescents between 10 and 19 years of age, in part because these were the children who, from a clinical perspective, seemed to be at risk for having serious problems in the classroom.

In our first large study we administered a comprehensive battery of neuropsychological tests to 125 diabetic children (mean age = 14.7 years) who had been diabetic for at least 3 years prior to testing, and who been diagnosed between the ages of 2 months and 14 years. In addition, 83 healthy nondiabetic children were also evaluated. Eighty percent of them were siblings of the diabetic subjects; the remainder were recruited from the families of the medical center staff. No child in any group had a past history of any neurologic or psychiatric disorder, and the three groups were comparable on demographic measures (parent educational and occupational level). Because of the relatively small number of black diabetic children in this catchment area (11%), we restricted our analyses to white teenagers. The 46 subjects who developed diabetes at or before 5 years of age were assigned to an "early onset" subgroup; the remaining 79 diabetics subjects diagnosed after that age were assigned to a "later onset" subgroup. An age at onset of 5 years was selected in part because of the earlier work by Ack and associates (1961), and in part because a preliminary discriminant function analysis made by us during the first year of data collection indicated that an age at onset of 5 years best differentiated "impaired" from "nonimpaired" diabetic subjects. The very large literature on the effects of other childhood chronic diseases (e.g., epilepsy) has also found that children diagnosed before age 5 have the greatest risk of manifesting cognitive impairments as adolescents or young adults (e.g., Dikmen, Matthews, & Harley, 1975).

Included in the test battery were subtests from the Wechsler Intelligence Scale for Children (WISC-R) or the Wechsler Adult Intelligence Scale (WAIS), the Wechsler Memory Scale (WMS), and the Wide Range Achievement Test (WRAT). In addition, a number of specialized neuropsychological tests were administered, including the Hooper Visual Organization Test, the Trail Making Test, the Grooved Pegboard Test, and several learning and memory tests. Factor analysis techniques were used to group the tests into five general cognitive domains: General Intelligence, Visuospatial Processes, Learning and Memory, Attention and School Achievement, and Mental and Motor Speed. Multivariate analysis of variance techniques were then used to compare the three groups on each of these five clusters.

We found that the group of early onset diabetic subjects was impaired, relative to the other two groups, in *every* cognitive domain. They learned new information less efficiently, they recalled less of that information after a 30-min delay, they tended to distort or omit details when copying geometric designs, they made more errors on a number of different visual information-processing tasks, and they performed more slowly (and often less accurately) on tasks that required rapid responding. Not surprisingly, they also earned significantly lower scores on subtests from the Wechsler IQ scales, and performed more poorly on standardized measures of school achievement. In contrast, on nearly all measures, the scores of the later onset diabetic subjects did not differ *statistically* from the nondiabetic control subjects, though there was a tendency for the diabetic group to earn scores that were somewhat lower than controls.

Finding statistically significant between-group differences does not necessarily mean that the magnitude of these differences is clinically significant. To determine the extent to which these early onset diabetic subjects were clinically impaired, we first established "cutting scores" for each of the 20 variables that best discriminated those subjects from the other two groups. This was done by classifying as "impaired" any score that was more than two standard deviations below the mean for the normal control group. We then determined the number of tests on which a subject fell in the "impaired" range. The subject was actually classified as having clinically significant neuropsychological impairment only if they fell in the "impaired" range on three or more measures. This latter criterion was adopted to reduce the possibility of capitalizing on change performance fluctuations on only one or two tests. Using these criteria, a significantly greater proportion of the early-onset subjects were clinically impaired (24%), as compared with the later onset (6%) and nondiabetic control (6%) subjects.

What is it about developing diabetes early in life that increases the risk of significant neuropsychological impairment? Two possible explanations come to mind. A view that remains popular, though is probably incorrect, suggests that these cognitive problems are primarily psychogenic in origin. It has been hypothesized that the stresses and psychosocial disruption that occurs in the family treating the very young diabetic child could interfere with the child's cognitive growth and development—perhaps by reducing, or otherwise modifying, the child's opportunities for stimulation (e.g., Cerreto & Travis, 1984). A more likely alternative explanation argues that the cognitive deficits of our early onset subjects are organic in origin. Not only is the brain of the young child particularly sensitive to any type of metabolic derangement or toxic/hypoxic event, but young diabetic children seem to be unusually susceptible to episodes of hypoglycemia (Ternand et al., 1982). Given the link between the occurrence of hypoglycemic seizures early in life and the development of neurological and neuroanatomical disorders (Hirabayashi, Kitahara, & Hishida, 1980; Ingram, Stark, & Blackburn, 1967), it would not be surprising to find a higher incidence of neuropsychological deficit in diabetic children who have had such episodes during the first 5 years of life.

With the right type of psychosocial and biomedical data, one should be able to differentiate empirically between these two alternative hypotheses. In our study, we did not collect detailed data on the psychosocial characteristics of the family and their child during the first 5 years of life. On the other hand, it is not clear that reliable data of that kind can *ever* be obtained retrospectively. Though we were able to obtain medical history information from the family on the number of serious metabolic crises (e.g., hypoglycemic seizure or coma; episode of ketoacidosis), our examination of those episodes (which ranged from 0 to 989) suggest that the ascertainment of this information is also extremely unreliable. Attempts to corroborate parent reports with information from medical charts were successful only in demonstrating remarkably little consensus. We concluded that the only way to unequivocally demonstrate a quantitative relationship between metabolic crises (and other biomedical and psychosocial events) is to follow diabetic children prospectively from the day they are diagnosed.

Because we suspected that parents' estimates of serious hypoglycemia were extremely inaccurate, we merely asked them whether their diabetic children had or had not *ever* experienced a hypoglycemic seizure. Although we found that a significantly greater proportion (42%) of our subjects with early onset of diabetes had one or more seizures, compared to our subjects with later onset of diabetes (25%), the correspondence between the occurrence of a seizure and the development of impairment was found to be less than perfect. Furthermore, because so few subjects in our study manifested clinically significant biomedical complications of diabetes (e.g., retinopathy), it was impossible to test the hypothesis generated by several adult neuropsychologists (Rennick et al., 1968; Skenazy & Bigler, 1984) that certain complications are risk factors for cognitive deficits. We did, however, examine the relationship between neuropsychological test scores and degree of metabolic control, as indexed by the glycosylated hemoglobin values, and found no significant relationship.

This study was the first to use a comprehensive battery of tests to demonstrate that children who develop diabetes early in life are at risk for manifesting *widespread* neuropsychological deficits. These results suggested that *if* a diabetic child is going to show evidence of cognitive impairment, those disturbances will be apparent by adolescence, and will affect virtually every cognitive domain. However, because different cognitive processes normally develop at very different rates, one might expect to find that diabetic children will display a somewhat variable pattern of results, depending on their age when evaluated. Three recent studies—two focusing on younger children, and one comparing younger and older adolescents—demonstrate how the behavioral expression of diabetes-related neuropsychological deficits varies at different ages.

Age at Onset and Spatial Information-Processing Skills in Younger Children

Using a somewhat different battery of tests and evaluating a younger group of diabetic subjects, Rovet and her associates in Toronto have also found support for the age at onset effect (Rovet, Ehrlich, & Hoppe, 1988). In their study, they evaluated a group of children, 6 to 14 years of age (mean = 10), comparing the performance of 27 early onset diabetic subjects with 24 later onset diabetic children and 30 nondiabetic control subjects, all of whom were siblings of the diabetic subjects. Approximately equal numbers of boys and girls were in each group. An age at onset of 4, rather than 5, years was used by Rovet and associates to differentiate the early and later onset subgroups.

Their neuropsychological test battery emphasized two different cognitive domains: verbal skills and spatial skills. Verbal processes were evaluated with the WISC-R Similarities and Vocabulary subtests, as well as the Primary Mental Abilities (PMA) Verbal Meaning Test. The WISC-R Block Design and Object Assembly subtests, the PMA Spatial Relations subtest, and the Beery–Buktenica Test of Visual Motor Integration were used to assess the spatial domain. In addition, academic achievement was evaluated with the WRAT. Using multivariate analysis techniques, they found that within the verbal domain, diabetic children—regardless of age at diagnosis—performed more poorly than the nondiabetic control group. In contrast, within the spatial domain, early onset diabetic children were more impaired than the later onset diabetic or control subjects. Further analysis revealed a significant Group × Sex interaction on spatial measures such that the early onset girls showed the greatest impairment. A similar interaction was not found with the verbal tests. On measures of academic achievement, the only between-group differences were found on the WRAT Arithmetic test, on which early onset diabetics earned significantly lower scores than later onset subjects.

Multiple regression techniques were used to determine whether performance on certain tests could be predicted from one or more diabetes-related biomedical variables (e.g., glycohemoglobin values; number of hypoglycemic seizures; etc.). A statistical model was constructed that was able to explain 14.4% of the variance on the spatial factor. Better performance was associated with a *longer* duration of illness, a later onset of diabetes, and few hypoglycemic convulsions. Of those three variables, duration of illness was the best predictor. For arithmetic achievement, a higher number of convulsions and poorer diabetic control (higher glycohemoglobin values) predicted lower test scores. Verbal scores were not related to any of the biomedical variables.

Why *shorter* rather than *longer* duration of diabetes should predict poorer scores on spatial tasks is somewhat puzzling. If level of performance were solely determined by CNS factors, I would have expected that those subjects with a longer duration of disease would have a greater degree of cognitive impairment. Rovet and her colleagues offer two possible explanations. On the one hand, they suggest that these results may be a statistical artifact and reflect the positive association between age at assessment and spatial skills, as well as a positive association between duration of diabetes and age at assessment. With their relatively small sample size, it becomes quite difficult to untangle this confound statistically. As an alternative explanation, they suggest that performance on spatial tasks may be particularly sensitive to ambient blood glucose fluctuations, and that children with diabetes of relatively long duration may have more stable blood glucose levels than recently diagnosed children. Unfortunately, this interesting speculation cannot be tested directly, as they did not measure blood glucose levels at the time of assessment. However, indirect evidence from their glycohemoglobin measures indicates that this possibility is unlikely. When they used the glycohemoglobin values to estimate recent blood glucose levels, they found no correlation between those values and duration of illness.

A third alternative explanation, which they did not entertain, is the possibility that their recently diagnosed diabetic children are having a psychosocial reaction to their disease (cf. Kovacs et al., 1985). Since anxiety (at least in adults) is known to adversely affect performance on tasks that requires rapid responding (King, Hannay, Mask, & Burns, 1978), it is this factor which could disrupt performance. As these youngsters begin to cope with their disease more effectively, however, their level of distress goes down (Kovacs et al., 1985). This reduction in anxiety could, in turn, be associated with improvement in their ability to perform certain tasks rapidly. Because Rovet's test battery confounds *spatial* information-processing and *rapid* information-processing, it would not be surprising to find the most recently diagnosed diabetic children (who are also most stressed) to be most impaired on those measures. Although intriguing, this scenario must be considered as speculative at the present time, in the absence of prospective data on both stress levels and spatial information-processing efficiency in newly diagnosed diabetic children.

A number of differences between Rovet's results and those reported by the Pittsburgh group deserve mention. First, the overall magnitude of the early onset effect tends to be quite small. Although a number of between-group comparisons were statistically significant, there is certainly little evidence that any of their early onset diabetic children manifested clinically significant neuropsychological impairments. Second, widespread cognitive impairment was not found. Rather, Rovet and associates found between-group differences to be limited to spatial measures. This failure to find impairments on verbal measures is most likely to be a consequence of age differences in the two samples, given the fact that verbal and visuospatial competencies mature at somewhat different ages. Third, the gender effects reported by Rovet et al. were not found by our group. This may reflect sex differences in vulnerability to cerebral insult. As Taylor (1969) has argued, young girls (who mature faster than boys and perform more poorly on spatial tasks) may manifest less complete hemispheric specialization which may, in turn, reduce the capacity of the right hemisphere for spatial processing. As a consequence, any electrophysiological or neurochemical disturbance will be more likely to impair those cognitive processes having a spatial component.

Despite those differences, Rovet's studies replicate our general findings: children who develop diabetes early in life have a heightened risk of manifesting deficits on certain cognitive tests. Again, serious hypoglycemia appears to be a factor that increases this risk, whereas level of recent metabolic control, ascertained from glycohemoglobin measurements, does not seem to be a potent predictor of poor neuropsychological outcome.

Age at Onset and Intelligence in Younger Children

In any group of diabetic children drawn from a relatively restricted age range, the variables "age at onset" and "duration of diabetes" are confounded: all other things being equal, a 12-year-old with an early onset of diabetes will have had the disease longer than a 12-year-old with a later onset of diabetes. Both the Pittsburgh group and the Toronto group used statistical procedures to "control" for that confound, though it is not clear how effective such procedures are at disentangling highly intercorrelated variables. A more elegant solution would be to stratify subjects into subgroups based on specific values of each of those variables. This approach has been taken by Holmes and Richman (1985) in their attempt to determine the independent contributions of age at onset and duration of diabetes on intelligence. They administered the WISC-R to 44 diabetic children, 6 to 16 years of age (mean = 12.3), and assigned them to one of four subgroups on the basis of age at onset (demarcated at 7 years) *and* duration of diabetes (demarcated at 5 years). For example, a subject with an age at onset of 7 years and a duration of diabetes of 5 years would be assigned to the "early onset/short duration" subgroup. Children were included only if their IQ scores fell in the "normal" range (85 to 129); using that criterion they excluded two subjects. We are not told whether these are early or late onset subjects.

Results from a two-way analysis of variance revealed that neither age at onset nor duration of diabetes had a statistically significant effect on Verbal IQ (VIQ) scores, although the age at onset factor approached significance ($p = .08$). In contrast, both a main effect of Age at Onset and an Onset × Duration interaction were found for Performance IQ (PIQ). That is, children with an age at onset before 7 years and a duration of diabetes greater than 5 years earned lower PIQs (mean = 95.6) than subjects in the other groups (range of means: 108–112). Moreover, this early onset/long duration subgroup also showed a clinically significant VIQ–PIQ discrepancy of 13 points (mean VIQ = 109; mean PIQ = 95.6). Not only was the mean VIQ–PIQ discrepancy for the other three subgroups much smaller (1 to 7), but it was in the opposite direction; that is, their PIQs were *higher* than their VIQs.

When individual subtest scores were compared, no statistically reliable differences were seen, though this is not surprising, given the small number of subjects in each subgroup (range = 9 to 12). It is interesting to note, however, that on all of the Performance subtests, the "early onset/long duration" subgroup tended to have the lowest age-scaled scores. In contrast, on the Verbal subtests, the lowest mean scores on Information, Vocabulary and Comprehension were found in the "late onset/long duration" subgroup.

This study provides additional support for the hypothesis that early onset of diabetes disrupts cognitive processes. Like Rovet and associates, Holmes and Richman focused on younger children and found nonverbal skills to be most affected. Again, the magnitude of this effect is clinically significant insofar as their "early onset/long duration" subjects manifested VIQ–PIQ discrepancies that were so large, on average, that they would be considered by many neuropsychologists to be pathognomonic of mild cerebral dysfunction.

Effects of Age at Onset and Age at Test on Short-Term Memory Efficiency in Adolescents

Taking a very different approach, we (Ryan, Morrow, Ecoff, & George, 1987) explicitly looked at short-term memory efficiency in our sample of diabetic and nondiabetic adolescents. Short-term memory was selected for several reasons. First, it appears that a child's performance on certain types of memory tasks continues to improve during adolescence (Rohwer & Bean, 1973). Second, this type of task mimics, in many ways, the sorts of mental operations normally carried out by high functioning individuals, insofar as the subject must process several types of information simultaneously. Although short-term memory has been operationally defined in a number of different ways, we employed the Brown–Peterson distractor technique (Peterson & Peterson, 1959) because it requires subjects to focus attention and carry out two mutually exclusive tasks simultaneously: remember a series of unrelated words, and count backwards by threes as accurately and as rapidly as possible.

In the present study, we administered the Four Word Short-Term Memory Test to 29 to early onset and 65 later onset diabetic youngsters, as well as to 65 demographically similar nondiabetic control subjects. All subjects were between 12 and 19 years of age. Virtually all of these subjects had been studied previously by us (Ryan, Vega, & Drash, 1985). Subjects younger than 12 years of age were not included because we had found in a pilot investigation that the task was so difficult that many of these youngsters simply could not complete it.

On each test trial, the subject hears four unrelated words (e.g., stain/lawn/cottage/angel) read at the rate of one word per second. They then hear a three-digit number from which they begin counting backwards by three until the examiner says "stop." At that point they attempt to recall the words. Three retention intervals were used: 5, 15, and 30 seconds. Five trials at each retention interval were randomly intermixed for a total of 15 trials.

To examine the effects of age on performance, subjects were stratified into younger (12.0 to 15.9 years) and older (16.0 to 19.0 years) subgroups. Figures 4.1 and 4.2 summarize the mean number of words correctly recalled by each group of subjects at each retention interval. For younger subjects, there were no statistically reliable differences between the three groups. However, among the older subjects, the early onset diabetics earned significantly lower scores than the other groups of subjects at each of the three retention intervals. This pattern of results suggests that early onset diabetic subjects may manifest a serious developmental delay, in terms of acquiring the complex cognitive skills that underlie efficient performance on this short-term memory test. It appears that as *non*diabetic teenagers get older, their performance on the Four Word Short-Term memory test improves. Exactly the same pattern appears in the later onset diabetic teenagers: the older later onset subjects performed at a level that is indistinguishable from the older nondiabetic controls, and significantly better than that of the younger later onset diabetic subjects. In contrast, no such age-associated improvement was seen in the early onset group. While the younger early onset subjects performed as well as the other two younger subgroups, their older counterparts did not perform like older control subjects; rather they perform like *younger* control subjects. It is as if the process of memory development has been arrested in these early onset diabetic youngsters. Unfortunately, because this is a cross-sectional, rather than a longitudinal, study, we cannot make a strong statement about the effects of early onset diabetes on developmental processes. These data do, however, suggest that prospective studies of diabetic children that specifically examine the rate of development in different cognitive domains could be a fertile area for future research.

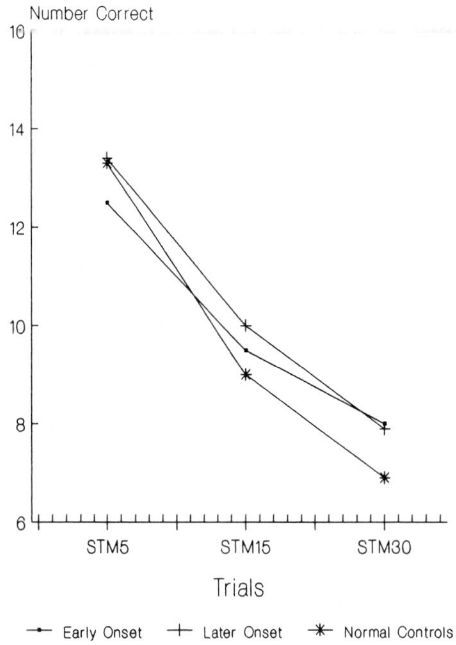

Figure 4.1. Short-term memory results. Younger subjects: 12–0 to 15–11.

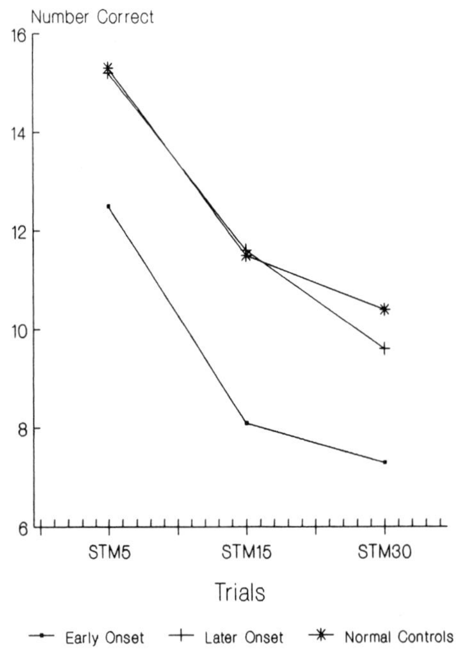

Figure 4.2. Short-term memory results. Older subjects: 16–0 to 19–0.

Age at Onset as a Risk Factor for Neuropsychological Impairment

Research to date suggests that the age at which a child develops diabetes may have a significant impact on that child's cognitive processes. The exact nature and extent of this relationship has not yet been clarified, in part because of differences in subject sampling, types of neuropsychological measures used, and operational definitions of diabetes-related variables, including "early" age at onset. Although there is a consensus that *groups* of early onset diabetic children perform more poorly on certain cognitive tests than groups of later onset diabetic or nondiabetic control subjects, these findings must be interpreted cautiously. Scrutiny of data from individual subjects will demonstrate that only a small subset actually show clinically significant impairments; the remainder show few meaningful decrements in performance. That is, age at onset must be considered only as a *risk factor* for neuropsychological impairment. Children who develop diabetes early in life are only *more likely* to manifest such impairments; there is no evidence that they will inevitably develop such deficits.

Furthermore, it is inaccurate to consider "age at onset" per se as a meaningful predictive variable. Rather, it should be thought of as only a surrogate for one or more variables that are more directly responsible for the development of neuropsychological deficit. Although we and others have speculated that the primary biomedical variable is serious hypoglycemia, the exact relationship between hypoglycemia and cognitive deficit has not yet been fully delineated. A review of data from Ryan, Vega, and Drash, 1985, and Rovet et al. will demonstrate that mere presence of a serious hypoglycemic episode is insufficient to predict clinically significant cognitive impairment. Our failure to find robust, statistically reliable relationships is hampered by the difficulty of quantitating severity of a hypoglycemic episode, particularly when many of these episodes occur nocturnally, and are unobserved or misinterpreted. Does one count only clinical seizures, or does one also include episodes in which the blood glucose value falls below a certain value (but what value, and for how long)? Because a reduction in blood glucose levels is associated with biochemical and electrophysiological changes at the neuronal level, one might expect to see a relationship between multiple episodes of low blood glucose values and the occurrence of cerebral dysfunction. Unfortunately, in order to use glucose readings as a predictor variable, one needs to monitor each child according to a regular, rigorously maintained schedule, or else there is a serious possibility of biased ascertainment: those children who monitor more will have more opportunities for recording both normal and abnormal blood glucose values.

The difficulties associated with the measurement of serious hypoglycemia provide an excellent example of the sorts of problems faced by researchers studying diabetes-related neuropsychological impairment.

Until these methodological problems are resolved, and until investigators are able to measure these variables prospectively over an extensive time period, we will have only an incomplete understanding of the age at onset effect in diabetic individuals.

Other Risk Factors for Neuropsychological Dysfunction in Diabetic Children

Based on studies described thus far, the reader may conclude that children who develop diabetes somewhat later in life are completely normal, from a neuropsychological perspective. To date, the only evidence contradicting that interpretation comes from a study from the Pittsburgh group (Ryan, Vega, Longstreet, & Drash, 1984) that focused on a group of youngsters who developed diabetes somewhat later in life —between 5 and 12 years of age (mean age at onset = 7.7 years). The 40 diabetic adolescents in this study were 12 to 19 years old (mean age = 15.5), and were compared with a group of 40 demographically similar nondiabetic control subjects who were closely matched in age (mean = 15.5). While all test scores were well within the normal range —that is, there was no evidence whatsoever of any type of clinically significant impairment in any subject—there were, nevertheless, a number of statistically reliable between-group differences. Somewhat unexpectedly, the diabetic teenagers were found to earn Wechsler Verbal IQ scores that were significantly lower than controls. This discrepancy was most apparent for those subjects aged 16 and older who received the Wechsler Adult Intelligence Scale (WAIS). An examination of individual subtest scores demonstrates that the diabetic subjects tended to earn lower scores than controls on the Information, Vocabulary, and Similarities subtests. A similar pattern of results was reported by Holmes and Richman for their subgroup of later onset/long duration diabetic children.

It is tempting to attribute these between-group differences to subtle brain dysfunction in the diabetic group—particularly in light of the additional finding that the diabetic group performed more poorly on several visual motor tests. If these differences were a consequence of acquired brain damage, however, we would have expected to find performance decrements on a wider range of measures, including tests of learning and memory ability. That was not the case. Although visuospatial deficits are frequently found in individuals with certain types of brain lesions, a qualitative analysis of those deficits demonstrated that our diabetic subjects earned lower scores only because they were slower than controls. They were, however, no less accurate. We have offered two alternative explanations for this pattern of results. The relatively lower scores earned by later onset diabetic children and adolescents on measures of verbal intelligence may be a consequence of their more erratic school attendance and/or a greater incidence of behavior problems in the classroom. On the other hand, their slower performance on a variety of visuomotor tasks may reflect a personality or response style characterized by extreme cautiousness and attention to detail.

School Attendance and Academic Achievement

Much of the information assessed on a test of verbal intelligence is information acquired in the classroom. Most children are able to answer questions like "Where is Panama?" or "What does the word 'seclude' mean?" primarily because they have been exposed to that information in school. For that reason, one might expect to find an association between Verbal IQ scores, results from standardized academic achievement tests, and school attendance records. In an early study, Weil and Ack (1964) administered the California Reading and Arithmetic Achievement Tests to a group of diabetic youngsters and their siblings, and found no statistically significant differences. Examining school grades, rather than formal achievement test scores, Sterky (1963) reached essentially the same conclusion, reporting no difference between diabetic and nondiabetic school children, and no relationship between school grades and age at onset, duration of diabetes, or degree of metabolic control—as determined by clinical ratings. More recently, however, several investigators have succeeded in finding evidence of academic deficiencies in diabetic youngsters, and at least one study has related those deficiencies to estimates of school attendance.

Focusing on "reading readiness," Gath and associates (1980) evaluated 70 diabetic and 70 nondiabetic children and found a greater proportion of diabetic youngsters to manifest a "reading backwardness." The best predictor of reading problems was not serious hypoglycemic episodes, but was the overall level of metabolic control, as determined by clinical ratings. Poor control was, in turn, associated with a greater level of family strife and psychosocial disruption. The number of school absences was not assessed by those investigators, and so it is impossible to determine whether the relationship between family problems and reading problems was mediated by school attendance.

In our own work (Ryan, Longstreet, & Morrow, 1985), we examined the association between academic achievement and school attendance more directly by interviewing a randomly selected sample of mothers of 62 adolescents who had participated in an earlier study (Ryan et al., 1984). To obtain detailed information about the child's school absence patterns over the last several years, we administered a structured school attendance history questionnaire that we modeled after those questionnaires used to assess lifetime drinking history (e.g., Skinner & Sheu, 1982). Not only did we find that diabetic children tended to miss twice as much school as their nondiabetic peers, but we found an association between estimates of lifetime school absences and performance on the Reading, Spelling, and Arithmetic subtests from the Wide Range Achievement Tests. This relationship between school absence and performance was specific to information most likely to be acquired in the classroom. When school attendance variables were used to predict performance on several visuomotor tasks, no statistically reliable correlations were found.

These results must be interpreted cautiously because of the retrospective nature of the data. There is always the possibility that a mother with a chronically ill child would be more likely to overestimate number of school absences. Nevertheless, a large number of studies, including those that have validated mothers' estimates by reviewing school records, have demonstrated that children with a chronic disease or with nonspecific health-related problems are likely to miss more school than their healthy peers, and that this may affect academic achievement scores (for review, see Weitzman, Klerman, Lamb, Menary, & Alpert, 1982). Moreover, unpublished data from a prospective study of newly diagnosed diabetic children (Kovacs et al., 1985) suggests that our results may *under*estimate school absences to some extent. Examining school records, Kovacs and her associates (personal communication) found that in the year *prior* to diagnosis these children missed an average of 9 days of school; in the year following diagnosis, they missed an average of 15 days of school—a figure that is quite close to the estimate obtained (13) in our cross-sectional study.

Further research on the link between school attendance and neuropsychological test performance is obviously needed. These preliminary findings, however, suggest that the somewhat lowered Verbal IQ scores obtained by later onset diabetic youngsters (e.g., Holmes & Richman, 1985; Ryan et al., 1984) may not necessarily have an organic etiology, but reflect the influence of psychosocial factors.

"Cautiousness" and Psychomotor Slowing

We have been repeatedly impressed by the fact that regardless of age at onset, diabetic youngsters perform a number of tasks more slowly than their nondiabetic peers (e.g., Ryan et al., 1984; Meuter et al., 1980). Although motor slowing is also an early sign of brain dysfunction, we have hypothesized that at least among later onset diabetic youngsters, another interpretation is equally plausible: this slowing reflects the development of a personality or response style characterized by extreme cautiousness and careful attention to detail. This possibility was first expressed by Brown in 1938. Observing the performance of diabetic children completing the Stanford–Binet, he reported that "carefulness, meticulousness, earnestness and conscientiousness were noted an unusual number of times. . . ." and could ". . . be attributed to the habit-training forced on the diabetic child by the regimen of the disease" (p. 181).

Like Brown, we have noted that later onset diabetic children are slower, but no less accurate, on a wide range of psychomotor tests. We could easily imagine that diabetic patients, burdened with a disease that requires them to monitor basic biological functions and balance their insulin dose with their food intake and exercise patterns, might develop a response style characterized by careful attention to detail. Indeed, a goal of many diabetes education programs is to develop in patients this type of "obsessive/compulsive" personality or response style. Although such a style is medically adaptive, it is likely to interfere with performance on any type of task that places a premium on rapid responding.

A series of recent studies by Holmes and associates have, however, provided a very different explanation for the response slowing seen in many diabetic patients. They found that when the blood glucose levels of diabetic young adults were experimentally manipulated, a significant decrement in performance was found in the hypoglycemic state (Holmes, Hayford, Gonzalez, & Weydert, 1983; Holmes, Koepke, Thompson, Gyves, & Weydert, 1984). Response speed, rather than accuracy, was most often affected, and these decrements were most likely to be found when subjects were asked to carry out less familiar, somewhat more complex, information-processing tasks.

Unfortunately, the lack of objective measures of a "cautious response style" has made it impossible to provide an empirical test of the cautiousness hypothesis. Similarly, because we (Ryan, et al., 1984) failed to record blood glucose values following each visuomotor test, it is not possible to determine whether the motor slowing we observed in our later onset diabetic youngsters is attributable to a reduction in ambient blood glucose values at the time of testing.

Juvenile-Onset Diabetes and Neuropsychological Dysfunction: Some Final Thoughts

During the past 10 years remarkable progress has been made in understanding the relationship between diabetes in childhood and neuropsychological functioning. As sampling strategies have become more sophisticated and as neuropsychological measures have become more sensitive to subtle cognitive impairment, researchers have begun to uncover changes in the information-processing efficiency of diabetic children and adolescents.

A small minority of diabetic children do indeed manifest clinically significant cognitive impairments. The exact nature of the impairment seems to differ, depending on the age of the subject, but the results from several different research groups, using diverse assessment instruments, suggests that the so-called age at onset effect is real. Children who develop diabetes in the first several years of life are—for whatever reason—more likely to manifest cognitive problems by school age, and as they grow older, these problems are likely to become increasingly severe. The incidence of these types of neuropsychological deficits is unknown; I would estimate that it encompasses less than 25% of the early onset diabetic population—which, in turn, represents only a very small proportion of all cases of juvenile-onset diabetes. If, as a number of writers have speculated, these deficits are largely a function of serious hypoglycemic episodes, they are obviously preventable. As Golden and his associates (1985) have demonstrated, careful blood glucose monitoring on the part of the parent can significantly reduce the number of serious hypoglycemic episodes in very young diabetic youngsters.

The vast majority of diabetic children do not show clinically significant impairments. In fact, in those instances when they do have difficulty on neuropsychological measures, their performance differs only slightly from that seen in their nondiabetic peers. These subtle between-group differences are most likely to appear on two very different types of measures: those requiring rapid responding, and those measuring "verbal intelligence" or academic achievement. The slight motor slowing seen on a number of tasks is not particularly alarming. Of greater concern, however, is the apparent difficulty many of these otherwise normal diabetic youngsters manifest on verbal intelligence tests. Is this finding (which needs to be replicated) merely a consequence of an increased number of school absences, or is another, yet unknown, variable responsible?

Future research on the neuropsychological consequences of diabetes in childhood is likely to move in the following directions. First, more of this work will take a longitudinal, rather than a cross-sectional, approach. A longitudinal methodology is the only way investigators will be able to unequivocally determine causal relationships between the occurrence of specific biomedical and psychosocial events and the development of neuropsychological impairment. Second, studies concurrently employing both neuropsychological and electrophysiological measures will need to be conducted if researchers are to determine the extent to which behavioral dysfunction is mediated by functional changes occurring within the CNS. This approach has recently been taken by our group, in a study of the transient effects of hypoglycemia on the individual (Kiss et al., 1989). Findings to date suggest that the interrelationships between metabolic, neuropsychological, and electrophysiological variables may be weaker than is commonly believed. Not only is there a wide degree of intersubject variability, but the correlation between behavioral and electrophysiological variables is relatively small in magnitude. Finally, neuropsychological research with children will need to explore more carefully the relationship between cognitive status and one specific biomedical variable: metabolic control. Although a number of investigators have reported that diabetic *adults* in poor metabolic control are more likely to show a variety of information-processing deficits than those adults in good metabolic control (for review, see Ryan, 1988), a similar relationship has not been noted in children—at least when glycohemoglobin values are used as the index of control. Although poor metabolic control may indeed be associated with cognitive dysfunction, it may be that cognitive dysfunction precedes or determines poor metabolic control, rather than the obverse. Patients who have mild cognitive impairments may have more difficulty adhering to an optimal diabetic regimen, and for that reason, be in relatively poor metabolic control. A longitudinal study of this important variable in a younger patient population will allow the determination of causal direction.

Acknowledgments. The preparation of this manuscript was supported in part by Grant DK 26069 from the National Institute of Diabetes and Digestive and Kidney Disease.

References

Ack, M., Miller, I., & Weil, W. (1961). Intelligence of children with diabetes mellitus. *Pediatrics, 28*, 764–770.

Amante, D., VanHouten, V., Grieve, J., Bader, C., & Margules, P. (1977). Neuropsychological deficit, ethnicity, and socioeconomic status. *Journal of Consulting and Clinical Psychology, 43*, 524–535.

Bale, R. (1973). Brain damage in diabetes mellitus. *British Journal of Psychiatry, 122*, 22–39.

Bestetti, G., & Rossi, G. (1982). Hypothalamic changes in diabetic Chinese hamsters. A semiquantitative, light and electromicroscopic study. *Laboratory Investigation, 47*, 516.

Breslau, N., Weitzman, M., & Messenger, K. (1981). Psychologic functioning of siblings of disabled children. *Pediatrics, 67*, 344–353.

Brown, G. (1938). The development of diabetic children, with special reference to mental and personality comparisons. *Child Development, 9*, 175–183.

Cerreto, M., & Travis, L. (1984). Implications of psychological and family factors in the treatment of diabetes. *Pediatric Clinics of North America, 31*, 689–710.

Cummings, J. (1985). *Clinical Neuropsychiatry*. New York: Grune & Stratton.

Dashiell, J. (1930). Variations in psycho-motor efficiency in a diabetic with changes in blood-sugar level. *Journal of Comparative Psychology, 10*, 189–197.

Dikman, S., Matthews, C., & Harley, J. (1975). The effect of early versus late onset of major motor epilepsy upon cognitive-intellectual performance. *Epilepsia, 16*, 73–81.

Drash, A., LaPorte, R., Becker, D., Orchard, T., Wagener, D., Rabin, B., & Kuller, L. (1983). Epidemiological studies in children with diabetes mellitus and their families: The Allegheny County Registry Experience. In G. Chiumello & M. Sperling (Eds.) *Recent Progress in Pediatric Endocrinology* (pp. 4, 125–136). New York: Raven Press.

Eeg-Olofsson, O., & Petersen, I. (1966). Childhood diabetic neuropathy: a clinical and neurophysiological study. *Acta Paediatrica Scandinavica, 55*, 163–176.

Fritsch, G., & Hitzig, E. (1870). Über die elektrische Erregbarkeit des Grosshirns. *Archiv für Anatomie und Physiologie*, 300–332.

Gath, A., Smith, M., & Baum, J. (1980). Emotional, behavioural, and educational disorders in diabetic children. *Archives of Disease in Childhood, 55*, 371–375.

Gilhaus, K., Daweke, H., Lülsdorf, H., Sachsse, R., & Sachsse, B. (1973). EEG-Veränderungen bei diabetischen kindern. *Deutsche Medizinische Wochenschrift, 98*, 1449–1454.

Golden, M., Russell, B., Ingersoll, G., Gray, D., & Humner, K. (1985). Management of diabetes mellitus in children younger than 5 years of age. *American Journal of Diseases of Children, 139*, 448–452.

Grishaw, W., West, H., & Smith, B. (1939). Juvenile diabetes mellitus. *Archives of Internal Medicine, 64*, 787–799.

Hamburg, B., Lipsett, L., Inoff, G., & Drash, A. (Eds.). (1980). *Behavioral and Psychosocial Issues in Diabetes.* Washington, DC: US Department of Health and Human Services.

Haumont, D., Dorchy, H., & Pelc, S. (1979). EEG abnormalities in diabetic children: Influence of hypoglycemia and vascular complications. *Clinical Pediatrics, 18*, 750–753.

Heaton, R., Grant, I., & Matthews, C. (1986). Differences in neuropsychological test performance associated with age, education, and sex. In Grant, I. & Adams, K. (Eds.), *Neuropsychological Assessment of Neuropsychiatric Disorders.* New York: Oxford University Press.

Hirabayashi, S., Kitahara, T., & Hishida, T. (1980). Computed tomography in perinatal hypoxic and hypoglycemic encephalopathy with emphasis on follow-up studies. *Journal of Computer Assisted Tomography, 4*, 451–456.

Holmes, C., Hayford, J., Gonzalez, J., & Weydert, J. (1983). A survey of cognitive function in different glucose levels in diabetic persons. *Diabetes Care, 6*, 180–183.

Holmes, C., Koepke, K., Thompson, R., Gyves, P., & Weydert, J. (1984). Verbal fluency in naming performance in type I diabetes at different blood glucose concentrations. *Diabetes Care, 7*, 454–459.

Holmes, C. & Richman, L. (1985). Cognitive profiles of children with insulin-dependent diabetes. *Developmental and Behavioral Pediatrics, 6*, 323–326.

Ingram, T., Stark, G., & Blackburn, I. (1967). Ataxia and other neurological disorders as sequels of severe hypoglycemia in childhood. *Brain, 90*, 851–862.

Joslin, E. (1935). Studies in diabetes mellitus. II. Its incidence, factors underlying its variation. *American Journal of the Medical Sciences, 187*, 433.

Junker, V., Jaggi, C., Bestetti, G., & Rossi, G. (1985). Basement membrane of hypothalmus and cortex capillaries from normotensive and spontaneously hypertensive rats with streptozocin-induced diabetes. *Acta Neuropathologica, 65*, 202.

Katz, P. (1957). Behaviour problems in juvenile diabetics. *Canadian Medical Association Journal, 76*, 738–743.

Kellerman, J., Zeltzer, L., Ellenberg, L., Dash, J., & Rigler, D. (1980). Psychological effects of illness in adolescence, I. Anxiety, self-esteem, and perception of control. *Journal of Pediatrics, 97*, 126–131.

King, G., Hannay, H., Mask, B., & Burns, J. (1978). Effects of anxiety and sex on neuropsychological tests. *Journal of Consulting and Clinical Psychology, 46*, 375–376.

Kiss, I., Ryan, C.M., Mitrakou, A., Jensen, T., Durrant, J., & Gerich, J. (1989). The effects of experimentally induced hypoglycemia on neuropsychological and electrophysiological indices of cognitive function. *Journal of Experimental Neuropsychology, 11*, 77.

Kovacs, M., Feinberg, T., Paulauskas, S., Finkelstein, R., Pollock, T., & Crouse-Novak, M. (1985). Initial coping responses and psychosocial characteristics of children with insulin-dependent diabetes mellitus. *Journal of Pediatrics, 106*, 827–834.

Luse, S., Gerritsen, G., & Dulin, W. (1970). Cerebral abnormalities in diabetes mellitus: An ultrastructural study of the brain in early onset diabetes mellitus in the Chinese hamster. *Diabetologia, 6*, 192.

McGavin, A., Schultz, E., Peden, G., & Bowen, B. (1940). The physical growth, the degree of intelligence, and the personality adjustment of a group of diabetic children. *New England Journal of Medicine, 223*, 119–127.

Meuter, F., Thomas, W., Grüneklee, D., Gries, F., & Lohmann, R. (1980). Psychometric evaluation of performance in diabetes mellitus. *Hormone and Metabolic Research, Suppl. 9*, 9–17.

Milberg, W., Hebben, N., & Kaplan, E. (1986). The Boston approach to neuropsychological assessment. In K. Adams & I. Grant (Eds.). *Neuropsychological Assessment of Neuropsychiatric Disorders* (pp. 65–86). New York: Oxford University Press.

Miles, W., & Root, R. (1922). Psychologic tests applied to diabetic patients. *Archives of Internal Medicine, 30*, 767.

Miller, W. (1975). Psychological deficit in depression. *Psychological Bulletin, 82 (2)*, 238–260.

Mooradian, A. (1988). Diabetic complications of the central nervous system. *Endocrine Reviews, 9*, 346–356.

Mukai, N., Hori, S., & Pomeroy, M. (1980). Cerebral lesions in rats with long-term streptozocin-induced diabetes mellitus. *Acta Neuropathologica, 51*, 79.

Peterson, L., & Peterson, M. (1959). Short-term retention of individual verbal items. *Journal of Experimental Psychology, 58*, 193–198.

Rennick, P., Wilder, R., Sargent, J., & Ashley, B. (1968). Retinopathy as an indicator of cognitive-perceptual-motor impairment in diabetic adults. *Proceedings of the 76th Annual Convention of the American Psychological Association, 3*, 473–474.

Reske-Nielson, E., Lundbaek, K., & Rafaelsen, O. (1965). Pathological changes in the central and peripheral nervous system of young long-term diabetics. *Diabetologia, 1*, 232–241.

Rohwer, W., & Bean, J. (1973). Sentence effects and noun-pair learning: A developmental interaction during adolescence. *Journal of Experimental Child Psychology, 15*, 521–533.

Rovet, J., Ehrlich, R., & Hoppe, M. (1988). Specific intellectual deficits associated with the early onset of insulin-dependent diabetes mellitus in children. *Child Development, 59*, 226–234.

Ryan, C. (1988). Neurobehavioral complications of type I diabetes. Examination of possible risk factors. *Diabetes Care, 11*, 86–93.

Ryan, C., Leahy, L., Morrow, L., & George, W. Effects of IDDM on the perceived quality of life of adolescents and young adults. Under editorial review.

Ryan, C., Longstreet, C., & Morrow, L. (1985). The effects of diabetes mellitus on the school attendance and school achievement of adolescents. *Child: Care, Health and Development, 11*, 229–240.

Ryan, C., Morrow, L., Ecoff, R., & George, W. Short term memory disturbances in diabetic adolescents. Paper presented at the Annual Meeting of the American Psychological Association, New York.

Ryan, C., Morrow, L., Bromet, E., & Parkinson, D. (1987). The assessment of neuropsychological dysfunction in the workplace: Normative data from the Pittsburgh Occupational Exposures Test Battery. *Journal of Clinical and Experimental Neuropsychology, 9*, 665–679.

Ryan, C., Vega, A., & Drash, A. (1985). Cognitive deficits in adolescents who developed diabetes early in life. *Pediatrics, 5*, 921.

Ryan, C., Vega, A., Longstreet, C., & Drash, A. (1984). Neuropsychological changes in adolescents with insulin-dependent diabetes. *Journal of Consulting and Clinical Psychology, 52*, 335–342.

Shirley, H., & Greer, I. (1940). Environmental and personality problems in the treatment of diabetic children. *Journal of Pediatrics, 16*, 775–781.

Skenazy, J., & Bigler, E. (1984). Neuropsychological findings in diabetes mellitus. *Journal of Clinical Psychology, 40*, 246–258.

Skinner, H., & Sheu, W.- J. (1982). Reliability of alcohol use indices: the lifetime drinking history and the MAST. *Journal of Studies on Alcohol, 43*, 1157–1170.

Stein, S., & Charles, E. (1971). Emotional factors in juvenile diabetes mellitus: A study of early life experience of adolescent diabetics. *American Journal of Psychiatry, 128*, 700–704.

Sterky, G. (1963). Family background and state of mental health in a group of diabetic schoolchildren. *Acta Paediatrica, 52*, 377–390.

Sullivan, B. (1978). Self-esteem and depression in adolescent diabetic girls. *Diabetes Care, 1*, 18–22.

Swift, C., Seidman, F., & Stein, H. (1967). Adjustment problems in juvenile diabetes. *Psychosomatic Medicine, 29*, 555–571.

Tavormina, J., Kastner, L., Slater, P., & Watt, S. (1976). Chronically ill children: A psychologically and emotionally deviant population. *Journal of Abnormal Child Psychology, 4*, 99–110.

Taylor, D. (1969). Differential rates of cerebral maturation between sexes and between hemispheres. Evidence from Epilepsy. *The Lancet, 2*, 140–142.

Ternand, C., Go, V., Gerich, J., & Haymond, M. (1982). Endocrine pancreatic response of children with onset of insulin-requiring diabetes before age 3 and after age 5. *Journal of Pediatrics, 101*, 36–39.

Vega, A. (1980). Neuropsychological correlates: Central nervous function in diabetes. In B. Hamburg, L. Lipsett, G. Inoff, & A. Drash (Eds.). *Behavioral and Psychosocial Issues in Diabetes* (pp. 189–192). Washington, DC: National Institutes of Health.

Weil, W., & Ack, M. (1964). School achievement in juvenile diabetes mellitus. *Diabetes, 13*, 303–306.

Weingartner, H., Cohen, R., Murphy, D., Martello, J., & Gerdt, C. (1981). Cognitive processes in depression. *Archives of General Psychiatry, 38*, 42–47.

Weitzman, M., Klerman, L., Lamb, G., Menary, J., & Alpert, J. (1982). School absence: A problem for the pediatrician. *Pediatrics, 69*, 739–746.

5

Diabetes and Adaptations in Family Systems

Barbara J. Anderson

The purpose of this chapter is to review theorietical perspectives and recent empirical investigations which address two basic questions:

1. What factors influence how *family systems adapt* to IDDM and NIDDM?
2. How do different patterns of *family adaptation* impact on the diabetic family member's *metabolic* and *psychological functioning?*

Very few empirical studies have examined the adult with diabetes within the context of the family (Edelstein & Linn, 1985). The scarcity of studies with diabetic adults which include family variables is well documented (Glasgow & Toobert, 1988) Accordingly, the literature covered in this chapter will necessarily focus more on children and adolescents and their families than on adults, and more on IDDM than on NIDDM.

It is also important to clarify the terms "family system" and "adaptation" used in the title of this chapter. The term "family system" indicates that we will be looking at the diabetes literature for its relevance to understanding the family as a complexly functioning system of parents, children, spouses, siblings, and parent–child subsystems, in which a change in any one member, such as the diagnosis of a serious chronic disease which requires adherence to a complex daily medical treatment plan, promotes change on the part of all other individual members and subsystems within the family group. The term "adaptation" refers to the process by which systems change in interaction with their environment, in ways that enhance control over the environment (White, 1976). It is clear that *both the individual diagnosed with diabetes as well as the family undergo a process of adaptation*, and the goal in this chapter is to review theories and empirical studies which have examined factors that impact on family adaptation to diabetes and have focused on how different patterns of family adaptation impact on the health and psychological adaptation of patients.

Why Study the Family's Role in Insulin-Dependent Diabetes Mellitus (IDDM) and Non-Insulin-Dependent Diabetes (NIDDM)?

What distinguishes diabetes from among other chronic physical diseases is the demand on the patient for self-care and for clinical decision-making responsibilities which require major life-style adjustments and which are transferred to diabetic patients almost immediately after diagnosis (Drash & Becker, 1978). Diabetes self-care affects many components of *family* life—food, physical activity, finances, and time. Because diabetes treatment impacts on many facets of family life, the family of the person with diabetes has been of increasing interest to researchers attempting to understand optimal patterns of family adaptation for patients as they attempt to adhere to the demands of the diabetic treatment regimen. Because the daily treatment required of persons with diabetes *impacts and intrudes upon* expectations for everyday behavior in the family, relationships between family members, and family routines, how the family handles these intrusions plays a central role in the effectiveness with which diabetes is managed at home (Hauser & Solomon, 1985).

Theories of the Family's Role in Diabetes

Linear Models of the Family's Role in Diabetes

In the pediatric literature, until the 1970s, investigations of family adaptation to diabetes in childhood were based on linear approaches. For example, maternal attitudes were seen as single causes of psychological and metabolic outcomes in the diabetic children (see Anderson & Auslander, 1980, for a review of these early approaches to the family of the diabetic child). There was no attention given to the impact of the disease process on the child, nor was recognition given to the impact of the diabetic child's age, disease severity, or the child's adjustment on the other family members' functioning. This approach parallels much of the work on child development conducted early in this century, in which family influences on developing children, in general, were seen as unidirectional, until the influence of the child's age, temperament, and unique personality were appreciated as stimuli for parental behavior. Over the past two decades, linear models of family influences in diabetes in which parental attitudes and personality variables were seen as single and unidimensional determinants of the child's adaptation of diabetes have been replaced with more complex systems approaches. Additional variables such as the disease process and developmental factors in both the child and the parents are now seen as potentially powerful influences shaping the family's response to the diagnosis and treatment of IDDM.

Family System Models

Family system means more than just a consideration of all of the members of the family. When we use the term family system, we are using it in the sense of family systems theorists such as Jackson (1957) and Watzlawick, Beavin, and Jackson (1967), who emphasize that individuals within families must be seen as members of a larger social context in which simple explanations or linear causes for behaviors must be replaced by understanding the behavior of an individual family member as a product of reciprocal interactions and circular causes within the family. As Turk and Kerns (1987) have summarized, a family system has a complex internal organizational structure which is self-regulating, in that it has homeostatic mechanisms to restore balance and is open to continuous interchange with the external social and physical environment.

One of the first theorists to apply a family systems approach in diabetes was Minuchin (Minuchin, Rosman, & Baker, 1978). Minuchin and colleagues applied the family systems model to children with what they termed "psychosomatic diabetes," a subset of children with IDDM who, despite the fact that they were taking their insulin as prescribed, had repeated episodes of diabetic ketoacidosis. When hospitalized and removed from their family environments, these children seemed to be effectively controlled without adjustment of their treatment regimen. Using an experimental procedure in which these children and their parents were subjected to stressful interviews and frequent blood draws in the laboratory, Minuchin and colleagues concluded that the physiological evidence supported the hypothesis that the psychosomatic symptom plays a role in family homeostasis. We have recently published a critique of the "psychosomatic family model" focusing on deficiencies in the data which Minuchin and colleagues presented in support of this model (Coyne & Anderson, 1988). What is most significant about this work, which was published in the classic text *Psychosomatic Families* (Minuchin et al., 1978), is that it articulated for the first time a theoretical model which called attention to the *interconnectedness* of the family and the management of diabetes in children.

Recently, another systems approach to understanding family influences in the management of diabetes in children has been developed by Newbrough and colleagues at Peabody College called "A Family Development Approach" (Newbrough, Simpkins, & Maurer, 1985). Newbrough and colleagues put the reciprocal influences within the family within the context of historic factors of both the family and the broader societal norms and values. Moreover, these authors have focused on the family within the context of stages of diabetes management from prediagnosis through long-term stabilization and have emphasized developmental level of the diabetic child and the parent's stage in the life cycle as important factors influencing the diabetes-related tasks with which families cope and the success with which diabetes management is implemented at home. This model identifies 13 interconnected variables that potentially impact on the effectiveness of the family system's adaptation to diabetes measuring child outcomes: (1) parent's history and developmental stage; (2) community and peer culture norms; (3) child's history and developmental stage; (4) family developmental level or stage; (5) parent's knowledge and perception of child and condition; (6) child's knowledge and perception of self and condition; (7) parent's physical and psychological state; (8) ongoing situation (life events and routines); (9) child's physical and psychological state; (10) parent's resources (instrumental and affective); (11) child's resources (instrumental and affective); (12) compliance behavior; and (13) metabolic control or functioning. The "Extended Family Development Model" is very complex and is the most comprehensive model, to date, of the family systems approach applied to diabetes in children.

In summary, as described earlier, until the 1970s, studies of families of diabetic children were based on a linear model. Subsequently, most studies of the families of diabetic children use a systems model as the appropriate framework within which to approach the role of the family in diabetes. In the following section, we will review these recent studies based on a systems model of the family's role in diabetes management, and we will focus on factors which have been identified as influencing the process of family, primarily parental, adaptation to diabetes.

Research on Family Adaptation to Diabetes in Childhood and Adolescence

Developmental Issues Influencing Family Adaptation

It is now widely recognized that the age and developmental level of the diabetic child influence responses of other family members toward the child, the disease, and treatment responsibilities (Anderson, 1984; Hauser & Solomon, 1985). There have been very few studies comparing parental and family responses to diabetic children of different ages, and although there are several important ongoing longitudinal studies of diabetic children and their families (Jacobson et al., 1986; Kovacs et al., 1985), findings from these prospective studies have not yet been published showing comparisons between family responses at different developmental stages of the diabetic child.

In the following sections we will look at studies which have addressed the question of how the age and developmental tasks of the diabetic child influence family adaptation. Across development, diabetes presents family members with the task of being sensitive to the balance between the patient's need for independence and mastery in terms of self-care and need for family support and involvement in the self-care tasks. This dilemma raises different issues for family adaptation at different stages of child and adult development. The struggle to balance independence and dependence in relationships between the person with diabetes and family members presents chronic coping tasks for families.

Infant and Toddler Years

When a child is diagnosed with IDDM during the first 3 years of life, the locus of responsibility is solely on the parents. Several investigations have identified difficult coping issues for parents with very young diabetic children. Leaverton (1979) reported that management problems facing parents with diabetic infants and toddlers include: monitoring diabetic control; establishing a meal schedule despite the child's "normally" irregular eating patterns; coping with the very young child's inability to understand the need for insulin injections; and managing conflicts with olders siblings due to the parental attention required by the very young diabetic child.

Children diagnosed before the age of 5 years may be at risk for severe hypoglycemic episodes (Rovet, Ehrlich, & Hoppe, 1987) This may be due to the difficulties in administering and adjusting the very small insulin doses needed by most young children, as well as the preverbal child's inability to reliably detect and communicate symptoms of hypoglycemia (Golden, Herrold, & Orr, 1983). It has recently been suggested by several researchers studying the relationship between the age of diagnosis and performance of diabetic adolescents on information-processing and memory tasks that children diagnosed before the age of 5 years are at increased risk for subtle neuropsychological problems (Hagen, Anderson, & Barclay 1986; Rovet et al., 1987; Ryan, 1988).

Michael Golden, pediatric endocrinologist at the University of Indiana Diabetes Research and Training Center, investigated the impact of a comprehensive treatment program for families with children diagnosed before the age of 5 years which focused on frequent blood glucose monitoring and individually designed insulin algorhythms for parental adjustment of the child's insulin. Although Golden and colleagues found that the diagnosis of diabetes in very young children created psychological trauma for the child and family, an aggressive insulin program seemed to benefit rather than further stress these families, by decreasing the frequency of hospitalizations and episodes of severe hypoglycemia (Golden, Russel, Ingersoll, Gray, & Hummer, 1985). Golden and colleagues emphasized the critical importance of the psychosocial support (ongoing contact with a psychiatric social worker and parent group educational meetings) provided to families participating in this intervention program.

There have been no studies of the role of family factors in the ability of infants and toddlers to cope with diabetes (Cerreto & Travis, 1984) Given the suggestion that children with early onset diabetes may be a group at increased risk for long-term behavioral, school, and neuropsychological problems (Ryan, 1988), additional prospective research examining the impact on families of diabetes in children at this young age as well as the relationship between different patterns of family adaptation and child health and behavioral outcomes should be given the highest priority.

Preschool and Early School Years (4 to 7 Years)

Similar to the infant and toddler periods of development, there have been very studies focused on 4- to 7-year-old children with diabetes in their family contexts. Bregani, Della Porta, Carbonne, Ongari, and diNatale (1979) reported that lack of cooperation with diet in the 4- to 7-year-old child with diabetes was often associated with overall emotional immaturity, whereas with 8- to 11-year-old diabetic children, compliance problems were more frequently due to the child's frustrations with following the diet in peer-group settings. Leaverton (1979) has suggested that "separation anxiety" is common for parents with 4- to 7-year-old diabetic children and that there are some appropriate fears and concerns which parents have as the diabetic child enters school. Anderson (1984) has suggested that school entrance by diabetic children may represent the first public context in which parents and children must cope with the social meaning of diabetes, including the tasks of educating others about the disease. Hagen and colleagues (1986) in a study comparing diabetic adolescents who were diagnosed before 5 years of age with diabetic adolescents diagnosed after age 5 reported that entering school with a chronic disease such as diabetes may put the diabetic youngster at increased risk for school problems. School entrance by diabetic children is an important area for further study and an area in which studying all facets of the problem—family reactions, the diabetic child's reactions, school personnel responses, and peer group responses—from a systems perspective is extremely important.

The Middle School Years (8 to 11 Years)

Family adaptation to diabetes during the middle school years is influenced by the rapid growth of children's skills and interests during this age period. The primary adaptation issue facing families is the gradual transfer of responsibility for diabetes care tasks from the parents to the child. In a study of 6- to 13-year-olds, Grey, Grenel, and Tamborlane (1980) investigated the relationships among family functioning, parental self-esteem, and the child's adjustment, self-esteem, and metabolic control. Children's and parents' self-esteem, family functioning, and metabolic control were all significantly better in the well-adjusted group of children. Nine of the "maladjusted" diabetic children were described by the parents as unhappy, passive, and dependent. These authors suggest that preadolescent diabetic children with adjustment problems may often be overlooked because they are not overtly rebellious and hostile but rather overdependent on family members and withdrawn from their peers. Bregani and colleagues (1979) also emphasized the importance of the peer group for 8- to 11-year-old diabetic children. Maternal interviews indicated that during this age period, diabetic children begin to feel a heightened sense of frustration and of social stigma from their diabetic diet restrictions, and the child's emerging self-awareness and ability to compare him/herself with peers make the diabetic child vulnerable to feelings of inadequacy.

It has been frequently suggested that transfer of responsibility for treatment tasks to the diabetic child should be initiated during the middle childhood years. Several age-related guidelines for the child's responsibility in managing diabetes have been proposed (e.g., Greydanus and Hofmann, 1979). Cerreto and Travis (1984) have reported that cohesive families which are "well-balanced between disengagement and enmeshment" and who have rules and procedures followed by all family members, and families in which both parents agree in general about family goals have children who are in good metabolic control. There are few other familiy studies of diabetic preadolescent children. Given the significant development of the child's sense of initiative and industry during these middle childhood years and the implications of this growth for division of responsibility for diabetes management tasks within the family, future studies are needed on the development of different patterns of negotiating responsibilities between parents and diabetic child and the impact of these different family patterns on the child's metabolic functioning and sense of self-efficacy with respect to diabetes management.

The Adolescent Years (12 to 19 Years)

As mentioned earlier, across child development the balancing of responsibility for diabetes management between parents and the diabetic child is the major issue defining family adaptation to this chronic disease. During adolescence, more than at any other stage of child development, the conflict inherent in the changing balance of responsibiltiy between the diabetic child and the family for diabetes management becomes more dramatic (Grossman, 1987). With respect to normal child development, adolescence is marked by dramatic biological, social, emotional, and cognitive changes and is usually divided into three phases —early (12–14 years), middle (14–16 years), and later (17–19 years) adolescence—based on different developmental issues which are prominent at each age period. The period between 12 and 14 years, early adolescence, is characterized by rapid physical growth and the sexual maturation. Young adolescents and their family members must begin to integrate these physical changes into their image of who the teenager is and must collectively acknowledge that the young teenager is no longer a child but is on the threshold of becoming an adult. It is common for families to change their expectations for a broad range of behaviors of the young adolescent at this time. Therefore, diabetes management is frequently "turned over" to the young teenager by parents who frequently maintain some well-meaning "parental watchfulness" (Cerreto & Travis, 1984), which often complicates the adolescent's assumption of responsibility. Another factor complicating this transition of responsibility for diabetes management within families is the new difficulty of controlling blood glucose levels during puberty. Several investigators have recently demonstrated that the physiological changes of puberty cause insulin resistance in both nondiabetic and diabetic adolescents, and that this reduction in insulin sensitivity contributes to hyperglycemia in young diabetic adolescents and may undermine self-care efforts (Amiel, Sherwin, Simonson, Lauritano, & Tamborlane, 1986; Bloch, Clemons, & Sperling, 1987).

During middle adolescence, 14–16 years, the adolescent continues to mature cognitively as well as physically and strives to define a more mature sex-role identity. Independence is increasingly sought from the family, and relationships with peers, including opposite-sex peers, become much more important. The family must continually adapt to this pulling away by the teenager, and "parental watchfulness" or the parents' needs to scrutinize their teenager's health and diabetes care tasks are increasingly frustrated by the adolescent's increasing autonomy in all areas of functioning. The widening sphere of independence by the adolescent coupled with the adolescent's normal drive to be accepted by peers and to "experiment" increases the concern of parents and often results in interaction patterns in which diabetes only elicits negative attention within the family—either concern and frustration over elevated blood glucose and urine ketone levels, or anger and blame over the adolescent's poor adherence to the treatment regimen (Cerreto & Travis, 1984). It has been suggested that parents and health care professionals frequently overestimate the teenager's conceptual understanding of diabetes (Cerreto & Travis, 1984), and parents likewise frequently overestimate adolescent's abilities to follow-through with diabetes care tasks without immediate positive reinforcements and support, mistakenly assuming that "long term good health" will provide sufficient motivation to "take good care of yourself" (Green & Horton, 1982).

Given the inherent conflicts between diabetes self-care and adolescent developmental tasks, it is no surprise that empirical studies document a relationship between problems with adolescent metabolic control and family conflict, lack of cohesion, and rigidity (Anderson, Miller, Auslander, & Santiago, 1981; Bobrow, AvEuskin, & Siller, 1985). Yet Hanson and colleagues (1987) have pointed out that it has been unclear if positive family relationships directly enhance the physical health of adolescents or if positive family interactions improve adherence which, in turn, promotes good metabolic control. To address this question, Hanson et al. (1987) examined the relationship between adherence and metabolic control of diabetic adolescents (mean age = 14.4 years) and family functioning, measured by mothers' and fathers' reports on a measure of marital satisfaction and FACES II, a standardized measure of family cohesion and adaptability, as well as by the adolescents' report on the Supportive subscale of the Diabetes Family Behavior Checklist (Schafer et al., 1986). Positive family relations were directly related to adolescent adherence but not to metabolic control, suggesting that family relations play an important role in the maintenance of adolescent adherence behaviors.

During adolescence, families also have to adapt to changes in their relationships with diabetes health care providers (Green & Horton, 1982). Many older teenagers now want privacy during clinic visits and examinations with doctors; in addition, many health care providers encourage adolescents to begin to telephone them directly rather than relying on parents to communicatie with the health care team (Cerreto & Travis, 1984). For many parents, these changes are very difficult and stressful. Given the importance of positive family relationships for adolescent adherence, more research is needed on how the health care delivery system can optimize the adaptation of families of diabetic adolescents during this period of dramatic shifts in family roles concerning communication with health care providers and shifts in controlling diabetes management at home.

During late adolescence, family adaptation to diabetes is influenced by how the adolescent is coping with other developmental tasks such as choosing a career and educational goals or establishing intimate relationships. If the adolescent has delayed choosing a career or educational goals after high school and is not prepared to assume independent living, the parents may have a difficult time encouraging their older adolescent toward appropriate independence. One of the central developmental tasks facing older diabetic adolescents is learning to develop a support system outside of the family with respect to diabetes and its management. There are no empirical studies of these important developmental issues which confront older diabetic teenagers and their families.

Additional Issues Influencing Family Adaptation to Diabetes

Throughout this section the focus has been on studies which have addressed the issue of family adaptation to diabetes at different stages of child development. Yet we know from the literature on normal child development that there are other powerful factors, such as the child's unique temperament (Chess, Thomas, & Birch, 1965) and level of cognitive functioning (Elkind, 1970), which will influence how the family adapts to the child, and therefore to the child's's diabetes and treatment requirements. Such individual characteristics of diabetic children have only very recently become the focus of research, although not with respect to their impact on family adaptation. With respect to temperament, Rovet and Ehrlich (1988) have recently reported that compared with sibling controls, children with IDDM did not reveal a characteristic temperament profile or show unique problem areas. However, children with higher activity levels, greater regularity in routines, milder reactions to external stimuli, distractibility, and negative moods had better glycemic control. Future work is needed to understand the impact on the family and on family implementation of the treatment regimen of different temperament profiles in diabetic youngsters. With respect to level of cognitive functioning, we have almost no evidence on how families would be impacted by variations in level of cognitive functioning in their diabetic child. Ingersoll, Orr, Herrold, and Golden (1986) have reported a relationship between level of cognitive maturity and ability to implement a self-management regimen in diabetic adolescents. Clearly the family would be affected very differently by teenagers' varying cognitive capabilities; expectations for adolescent behavior and division of responsibility within the family would have to take into account the adolescent's ability to understand the complexities of most insulin regimens. This pioneering work of Ingersoll and colleagues should be extended to an examination of the implications for the family of varying levels of cognitive maturity in children with diabetes, as well as the family's role in the development of cognitive maturity of the diabetic child.

Parental Roles and Responses to Diabetes

The literature on family adaptation to diabetes is very consistent in reporting that the primary responsibilitty for diabetes management at home is assumed by mothers and that fathers' roles with respect to diabetes management at home are less intense than mothers' roles (Zrebiec, 1987). In this respect, diabetes is no different than other chronic diseases in its impact on the family. Investigators have reported that mothers frequently have the primary responsibility for clinical decision making and for implementation of treatment regimens at home and that, in addition, mothers also often experience the most personal distress with respect to their child's condition and treatment (Sabbath, 1974). It should be pointed out, however, that most of the literature on the impact of chronic childhood illness on families has focused on the mother's experiences; much less is known about the impact of chronic childhood illness on fathers (Sabbath, 1974).

Similarly, in studies of diabetes and the family, few investigators have studied fathers directly. Sullivan (1979) reported that for teenage girls with IDDM the report of a positive father–daughter relationship was related to the daughter's good metabolic control. Several investigators have reported that concordance between the father and the mother in terms of diabetes care issues is related to good metabolic control in the child (Anderson & Auslander, 1980). However, cause–effect cannot be assumed here, for children with well-controlled diabetes may prompt concordance between parents in their approach to diabetes management. The past exclusive focus on mothers of diabetic children has resulted in a very limited understanding of how fathers adapt to diabetes and the impact of different paternal coping styles on the child's metabolic and psychosocial functioning.

Research on the Impact of Diabetes on Siblings

For a long time in the literature on childhood diabetes, siblings were used as "healthy comparison subjects" for the diabetic child in the family, rather than being studied in their own right with respect to the special coping issues confronting the sibling of a child with diabetes. Similar to fathers, the experiences of siblings of diabetic children have also been overlooked in past research (Hauser & Solomon, 1985). One recent study (Beit-Halachimi, Kaplan, Laron, Karp, & Galatzer, 1982) suggested that siblings of children with diabetes may experience subtle emotional and interpersonal burdens because of their sibling's diabetes. As investigators begin to utilize more complete family systems models, siblings, like fathers, will begin to play a more prominent role in research on family adaptation (Hauser & Solomon, 1985)

The Broader Context Within Which Families Raise Diabetic Children

The extent to which the family of a diabetic child has additional stresses influences adjustment (Turk & Kerns, 1987). Several investigators have reported that the diabetic child's control deteriorates in families which experience significant financial stress, death of a family member, divorce or separation of parents (Koski, Ahlas, & Kumento, 1976). Moreover, diabetes frequently adds to the financial and social stresses of families (Hamburg & Inoff, 1983). We have very little systematic information about how the broader contextual factors which are identified in the Family Development Model of Newbrough and colleagues (see discussion above) influence the adaptation of families to diabetes.

Research on Family Adaptation to Diabetes in Adulthood

The literature on the adaptation of families to diabetes in an adult is quite small, and studies have not been undertaken from specific theoretical perspectives. Rather, it appears as if the issue driving most of the family research on adults with diabetes is understanding how perceptions of spouse support relate to adherence by adult diabetic patients and to metabolic control. As compared to family studies in the adolescent period, few research studies have addressed the next developmental period of young adulthood, nor have they studied the young adult with IDDM within the family context (Ahlfield, Norman, Soler, & Marcus, 1985). When this age period has been the focus of study, interest has centered on spouse support and decisions about having children. There has been no empirical work and little discussion of the impact of a *parent's* diabetes on the family environment of young children (Anderson & Kornblum, 1984). Based on a small pilot survey of young adults with IDDM, Anderson and Kornblum (1984) identified several family issues that were repeatedly raised by the patients: (1) the uncontrollable moodiness and irritability that occur when the patient's blood sugar level is low or chronically high negatively affect other family members and family interactions and (2) the diabetic parent's constant additional responsibility for self-care frequently conflicts with the needs of other family members. Anderson and Kornblum report that every diabetic adult reported that the cooperation and support of their spouse in managing their disease were essential. Spouse support in diabetes was also studied by Ahlfield et al. (1985) who surveyed 50 young adults with IDDM as to the impact of the disease on their marriage, quality of daily life, and plans for having children. Twenty-six of the young adults with IDDM were married and 22 of these spouses also participated in this research. In terms of agreement between spouses, high agreement was reported between diabetic adults and their spouses concerning the spouse's behaviors which are supportive of the patient's adherence to the diabetic regimen. While most of the couples agreed that diabetes did not interfere with daily tasks (82%) or with socialization with friends (82%), they agreed much less on the impact of diabetes on finances (55%) and family activities (50%). Invariably, diabetic patients perceived that the disease interfered more with these aspects of their lives than did their spouses. Significantly more men than women found diabetes a source of friction in their marriage. Women, however, were more likely to report that diabetes caused a financial burden. None of the young diabetic adults surveyed reported making a conscious decision to remain unmarried. However, 30% of the women and 23% of the men had decided not to have children. The authors conclude that health care professionals treating young adult patients need to be sensitive to these family-related issues.

Spouse support and its relationship to metabolic control and to the adherence of diabetic patients to their medical regimen has been studied systematically by Schafer, McCaul, and Glasgow (1986). An objective system was developed for assessing the frequency with which family members engage in behaviors defined as supportive (e.g., "plan family activities so that they will fit in with your diabetes self-care schedule") or nonsupportive (e.g., "eat foods that are not part of your diabetic diet"). All subjects were free of major diabetic complications. A parent or spouse was also asked to complete this Family Behavior Checklist. In an initial study with 54 adults and 18 adolescents with IDDM, all patients and family members completed this Family Behavior Checklist on two occasions, 6 months apart. Results indicated that adolescents and their family members perceived negative family behaviors as occurring more frequently than did adult patients and their family members. For adults, more perceived negative family interactions were associated with poorer adherence, whereas for adolescents there were no consistent patterns between the report of positive or negative family behavior and adherence. Moreover, perceptions of greater negative but not positive family interaction were marginally associated with poorer metabolic control for adults, also relationships between adherence measures and control were negligible.

Glasgow and colleagues extended this work to include patients with non-insulin-dependent diabetes and their families (Glasgow & Toobert, 1988). In this study, measures of perceived stress and satisfaction with their health care system were also collected. The mean age of the patients in this second study was 60 years, with women constituting 66% of the sample. Patients with major complications of diabetes were not eligible. Unlike the findings for IDDM adults, with NIDDM patients no relationship was found between frequency of negative family behaivor and adherence to the diabetic regimen. Regimen-component-specific measures of family support were stronger predictors than were the overall positive or negative summary scores. Moreover, measures of stress and medical care satisfaction improved the prediction of adherence. The investigators concluded that interventions to improve adherence must be multifaceted and target families as well as other aspects of the social environment.

Edelstein and Linn (1985) studied diabetic men, mean age of 55 years, who had been on insulin at least 1 year. Using the standardized family inventory, the Family Environment Scale (Moos, 1974), the authors concluded that perception of the family environment was associated with degree of metabolic control. An orientation toward achievement in the family most predicted good control in this sample. A family environment which was not highly organized and controlled was also predictive of good control. Perceived lower levels of family conflict, criticism, and tension also predicted good metabolic control. The authors suggested: "Even with the team approach to care of diabetes, the family is sometimes forgotten. Family members need to be included not only in the early aspects of treatment, such as education concerning the disease, but in the ongoing treatment process" (p. 544).

Priorities for Future Research on Families and Diabetes

In this chapter, several methodological and measurement limitations of existing family research in diabetes have been discussed. In summary, future research should give priority to the following:

1. Direct observation of naturally occurring family interactions between different dyads and triads in the family system, as opposed to exclusive use of self-report, standardized family inventories.
2. Assessment of the impact of different temperamental and cognitive styles of diabetic children on family adaptation.
3. Stages of the family life cycle, and the adaptational tasks demanded at different phases in the evolution of the family unit.
4. Longitudinal studies across critical developmental transition periods, such as the toddler years to school entry; late adolescence to young adulthood.
5. Increased focus on fathers and siblings and adaptions in other family dyads besides the mother–diabetic child pair.
6. Broaden the family system to include financial and other resources of the family such as social support networks and availability of extended family.
7. Expand beyong the conventional spouse role to study the impact of diabetes on adaptation in other adult roles, e.g., how is adherence to the diabetic regimen influenced by being a parent or by relationships with grandparents?

In addition to strengthening basic research in this field, it is appropriate to begin to apply existing research and knowledge to health care delivery systems (Turk & Kerns, 1987). As stated by Edelstein and Linn (1985) "the family is sometimes forgotten" in the delivery of health care by systems which cling tenaciously to the individual model. Although it has been repeatedly documented that there is a strong linkage between family adaptation and metabolic functioning, and adherence to the diabetic regimen by children, adolescents, and adults, health care in diabetes continues to be delivered within the confines of an individual model. As health care delivery and interventions expand to use family members strategically in planning and implementing diabetes treatment, health care providers can identify more empirically the significant interconnections between patient and family adaptation.

References

Ahfield, J.E., Norman, R.D., Soler, G., & Marcus, S.D. (1985). The young adult with diabetes: Impact of the disease on marriage and having children. *Diabetes Care, 8*, 52–56.

Amiel, S.A., Sherwin, R.S., Simonson, D.C., Lauritano, A.A., & Tamborlane, W.V. (1986). Impaired insulin action in puberty: A contributing factor to poor glycemic control in adolescents with diabetes. *New England Journal of Medicine 315*, 215–219.

Anderson, B.J. (1984). The impact of diabetes on the developmental tasks of childhood and adolescence: A research perspective. In M. Nattrass & J. Santiago (Eds.), *Recent advances in diabetes* (pp 165–171). London: Churchill Livingston.

Anderson, B.J., & Auslander, W.F. (1980). Research on diabetes management and the family: A critique. *Diabetes Care 3*, 696–702.

Anderson, B.J., & Kornblum, H. (1984). The family environment of children with a diabetic parent: Issues for research. *Family Systems Medicine 2*, 17–27.

Anderson, B.J., Miller, J.P., Auslander, W.F., & Santiago, J.V. (1981). Family characteristics of diabetic adolescents: Relationships to metabolic control. *Diabetes Care, 4*, 586–594.

Beti-Halachmi, N., Kaplan Y., Laron, Z., Karp, M., & Galatzer, A. (1982). Impact of diabetes mellitus on healthy siblings. In Z. Laron & A. Galatzer (Eds.). *Psychosocial aspects of diabetes in children and adolescents*. Basel: Karger.

Bloch, C.A., Clemons, P.S., & Sperling, M.A. (1987). Puberty decreases insulin sensitivity. *Journal Pediatrics 110*, 481–87

Bobrow, E.S., AvEuskin, T.W., & Siller, J. (1985) Mother-daughter interaction and adherence to diabetes regimens. *Diabetes Care 8*, 145–156.

Bregani, P., Della Porta, V., Carbonne, A., Ongari, B., & diNatale, B. (1979). Attitudes of juvenile diabetics and their families towards dietetic regimen. *Pediatric and Adolescent Endocrinology, 7*, 159–163.

Cerreto, M.C., & Travis, L.B. (1984). Implications of psychological and family factors in the treatment of diabetes. *Pediatric Clinics of North America, 31*, 689–710.

Chess, S., Thomas, A., & Birch, H. G. (1965). *Your child is a person*. New York: Viking.

Coyne, J.C., & Anderson, B.J. (1988). The "psychosomatic family" reconsidered: Diabetes in context. *Journal of Marital and Family Therapy, 14*, 113–123.

Drash, A.L., & Becker, D. (1978). Diabetes mellitus in the child: Course, special problems, and related disorders. In H. Katzen and R. Mahler (Eds.). *Diabetes, obesity, and vascular disease. Advances in modern nutrition*, Vol. 2. (pp. 615–643). New York: Wiley.

Edelstein, J., & Linn, M.W. (1985). The influence of the family on control of diabetes. *Social Science in Medicine. 21*, 541–544.

Elkind, D. (1970). *Children and adolescents: Interpretive essays on Jean Piaget*. New York: Oxford University Press.

Glasgow, R.E., & Toobert, D.J. (1988). Social environment and regimen adherence among Type II diabetic patients. *Diabetes Care, 11*, 377–386.

Golden, M., Herrold, A., & Orr, D. (1983). An approach to prevention of recurrent diabetic ketoacidosis in the pediatric population. *Journal of Pediatrics, 107*, 195–200.

Golden, M.P., Russell, B.P., Ingersoll, G.M., Gray, D.L., & Hummer, K.M. (1985). Management of diabetes mellitus in children younger than 5 years of age. *American Journal of Diseases of Children, 139*, 448–452.

Green, L.W., & Horton, D. (1982). Adolescent health: Issues and challenges. In T. Coates, A. Peterson, & P.C. Perry (Eds.). *Promoting adolescent health* (pp. 23–45). New York: Academic Press.

Grey, M.J., Grenel, M., & Tamborlane, W.V. (1980). Psychosocial adjustment of latency age diabetes: Determinants and relationships to control. *Pediatrics, 65*, 69–73.

Greydanus, D.E., & Hofmann, A.D. (1979). A perspective on the brittle teenage diabetic. *Journal of Family Practice, 9*, 1007–1012.

Grossmann, H.Y. (1987). The adolescent with insulin-dependent diabetes mellitus: Psychological considerations. In S. Brink (Ed.). *Pediatric and adolescent diabetes mellitus* (pp.139–149). Chicago: Year Book Medical Publishers.

Hagen, J.W., Anderson, B.J., & Barclay, C.R. (1986). Issues in research on the young chronically ill child. *Topics in Early Childhood Special Education, 5* (4), 49–57.

Hamburg, B.A., & Inoff, G.E. (1983). Coping with predictable crises of diabetes. *Diabetes Care, 6*, 408–416.

Hanson, C.L., Henggeler, S.W., & Burghen, G.A. (1987). Model of associations between psychosocial variables and health-outcome measures of adolescents with IDDM. *Diabetes Care, 10*, 752–758.

Hauser, S., & Solomon, M.L. (1985). Coping with diabetes: Views from the family. In P. Ahmed & N. Ahmed (Eds.), *Coping with juvenile diabetes* (pp. 234–266). Springfield, IL: Charles C Thomas.

Ingersoll, G.M., Orr, D.P., Herrold, A.J., & Golden, M.P. (1986). Cognitive maturity and self-management among adolescents with insulin-dependent diabetes mellitus. *Journal of Pediatrics, 108*, 620–623.

Jackson, D.C. (1957). The question of family homeostasis. *Psychiatric Quarterly, 31*, 79–90.

Jacobson, A.M., Hauser, S.T., Wertlieb, D., Wolsdorf, J., Orleans, J., & Vieyra, M. (1986). Psychologiscal adjustment of children with recently diagnosed diabetes mellitus. *Diabetes Care, 9*, 323–329.

Koski, M.L., Ahlas, A., & Kumento, A.A. (1976). A psychosomatic follow-up study of childhood diabetics. *Acta Peadopsychoiatrice, 42*, 12–25.

Kovacs, M., Feinberg, T., Pavlavskas, S., Finkelstein, R., Pollack, M., & Crosse-Novac, M. (1985). Initial coping response and psychosocial characteristics of children with IDDM. *Journal of Pediatrics, 106*, 827–834.

Leaverton, D.R. (1979). The child with diabetes mellitus. In J.D. Call, J.D. Nosphpize, R.I. Cohen, & I. Berlin (Eds.). *Basic handbook of child psychiatry*, Vol 1. New York: Basic Books.

Minuchin, S., Rosman, B.L., & Baker, L. (1978). *Psychosomatic families*. Cambridge, MA: Harvard University Press.

Moos, R. (1974). *The family environment scale*. Palo Alto, CA: Consulting Psychologist Press.

Newbrough, J.R., Simpkins, C.G., & Maurer, H. (1985). A family development approach to studying factors in the management and control of childhood diabetes. *Diabetes Care*, 8, 83–92.

Norman, D.K. (1987). Psychosocial commentary on insulin-dependent diabetes mellitus. Infancy to age 5 years. In. S. Brink (Ed.). *Pediatric and adolescent diabetes mellitus* (pp. 33–42). Chicago: Year Book Medical Publishers.

Rovet. J.F., & Ehrlich, R.M. (1988). Effect of temperament on metabolic control in children with diabetes mellitus. *Diabetes Care, 11*, 77–82.

Rovet, J.F., Ehrlich, R.M., & Hoppe, M. (1987). Intellectual deficits associated with early-onset of insulin dependent diabetes mellitus in children. *Diabetes Care, 10*, 510–515.

Ryan, C.M. (1988). Neurobehavioral complications of Type I diabetes: Examination of possible risk factors. *Diabetes Care, 11*, 86–93.

Sabbath, B. (1984). Understanding the impact of chronic childhood illness on families. *Pediatric Clinics of North America, 31* (1), 47–57.

Schafer, L.C. McCaul, K.D., & Glasgow, R.E. (1986). Supportive and non-supportive family behaviors: Relationships to adherence and metabolic control in persons with type I diabetes. *Diabetes Care, 9*, 179–185.

Sullivan, B.J. (1978) Self-esteem and depression in adolescent diabetic girls. *Diabetes Care, 1*, 18–22.

Turk, D.C., & Kerns, R.D. (1987). The family in health and illness: A life-span perspective. In D.C. Turk & R.D. Kerns (Eds.) *Health, illness and families* (pp. 1–22). New York: Wiley.

Watzlawick, P. Beavin J.H., & Jackson, D.C. (1967). *Pragmatics of human communication: A study of interactional patterns, pathologies, and paradoxes*. New York: Norton.

White, R.W. (1976). Strategies of adaptation: An attempt at systematic description. In R. Moos (Ed.). *Human adaptation* (pp. 17–32). Lexington, MA: D.C. Heath and Co.

Zrebiec, J.F. (1987). Psychosocial commentary on insulin-dependent diabetes mellitus in 5- to 9-year-old children. In S.J. Brink (Ed.). *Pediatric and adolescent diabetes mellitus* (pp. 79–88). Chicago: Year Book Medical Publishers.

6

Eating Disorders and Diabetes

Marsha D. Marcus and Rena R. Wing

There is a growing awareness of the importance of disordered eating behavior among patients with insulin-dependent diabetes mellitus (IDDM), and several studies have suggested that the eating disorders anorexia nervosa and bulimia nervosa are more common among IDDM patients than in the population at large. Disturbed patterns of eating that do not meet criteria for the diagnosis of an eating disorder are apparently common among IDDM patients as well. The behaviors associated with disordered eating (e.g., binge eating, purge behaviors) may also seriously affect glycemic control and complicate the management of IDDM.

In this chapter, we will discuss evidence related to the prevalence of these disorders and their milder variants among IDDM patients and examine the implications of these problems for the treatment of IDDM.

Anorexia Nervosa and Bulimia Nervosa

Anorexia nervosa and bulimia nervosa are disorders characterized by gross disturbances in eating behavior. The criteria for these disorders, which are presented in Table 6.1, have been recently revised by the American Psychiatric Association (1987) in its Diagnostic and Statistical Manual (Third Edition-Revised) (DSM-III-R).

According to the DSM-III-R (American Psychiatric Association, 1987), the essential features of anorexia nervosa are refusal to maintain body weight over minimal normal levels, an intense fear of gaining weight or becoming fat, a distorted body image, and amenorrhea (in females).

Table 6.1. DSM-III-R Diagnostic Criteria for Eating Disorders

Anorexia Nervosa

A. Refusal to maintain body weight over minimal normal weight for age and height, e.g., weight loss leading to maintenance of body weight 15% below that expected; or failure to make expected weight gain during period of growth, leading to body weight 15% below that expected.

B. Intense fear of gaining weight or becoming fat, even though underweight.

C. Disturbance in the way in which body weight, size, or shape is perceived, e.g., person claims to "feel fat" even when emaciated or believes that one area of body is "too fat" even when obviously underweight.

D. In females, absence of at least three consecutive menstrual cycles when otherwise expected to occur (primary or secondary amenorrhea). (A woman is considered to have amenorrhea if her periods occur only following hormone, e.g., estrogen, administration).

Bulimia Nervosa

A. Recurrent episodes of binge eating (rapid consumption of a large amount of food in a discrete period of time).

B. A feeling of lack of control over eating behavior during the eating binges.

C. The person regularly engages in either self-induced vomiting, use of laxatives, or diuretics, strict dieting or fasting, or vigorous exercise in order to prevent weight gain.

D. A minimum average of two binge eating episodes a week for at least three months.

E. Persistent overconcern with body shape and weight.

The major difference between the DSM-III-R criteria for anorexia nervosa and the criteria used in the DSM-III (American Psychiatric Association, 1980) is that the DSM-III weight loss criterion of 25% was found to be too restrictive and was changed to 15%. In addition, for females, the absence of three or more consecutive menstrual cycles was added as a criterion.

Bulimia nervosa is characterized by recurrent episodes of binge eating, a feeling of lack of control over eating behavior during binge episodes, self-induced vomiting or the use of laxatives, diuretics, strict dieting, fasting or vigorous exercise to prevent weight gain, and persistent overconcern with weight and shape. In contrast to the DSM-III criteria, the revised criteria specify a minimum frequency of binge episodes for the diagnosis and the criterion of depressed mood and self-deprecating thoughts after episodes has been excluded. Finally, the term bulimia nervosa is used in the DSM-III-R instead of the DSM-III term, bulimia, as the newer term emphasizes the relationship of the disorder to anorexia nervosa. In both disorders, patients demonstrate preoccupation with food, shape, and weight. Furthermore, approximately half of anorexia nervosa patients suffer bulimic episodes (Casper, Eckert, Halmi, Goldberg, & Davis, 1980). The presence of bulimic episodes in anorexia nervosa patients is believed to be associated with longer duration of illness and a negative prognosis (Beumont, George, & Smart, 1976).

Estimates of the prevalence of anorexia nervosa range from 0.001% to 1% of adolescent females, the population at highest risk (American Psychiatric Association, 1987). Depending on the criteria used to define the disorder, prevalence rates of bulimia have ranged from 1.3 (Schotte & Stunkard, 1987) to 19% (Halmi, Falk, & Schwartz, 1981) of young adult women. In general, studies that have used stricter diagnostic criteria have yielded prevalence rates of 1.3 to 5% (Mitchell & Pyle, 1985).

The etiology of eating disorders is unknown. However, recently theorists (Andersen, 1985; Garfinkel & Garner, 1982; Johnson & Maddi, 1986) have agreed that anorexia nervosa and bulimia nervosa are best understood as multidetermined disorders representing a final common pathway of any number of different developmental routes. Biological, psychological, familial, and social factors have been implicated in both the development and maintenance of eating disorders with the relative importance of these factors varying among individuals.

Despite the fact that an eating disorder in a given individual is the result of a complex interplay of multiple factors, there is general consensus that eating disorders are associated with efforts to diet (Garner, Rockert, Olmsted, Johnson, & Coscina, 1985). In fact, it appears that the prevalence of eating disorders is increasing, and it has been argued that this increase is secondary to the undisputed sociocultural emphasis on slimness (Garner, Garfinkel, Schwartz, & Thompson, 1980). Although, recent investigators have questioned whether prevalence rates have actually increased (Schotte & Stunkard, 1987), available data suggest that behaviors associated with eating disorders i.e., binge eating, self-induced vomiting, strict dieting, and preoccupation with shape and weight are widespread. For example, as many as 70% (Hawkins & Clement, 1980) of college students report episodes of binge eating. Therefore, while DSM-III-R eating disorders pose a serious problem, many more individuals report milder disturbances.

Subclinical Eating Disorders

In a society where both dieting and "pigging out" are ways of life, what constitutes abnormal eating behavior? Although few would argue that culturally sanctioned overeating on holidays (e.g., Thanksgiving or

Christmas) reflect disordered eating, it is less clear when eating and diet behaviors become clinical concerns. The issue of "abnormal" eating is particularly salient in individuals with IDDM, where even occasional (presumably "normal") binge episodes may affect diabetic control.

Although there is no consistent agreement on what defines a "subclinical," "partial," or "mild" eating disorder, generally these terms refer to cases where an individual meets some but not all of the criteria for a diagnosis of an eating disorder. Some researchers (Fairburn, 1987) argue that any definition of a partial syndrome must include undue importance attached to weight and shape as a criterion, plus other symptoms. In addition, it appears that increased frequency of disordered eating behaviors such as binge eating and self-induced vomiting are associated with clinical severity. Schotte and Stunkard (1987) reported data which indicate that binge and purge behaviors occurring more frequently than once a month suggest clinically significant eating problems. In summary, there is no generally accepted definition of subclinical eating disorder, nor is there a clear deliniation between abnormal and normal eating behavior.

Eating Disorders and IDDM—Clinical Reports

Reports of eating disorders among IDDM patients have proliferated in the literature during the last decade. Table 6.2 summarizes relevant clinical characteristics of 57 reported cases of co-occurring IDDM and eating disorders. Hillard and Hillard (1984), appropriately noting the problems of generalizing from case reports, drew some preliminary conclusions from 22 reported cases in their excellent review. Their observations appear equally valid after examination of the data from the now larger series:

1. Although early observers (Crisp, 1977; Fairburn & Steel, 1980) noted that the association of IDDM and eating disorders was rare, it is clear from the number of reports that co-occurrence of these disorders is not uncommon.
2. The diagnosis of IDDM occurs before that of an eating disorder in the preponderance (90%) of the cases. This, of course, is consistent with the notion that IDDM is a risk factor for the development of an eating disorder. However, as Hillard and Hillard (1984) noted, the average age of onset for IDDM is earlier than for eating disorders.
3. Ninety-five percent of cases of eating disorders among IDDM patients have occurred in women. This parallels sex ratio findings in the general population (American Psychiatric Association, 1987).

Table 6.2. IDDM and Eating Disorders: A Summary of Reported Cases

Clinical Reports	No. of Cases	Onset of IDDM Before Eat. Dis.	Sex	AN	AN + BUL	BN	Self-Induced Glycosuria	Poor Metabolic Control	Major Diabetic Complications
Fairburn & Steel, 1980	3	3	3F	2	1		NR[a]	0	0
Garner, 1980	1	1	1F	1			1	1	NR
Gomez, Dally, & Isaacs, 1980	2	1	2F	2			NR	1	NR
O'Gorman & Eyre, 1982	1	1	1F		1		1[b]	0	NR
Roland & Bhanji, 1982	3	3	2F,1M	1	2		NR	3	1
Hillard, Lobo, & Keeling, 1983	1	1	1F			1	0	1	NR
Hudson, Hudson, & Wentworth, 1983	1	1	1F			1	1	1	0
Hudson, Wentworth, & Hudson, 1983	6[c]	NR	5F,1M		2	4	4	5	3
Powers, Malone, & Duncan, 1983	4	4	4F	2	2		3	NR	NR
Szmukler & Russell, 1983	3	3	2F,1M		2	1	3	3	2
Brooks, 1984	2	2	2F		2		NR	2	NR
Featherstone & Beitman, 1984	1	1	1F			1	1	1	NR
Hardoff, Shenker, & Nussbaum, 1984	1	1	1F	1			0	0	NR
Sreenivasan, 1984	2	1	2F	1	1		NR	1	NR
Szmukler, 1984	3[c]	3	3F	1	2		2	3	0
Malone & Armstrong, 1985	1	1	1F	1			1	1	NR
Schechter, 1985	1	1	1F		1		0	NR	NR
Nielsen, Borner, & Kabel, 1987	5	4	5F	4	1		1	4	2
Steel, Young, Lloyd, & Clarke, 1987	15	13	15F	4	8	3	9	11	11
Newman, Schlefer, & Abraham, 1988	1	1	1F		1		1	1	1
Totals	57	46	54,3	20	26	11	28	39	20
Total Reported		51	57	57	57	57	45	52	42
% of Cases Reported		90%	95%F 5%M	35%	46%	19%	62%	75%	48%

[a]NR = not reported.
[b]Probable self-induced glycosuria.
[c]Number of cases refers to new cases reported.

4. IDDM patients have available a purge technique specific to diabetes, i.e., underdosing or omission of insulin. Sixty-two percent of eating disordered IDDM patients reported deliberate manipulation of insulin to promote weight loss. Regular elimination of insulin doses would be predicted to have negative consequences for glycemic control.
5. Poor glycemic control was reported in 75% patients with eating disorders, and although few studies reported on complications, a recent report (Steel, Young, Lloyd, & Clarke, 1987) indicated that major diabetic complications may be prevalent as well.
6. The management of IDDM is complicated by the presence of an eating disorder and vice versa. In fact, it appears that the disorders exacerbate one another. Szmukler (1984) commented that "the relationship between diabetes and anorexia nervosa/bulimia shows a kind of synergism in which one disorder worsens the other and where successful therapeutic interventions may consequently prove exceedingly difficult" (p. 368).

Prevalence of Eating Disorders in IDDM Patients

The prevalence of eating disorders among IDDM patients is not known because there have been no controlled studies utilizing rigorous diagnostic criteria. However, several recent studies have suggested increased prevalence rates of eating disorders among IDDM patients. Rosmark, Berne, Holmgren, Lago, Renholm, and Sohlberg (1986) studied 86 IDDM patients under 40 years of age and 93 normal control subjects. Patients were asked to complete the Eating Attitudes Test (EAT) (Garner, Olmsted, Bohr, & Garfinkel, 1982), a self-report questionnaire that assesses the symptoms of anorexia nervosa. Four items of the EAT that describe behaviors appropriate for IDDM patients (e.g., "display self-control around food," "feel uncomfortable eating sweets") were excluded from scoring. Female IDDM patients had significantly higher total scores on the adjusted EAT than controls. Further, based on questionnaire scores and clinical information, the authors concluded that a significantly greater proportion (9%) of the female IDDM patients than controls (0%) had an eating disorder.

Hudson, Wentworth, Hudson, and Pope (1985) also reported a high prevalence rate of anorexia nervosa and bulimia among female IDDM patients aged 14–25. Subjects were 264 women treated at a large urban diabetes referral center ($N = 100$) and a small town rural practice ($N = 164$). Patients were mailed a questionnaire based on DSM-III criteria for anorexia nervosa and bulimia. Unfortunately, only 38% of the urban sample and 25.6% of the rural sample responded to the questionnaire. However, of the respondents, two subjects met criteria for "borderline" anorexia nervosa (all DSM-III criteria except 75% of predicted weight for height), and 17 met DSM-III criteria for a history of bulimia (plus additional criteria of binge eating at least once a week as well as self-induced vomiting or laxative abuse). Extrapolating from these findings and using the unsubstantiated, but conservative, assumption that none of the nonresponders had eating disorders, this study suggests an overall prevalence rate of eating disorders of 7.2% among this group of IDDM patients. The Rosmark et al. (1986) and Hudson et al. (1985) studies rely on self-report data which make the data difficult to interpret since an eating disorder can only be diagnosed by clinical interview.

However, in another study, Steel et al., (1987), using medical records, examinations, and interviews, identified 15 cases of anorexia nervosa or bulimia among 208 women aged 16–25 who attended a diabetic clinic at the Royal Infirmary of Edinburgh. The 7% rate of clinically apparent eating disorders among this group is consistent with the findings from questionnaire studies.

Finally, in the most rigorous study to date, Rodin, Johnson, Garfinkel, Daveman, and Kenshole (1986) screened 58 women, aged 15–22 who had IDDM for 1 year or more using the Eating Attitudes Test-26 (Garner, et al., 1982) and the Eating Disorders Inventory (Garner, Olmsted, & Polivy, 1982). Subjects who scored above predetermined cut-off points suggestive of eating problems were interviewed using DSM-III criteria for anorexia nervosa and bulimia. Rodin et al. (1986) diagnosed "partial syndromes" in individuals who did not meet DSM-III criteria for an eating disorder, but who demonstrated similar psychopathology that significantly impaired adjustment. In total, 12 women (20.7%) were diagnosed as having clinically significant eating disorders. Anorexia nervosa was diagnosed in four (6.9%) patients and "partial" anorexia nervosa was identified in two additional subjects (3.4%), while bulimia was found in four women (6.9%) and "partial" bulimia was diagnosed in two women (3.4%). Thus, in the only study to date utilizing clinical interviews, nearly 14% of the female patients had eating disorders.

One additional line of evidence suggests an association between IDDM and eating disorders. Nielsen, Borner, and Kabel (1987) identified 5 cases of IDDM among 242 patients treated for eating disorders at the Child Psychiatric and Psychiatric Clinics at Rigshospitalet in Copenhagen over a 25-year period. The authors concluded that since the prevalence of IDDM in Denmark is approximately 3.2/1000, the finding of 5 cases of IDDM in a series of 242 eating disorder patients represents a sixfold increase in expected prevalence. However, Righospitalet is a tertiary care center, likely to receive the most difficult eating disorder cases for care, and there are no epidemiological data on the prevalence of eating disorders in Denmark.

In the aggregate, available data strongly suggest that adolescent and young adult women with IDDM may be at increased risk for the development of eating disorders. However, these findings require corroboration. In addition to methodological limitations previously noted, extant studies have relied heavily on patient groups from specialty care centers that may not be representative of the IDDM patient population as a whole. The determination of whether IDDM patients are particularly vulnerable to eating disorders will require careful screening of community-based samples of IDDM patients and appropriate age- and sex-matched control groups who do not have IDDM. Diagnoses of eating disorders and their partial syndromes should be made using carefully defined criteria by interviewers who are blind to the metabolic control and/or self-reported eating problems of subjects. Despite the need for additional research, however, there is little doubt that eating disorders are a significant problem among IDDM patients.

Eating Disorders and Medical Consequences

Eating disorders are associated with numerous serious medical consequences. The medical complications of anorexia nervosa are largely secondary to starvation and can affect virtually every organ system (Mitchell, 1985). The disorder can be fatal and reported mortality in recent series ranges from 0 to 2% (Andersen, 1985). Bulimia nervosa is also associated with numerous medical consequences including salivary gland hypertrophy, dental enamel erosion, and electrolyte abnormalities. Esophageal and gastric irritation and tears, gastric dilatation and rupture, and alterations in neuroendocrine systems have also been reported (Mitchell, 1985).

The patient with IDDM and anorexia and/or bulimia faces additional risks as the combination of IDDM and an eating disorder is associated with unstable (Szmukler & Russell, 1983) and poor (Szmukler, 1984) glycemic control as well as major diabetic complications (Steel et al., 1987). The preponderance of clinical reports of eating disorders in IDDM patients have noted frequent bouts of hypoglycemia (Roland & Bhanji, 1982), ketoacidosis (Hudson, Hudson & Wentworth, 1983), as well as frequent hospitalizations (Sreenivasan, 1984) in these individuals. Although patients with the restricting type of anorexia nervosa may be less likely to evidence poor control (Fairburn & Steel, 1980), anorexia with bulimic episodes and bulimia nervosa have been consistently associated with poor control and may also be associated with major diabetic complications. As already noted, the majority of patients described in clinical reports had poor metabolic control. For example, in the series of six bulimic patients with IDDM reported by Hudson et al. (1983) the average total glycosylated hemoglobin was 16% and four of the six patients had major complications.

Similarly, Steel et al. (1987) reported severe hyperglycemia in 11 of 15 IDDM patients with eating disorders before, during, and after the eating disorder. Further, of this group of patients who were 17–30 ($M = 24.5$) years of age with an average duration of diabetes of 12.5 years, only 4 of 15 were free of clinical diabetic complications. Eleven patients had retinopathy, six had proliferative changes, and one was blind. Four of the 10 patients with anorexia nervosa reported painful polyneuropathy, while no other young female patient in the same clinic developed painful neuropathy. The pain started after the initial loss and remitted with weight gain in three of four patients. An additional two of the patients had chronic neuropathy whose symptoms appeared after the onset of the eating disorder. Finally, 6 of 15 patients had some degree of nephropathy.

The direction of the association between eating disorders and poor glycemic control in IDDM patients is not known. Most investigators have speculated that binge and purge behaviors may directly compromise diabetic control (Hillard & Hillard, 1984). However, Steel et al. (1987), noting that their group of IDDM patients evidenced poor glycemic control prior to the diagnosis of an eating disorder, concluded that poorly controlled young women were at risk for the development of an eating disorder. With regard to complications, it has been argued that poor glycemic control (Steel et al., 1987) and/or nutritional factors (Alloway, Reynolds, Spargo, & Russell, 1985) among IDDM patients with eating disorders may contribute to the onset of diabetic complications in these patients. Taken together, available evidence suggests that eating disorders in IDDM patients are associated with poor control and diabetic complications in young women. However, comparisons of IDDM patients with diagnosed eating disorders with IDDM controls matched for age, sex, SES, and duration of diabetes are needed to confirm these findings.

Subclinical Eating Problems in Patients with IDDM

Behaviors and attitudes associated with eating disorders are reported frequently among female IDDM patients as they are among young women who do not have diabetes. Schwarz and Citrin (1986) interviewed 30 women with IDDM aged 15–35 and reported that more than one third felt that they had an "eating problem." In another study, Stancin and Reuter (1987) recruited 59 women with IDDM between 18 and 30 years of age. On the basis of a bulimia screening form based on DSM-III criteria for bulimia, 58% of respondents reported binge eating. Seventeen percent reported self-induced vomiting following binge episodes, and 40% acknowledged reducing or omitting insulin for the purpose of weight loss. Finally, defining a binge as the ingestion of ≥ 500 calories in one sitting not as part of a meal, LaGreca, Schwarz, and Satin (1987) reported that 85% of a group of 30 female adolescents and young adult IDDM patients reported at least occasional binges, with an average of seven binges per month. Forty percent of this group reported manipulation of insulin to cope with overeating.

Several studies have indicated that such subclinical eating disturbances may compromise glycemic control. Schwarz and Citrin (1986) reported that poorly controlled patients ($HbA_1 \geq 9\%$) reported an average of 9 binge episodes/month compared to 1.2 episodes/month for well-controlled patients ($HbA_1 < 9\%$). Further, 55% of the poorly controlled patients, but none of the well-controlled patients believed that they had eating problems.

LaGreca et al. (1987) utilized a structured interview to obtain information from their sample of 30 women with IDDM. The group was divided into three groups on the basis of HbA_1 levels: good control (<9%), fair control (9–11%), and poor control (>12%). The average number of binge eating episodes/month reported was 1.2, 7.0, and 12.7 for the good, fair, and poor glycemic control groups, respectively. Further, many women in the fair (50%) and poor (70%) control groups reported manipulation of insulin dosages to cope with overeating, while no individual in the good control groups reported the omission or reduction of insulin.

Our research group studied a group of 202 adolescents aged 12–18 seen at the Diabetes Clinic at Children's Hospital of Pittsburgh (Wing, Nowalk, Marcus, Koeske, & Finegold, 1986). All patients completed the Binge Eating Scale (BES) (Gormally, Black, Daston, & Rardin, 1982), a measure of binge eating severity. Patients who scored two standard deviations above the mean ($N = 15$) on the BES were compared with age- and sex-matched patients who scored at the 50th percentile for their age and sex ($N = 15$) and the lowest 10% of BES scores ($N = 15$). The average HbA_1 of subjects with high BES scores was 13.17% compared to 11.8% and 10.8% for medium and low scoring patients.

When patients with the highest questionnaire scores were interviewed, they frequently reported eating patterns that markedly contrasted from recommended diabetes diet regimens. For instance, one patient who was quite preoccupied with her weight and shape reported a regular routine of skipping breakfast, having only a glass of milk for lunch, and then overeating all evening. The team responsible for this patient's diabetes care was unaware of this pattern, and insulin was prescribed on the assumption that the patient was compliant with the recommended diet. The inappropriate match of insulin and intake in this patient would be expected to have marked effects on glycemic control.

IDDM and Vulnerability to Eating Disorders

Although it does appear that IDDM patients may be particularly vulnerable to the development of eating disorders, it is unclear why this may be. IDDM patients may be at increased risk because of factors specific to diabetes. Alternatively, IDDM patients may be at increased risk for eating disorders because of factors involved in coping with chronic illness. These possibilities will be considered, in turn.

The treatment of IDDM may enhance the likelihood of disordered eating behavior. First, young IDDM patients are required to focus on diet and limit weight gain as one aspect of their medical regimen. They are often asked to limit or avoid particular foods, especially simple carbohydrates and/or fats and must consistently time meals so as to coordinate insulin with blood sugar changes. This intensive emphasis on weight, diet, and food may render IDDM patients particularly vulnerable to the development of eating disorders. Habitual dietary restraint has been consistently associated with binge eating severity among college populations (Hawkins & Clement, 1983) and some investigators have concluded that once any degree of overconcern with food and weight develops, disordered eating patterns almost inevitably follow (Wooley & Wooley, 1981). Preadolescent and adolescent female IDDM patients, like their non-IDDM peers, are likely to be more affected than males by considerable societal pressures to be thin and therefore are at greater risk than males to develop disordered eating patterns (Garner et al., 1980).

Insulin therapy may also be involved in the vulnerability of IDDM patients to eating disorders. The belief that insulin use leads to weight gain is apparently a common one (Szmukler, 1984), and the omission of insulin to promote weight loss seems to be prevalent among young women (Brink, 1988). Some research has indicated that glycemic control is poorer in adolescent females than their male age-mates (Anderson, Miller, Auslander, & Santiago, 1981; Daneman, Wolfson, Becker, & Drash, 1981), although such differences are not observed at other ages. Hormonal, compliance, and/or psychological factors may account for these differences. However, if physicians respond to such changes by increasing insulin dosages, additional weight gain and renewed attempts at stringent dieting may result. Further, intensive insulin regimens are being used increasingly in efforts to normalize blood glucose levels in IDDM patients (Brink, 1988). Recent findings have documented that intensive insulin therapy is associated with significant weight gain (DCCT Research Group, 1988). Thus, efforts to promote optimal glycemic control in adolescent females may lead to weight gain, thereby increasing the risk of disordered eating behavior. Conversely, poor control per se may be a risk factor in the development of eating disorders as poorly controlled adolescent females may face increased pressure from medical personnel and family members to diet.

Unlike other eating disorder patients, IDDM patients have available to them a purge technique specific to diabetes. The intentional induction of glycosuria to undo the effects of binge eating or to avoid weight gain is likely to contribute to poor glycemic control and to episodes of ketoacidosis. Szmukler (1984) reported that some IDDM patients with eating disorders welcomed queasy feelings secondary to hyperglycemia as this led to diminished appetite and that polydypsia after binge episodes facilitated self-induced vomiting.

Other aspects of IDDM may also increase the risk of eating disorders. Although IDDM has not been consistently associated with behavioral or psychological problems, IDDM may pose a challenge to the psychological well-being of adolescents. In fact, it has been noted (Tattersall & Lowe, 1981) that diabetes can interfere significantly with adolescent development by affecting body image, causing feelings of being different, and/or exacerbating dependence/independence conflicts. These problems, in combination with treatment-related factors described above, may contribute to enhanced risk of eating disorders among IDDM patients.

IDDM also places considerable demands upon family members. There may be a tendency among some parents to be overprotective or overinvolved with their youngsters with IDDM, thus exacerbating difficulties associated with the normal adolescent need to separate from parents in the process of identity formation. In fact, Minuchin and colleagues (Minuchin, Rosman, & Baker, 1978) described maladaptive characteristics that they found to apply both to families of poorly controlled diabetic patients and anorexia nervosa patients. These included enmeshment or overinvolvement of family members with one another, overprotectiveness, rigidity, and a lack of conflict resolution. Therefore, dysfunctional diabetes-related family interactions may contribute to an environment that may also foster the development of eating disorders.

Although it appears that many factors related to IDDM may increase the risk of eating disorders, for the most part it is unclear whether increased risk is related to IDDM specifically or more generally to problems associated with dealing with chronic or severe illness. For example, Patton, Wood, and Johnson-Sabine (1986) have reported that physical illness predisposes individuals to the development of anorexia nervosa. They compared 326 anorexia nervosa patients, 105 general practice patients, and 61 schizophrenic patients for history of physical illness. The anorexia nervosa patients were significantly more likely to have a history of severe physical illnesses of all types. Similarly, there have been reports of eating disorders associated with several specific medical conditions including cystic fibrosis (Goldbloom, 1988), Turner's Syndrome (Pitts & Guze, 1963) and urogenital malformations (Halmi & Rigas, 1973). Damlouji and Ferguson (1985) also described three patients who developed anorexia nervosa after physical traumas that affected body image. Therefore, a variety of medical problems may increase risk for the development of eating disorders.

The mechanisms through which this occurs are not known but there are several possibilities. Illness may cause chronic stress, lead to lower self-esteem, affect body image, feelings of mastery or competence, necessitate changes in diet, and/or affect family environment. One or more of these factors in concert with individual psychological variables may lead to an increased risk of developing an eating disorder. Further research comparing prevalence rates of eating disorders in adolescent IDDM patients to rates in age- and sex-matched controls who suffer from other illnesses is needed to elucidate the relationship between IDDM and eating disorders.

Additional research may also clarify the potential relation of other IDDM related factors to the onset of eating disorders. For example, recent research (Rovet, Ehrlich, & Hoppe, 1987; Ryan & Morrow, 1986) has suggested that psychological and behavior problems among young IDDM patients may vary as a function of age of onset of diabetes. Ryan and Morrow (1986) reported that adolescent girls with early onset IDDM (before 5 years) had poor self-concepts related to physical appearance. Since low self-esteem has also been implicated in the etiology of eating disorders (Fairburn, 1987), it might be expected that early onset IDDM patients would be likelier than later onset patients to develop eating disorders. On the other hand, Schriock, Winter, and Traisman (1984) noted that onset of IDDM closer to puberty is likelier to disrupt the hypothalamic-pituitary-gonadal axis and cause delayed menarche than prepubertal onset IDDM. Since disturbances of this axis are prominent in eating disorders as well, there could be increased risk for eating disorders among puberty-onset IDDM patients. Thus, further research may reveal that factors such as age of IDDM onset may mediate the relationship between IDDM and eating disorders.

Treatment of Eating Disorders

The first step in treatment is the accurate diagnosis of the eating disorder. This can be particularly difficult in IDDM patients because there may be a confound between the symptoms of poor glycemic control and eating disorders, for example, rapid weight loss (Hillard & Hillard, 1984). In addition, symptoms of depression that frequently accompany eating disorders, such as difficulty concentrating, sleep disturbance, and a lack of energy, can also be secondary to poor control of IDDM. Therefore, differential diagnosis may require consultation with a psychiatrist or clinical psychologist experienced in the assessment and treatment of eating disorders.

If an eating disorder is diagnosed in an IDDM patient, intensive interdisciplinary treatment is required because each disorder may exacerbate the other. Hillard and Hillard (1984) have suggested a three-step plan for the treatment of these patients. First, it is necessary to achieve a minimally acceptable level of glycemic control so that the patient is medically stable. The next step is treatment of the eating disorder to achieve stabilization of disordered eating behavior and concomitant improvement of diabetes. The final step is to focus on optimal control of diabetes and ongoing treatment of the eating disorder.

Inpatient treatment may be necessary to stabilize diabetes and/or the eating disorder. Indications for hospitalization include dangerously low body weight, binge and purge behaviors that compromise medical status, significant risk of suicide, inability to provide self-care, or need for differential diagnosis. It is preferable to arrange admission to a psychiatric or pediatric unit where the staff is trained and experienced in dealing with eating disordered patients as they are frequently hard to manage. Patients may hoard food for binges, dispose of food, secretly vomit, misrepresent calorie intake, and conceal disordered eating behavior. IDDM patients may refuse to eat after injection of insulin, fail to produce urine samples, and/or use the fact of their diabetes to manipulate the psychiatric team (Powers, Malone, & Duncan, 1983). Because of the potential difficulties involved in the management of these patients, close collaboration of the medical and psychiatric personnel responsible for care is imperative.

The treatment of eating disorders requires a balance between attending to relevant psychological issues and the impact of biological changes due to disturbed eating patterns (or poor control of IDDM). Therefore, Garner, Garfinkel, and Irvine (1986) have recommended that therapy include a focus on issues related to shape, binge eating, purge, and weight control behaviors as well as the psychological context of the disorder (i.e., developmental, personality, and familial themes).

Individual or group psychotherapy, family therapy, the use of medication, or a combination of these modalities have all been used in the treatment of these disorders. Cognitive behavioral therapy appears to have particular promise in the treatment of eating disorders (Garner, Fairburn, & Davis, 1987). This treatment utilizes behavioral techniques (e.g., self-monitoring, goal setting, stimulus control) to achieve and maintain control of disordered eating behavior. Cognitive strategies are used to address psychological issues, particularly the maladaptive thoughts and beliefs about diet, shape, and weight that are characteristic of eating disordered patients. Patients are taught to identify maladaptive cognitions (e.g., "I am too fat") and to recognize the connection between these thoughts and dysfunctional behaviors (e.g., strict dieting). The patient is then helped to substitute more realistic and adaptive thoughts (e.g., "I weigh 5 lb more than I want to, but I look fine.") for maladaptive ones. Finally, patients are taught problem-solving techniques to modify situations that may contribute to the eating problem, to anticipate future setbacks, and to develop a plan to cope with such problems.

Family therapy may also be helpful for IDDM patients with eating disorders particularly if the assessment indicates that parents are over-involved and/or overprotective of their youngster. The goal of the family work is to identify and limit maladaptive interactions and encourage interactions that promote the healthy development of the patient and family. Whether the family is actively involved in treatment or not, it is important that family members be provided information about eating disorders and supported in dealing constructively with their adolescent.

Finally, the use of medication may be indicated in the treatment of the eating disorder. To date, results of trials of pharmacotherapy in the treatment of anorexia nervosa have been disappointing, but there is some evidence that amitryptyline or cyproheptadine may be useful for selected patients (Halmi, Eckert, LaDu, & Cohen, 1986). However, antidepressants appear to be a helpful adjunct to the treatment of bulimia nervosa patients (Agras & McCann, 1987). A variety of tricyclic and other antidepressants as well as monoamine oxidase inhibitors have been utilized successfully in the short-term treatment of bulimia nervosa. Care is required in the treatment of IDDM patients with tricyclic antidepressants because the cardiac changes associated with these drugs may be more problematic in IDDM patients with microvascular or autonomic dysfunction (Newman, Schlefer, & Abraham, 1988). Further, there are no long-term outcome data on antidepressant treatment of bulimia nervosa. Therefore, it is advisable for pharmacotherapy to be used in conjunction with treatment that addresses psychological, family, and social problems of eating disorder patients.

There is little information on the long-term outcome of eating disorders, and particularly of patients with co-occuring IDDM. Certainly, the outcome of eating disorders is heterogeneous and dependent, at least in part, on individual clinical factors (e.g., duration of disorder, co-occurring character pathology). However, it is known that a significant proportion of patients will develop chronic problems (Andersen, 1985). Clinical reports have noted that some patients with IDDM and eating disorders recovered, but others have suggested that these patients fared poorly in treatment (Szmukler, 1984). However, the combination of disorders may complicate course and outcome and, therefore, the prevention of disorder would appear to be of primary importance.

Prevention of Eating Disorders

Physicians, nurses, and dietitians working with preadolescent and adolescent IDDM patients have an important role to play in preventing eating disorders. It is crucial to promote the development of a strong therapeutic relationship in which patients are encouraged to discuss their concerns about shape and weight. Clinicians should routinely inquire about diet behavior, stress-related eating, and binge episodes. It is important to acknowledge confessions of noncompliance with the diet regimen in a nonjudgmental manner so that the patient and health care team member can work together to adjust exercise and insulin regimens to accommodate some deviations from the meal plan. Diabetes patients need sound information about weight regulation. The dangers of strict dieting should be discussed and myths about diet and weight loss explored. Further, adolescent IDDM patients need special help in learning to eat and drink in social situations with a view to minimizing feelings of being different. Clinicians also need to be sensitive to indications that patients are adjusting insulin to promote weight loss and to provide sound information and practical advice or alternate methods of weight management. Emotional support and effective information in the context of a sound relationship may prevent problems as well as ameliorate mildly disturbed eating behavior.

The use of support groups to help IDDM patients deal with dietary compliance issues has also been suggested (Brink, 1988). Support groups have been used effectively as adjunctive treatment for eating disorders (Enright, Butterfield, & Berkowitz, 1985), and it would seem that peer support groups might be particularly helpful in aiding adolescent IDDM patients deal with their common problems. Group members could provide one another with information, practical assistance, social affirmation, and emotional support.

Finally, it may be helpful to identify patients at risk for the development of eating disorders (e.g., overweight female patients, poorly controlled patients, patients who self-report concerns about shape and weight) and intervene to prevent clinical disturbance. Psychoeducational programs focusing on attitudes about shape and weight and incorporating cognitive behavioral strategies to cope with these problems have been used successfully with eating disorder patients and with adolescent females at risk for these disorders. However, to date, there has been no effort to develop similar programs for IDDM patients. Such programs would then need to be tested to assess their effects on self-esteem, mood, eating behavior, compliance to the diabetes regimen, and glycosylated hemoglobin.

Conclusion

Eating disorders pose a significant problem among adolescent and young adult IDDM patients. Although additional research is necessary to determine the extent of the problem as well as the course and outcome of these disorders among IDDM patients, it is crucial for health care professionals to be aware of these disorders to promote early diagnosis and effective treatment.

Furthermore, binge eating, stringent dieting, concerns with shape and weight, and insulin manipulation are prevalent among young female IDDM patients and these behaviors and attitudes also appear to affect glycemic control. These findings strongly suggest the importance of developing and evaluating methods to ameliorate such subclinical eating problems before they seriously compromise diabetes management and/or develop into clinical eating disorders.

References

Agras, W.S., & McCann, U. (1987). The efficacy and role of antidepressants in the treatment of bulimia nervosa. *Annals of Behavioral Medicine, 9*, 18–22.

Alloway, R., Reynolds, E.H., Spargo, E., & Russell, G.F.M. (1985). Neuropathy and myopathy in two patients with anorexia and bulimia nervosa. *Journal of Neurology, Neurosurgery, and Psychiatry, 48*, 1015–1020.

American Psychiatric Association (1980). *Diagnostic and statistical manual of mental disorders* (3rd ed.). Washington, DC: Author.

American Psychiatric Association (1987). *Diagnostic and statistical manual of mental disorders* (3rd ed.—revised). Washington, DC: Author.

Andersen, A.E. (1985). *Practical comprehensive treatment of anorexia nervosa and bulimia.* Baltimore: Johns Hopkins University Press.

Andersen, B.J., Miller, J.P., Auslander, W.F., & Santiago, J.V. (1981). Family characteristics of diabetic adolescents: Relationship to metabolic control. *Diabetes Care, 4*, 586–594.

Beumont, P.J.V., George, C.G.W., & Smart, D.E. (1976). Dieters and vomiters and purgers in anorexia nervosa. *Psychological Medicine, 6*, 617–622.

Brink, S.J. (1988). Pediatric, adolescent, and young adult nutrition issues in IDDM. *Diabetes Care, 11*, 192–200.

Brooks, S.A. (1984). Diabetes mellitus and anorexia nervosa: Another view. *British Journal of Psychiatry, 144*, 640–642.

Casper, R.C., Eckert, E.D., Halmi, K.A., Goldberg, S.C., & Davis, J.M. (1980). Bulimia: its incidence and importance in patients with anorexia nervosa. *Archives of General Psychiatry, 37*, 1030–1035.

Crisp, A.H. (1977). The differential diagnosis of anorexia nervosa. *Proceedings of the Royal Society of Medicine, 7D*, 686–690.

Damlouji, N.F., & Ferguson, J.M. (1985). Three cases of posttraumatic anorexia nervosa. *American Journal of Psychiatry, 142*, 362–363.

Daneman, D., Wolfson, D.H., Becker, D.J., & Drash, A.L. (1981). Factors affecting glycosylated hemoglobin values in children with insulin-dependent diabetes. *The Journal of Pediatrics, 99*, 847–853.

DCCT Research Group. (1988). Weight gain associated with intensive therapy in the diabetes control and complications trial. *Diabetes Care, 11*, 567–573.

Enright, A.B., Butterfield, P., & Berkowitz, B. (1985). Self-help and support groups in the management of eating disorders. In D.M. Garner & P.E. Garfinkel (Eds.). *Handbook of Psychotherapy for anorexia & bulimia* (pp. 491–512). New York: The Guilford Press.

Fairburn, C.G. (1987). The definition of bulimia nervosa: Guidelines for clinicians and research workers. *Annals of Behavioral Medicine, 9*, 3–7.
Fairburn, C.G., & Steel, J.M. (1980). Anorexia nervosa in diabetes mellitus. *British Medical Journal, 280*, 1167–1168.
Featherstone, H.J., & Beitman, B.D. (1984). Diabetic hyperglycemia and glycosuria as a manifestation of bulimia. *Southern Medical Journal, 77*, 936–937.
Garfinkel, P.E., & Garner, D.M. (1982). *Anorexia nervosa: A multidimensional perspective*. New York: Bruner/Mazel.
Garner, D.M., Fairburn, C.G., & Davis, R. (1987). Cognitive behavioral treatment of bulimia nervosa. *Behavior Modification, 11*, 398–431.
Garner, D.M., Garfinkel, P.E., & Irvine, M.J. (1986). Integration and sequencing of treatment approaches for eating disorders. *Psychotherapeutic Psychosomatica, 46*, 67–75.
Garner, D.M., Garfinkel, P.E., Schwartz, D.M., & Thompson, M.M. (1980). Cultural expectations of thinness in women. *Psychological Reports, 11*, 483–491.
Garner, D.M., Olmsted, M.P., Bohr, Y., & Garfinkel, P.E. (1982). The eating attitudes test: Psychometric features and clinical correlates. *Psychological Medicine, 12*, 871–878.
Garner, D.M., Olmsted, M.P., & Polivy, J. (1983). Development and validation of a multidimensional eating disorder inventory for anorexia nervosa and bulimia. *International Journal of Eating Disorders, 2*, 15–34.
Garner, D.M., Rockert, W., Olstead, M.P., Johnson, C.L., & Coscina, D.V. (1985). Psychoeducational principles on the treatment of bulimia and anorexia nervosa. In D.M. Garner & P.E. Garfinkel (Eds.). *Handbook of psychotherapy for anorexia nervosa and bulimia* (pp. 513–572). New York: The Guilford Press.
Garner, S. (1980, October). Anorexia nervosa in diabetes mellitus [Letter to the editor]. *British Medical Journal, 281*, 1144.
Goldbloom, D.S. (1988). Anorexia nervosa and cystic fibrosis: A case report. *International Journal of Eating Disorders, 7*, 433–437.
Gomez, J., Dally, P., & Isaacs, A.J. (1980, July). Anorexia nervosa in diabetes mellitus [Letter to the editor]. *British Medical Journal, 281*, 61–62.
Gormally, J., Black, S., Daston, S., & Rardin, D. (1982). The assessment of binge eating severity among obese persons. *Addictive Behaviors, 7*, 47–55.
Halmi, K.A., Eckert, E., LaDu, T.J., & Cohen, J. (1986). Anorexia nervosa: Treatment efficacy of cyproheptadine and amitriptyline. *Archives of General Psychiatry, 43*, 177–181.
Halmi, K.A., Falk, J.R., & Schwartz, E. (1981). Binge-eating and vomiting: A survey of a college population. *Psychological Medicine, 11*, 697–706.
Halmi, K.A., & Rigas, C. (1973). Urogenital malformations associated with anorexia nervosa. *British Journal of Psychiatry, 122*, 79–81.
Hardoff, D., Shenker, I.R., & Nussbaum, M. (1984, February). Anorexia nervosa in a patient with juvenile diabetes. *New York State Journal of Medicine, 84*, 61.
Hawkins, R.C., & Clement, P.C. (1980). Development and construct validation of a self-report measure of binge eating tendencies. *Addictive Behaviors, 5*, 219–226.
Hawkins, R.C., III, & Clement, P.F. (1983). Binge eating syndrome: The

measurement problem and a conceptual model. In R.C. Hawkins, III & P.F. Clement (Eds.). *Binge eating: Theory, research, and treatment*. New York: Springer.

Hillard, J.R., & Hillard, J.A. (1984). Bulimia, anorexia nervosa, and diabetes: Deadly combinations. *Psychiatric Clinics of North America 7*, 367–378.

Hillard, J.R., Lobo, M.C., & Keeling, R.P. (1983). Bulimia and diabetes: A potentially life-threatening combination. *Psychosomatics, 24*, 292–295.

Hudson, J.I., Hudson, M.S., & Wentworth, S.M. (1983). Self-induced glycosuria: A novel method of purging in bulimia. *Journal of the American Medical Association, 249*, 2501.

Hudson, J.I., Wentworth, S.M., Hudson, M.S., & Pope, H.G. (1985). Prevalence of anorexia nervosa and bulimia among young diabetic women. *Journal of Clinical Psychiatry, 46*, 88–89.

Hudson, M.S., Wentworth, S.M., & Hudson, J.I. (1983, August). Bulimia and diabetes [Letter to the editor]. *The New England Journal of Medicine*, 309, 431–432.

Johnson, C.L., & Maddi, K. (1986). The etiology of bulimia: Biopsychosocial perspectives. *Annals of Adolescent Psychiatry, 13*, 253–273.

LaGreca, A.M., Schwarz, L.T., & Satin, W. (1987). Eating patterns in young women with IDDM: Another look [Letter to the editor]. *Diabetes Care, 10*, 659–660.

Malone, G.L., & Armstrong, B.K. (1985). Treatment of anorexia nervosa in a young adult patient with diabetes mellitus. *The Journal of Nervous and Mental Disease, 173*, 509–511.

Minuchin, S., Rosman, B., & Baker, L. (1978). *Psychosomatic families: Anorexia nervosa in context*. Cambridge: Harvard University Press.

Mitchell, J.E. (1985). Medical complications of anorexia nervosa and bulimia. In J.E. Mitchell (Ed.). *Anorexia and bulimia: Diagnosis and treatment* (pp. 48–77). Minneapolis: University of Minnesota Press.

Mitchell, J.E., & Pyle, R.L. (1985). Characteristics of bulimia. In J.E. Mitchell (Ed.). *Anorexia nervosa and bulimia: Diagnosis and treatment* (pp. 29–47). Minneapolis: University of Minnesota Press.

Newman, M.M., Schlefer, E., & Abraham, S. (1988). Nortriptyline and atenolol for the treatment of bulimia in a diabetic woman. *International Journal of Eating Disorders*, 7, 429–432.

Nielsen, S., Borner, H., & Kabel, M. (1987). Anorexia nervosa/bulimia in diabetes mellitus: A review and a presentation of five cases. *Acta Psychiatrica Scandinavica, 75*, 464–473.

O'Gorman, E.C., & Eyre, D.G. (1980). A case of anorexia nervosa and diabetes mellitus. *British Journal of Psychiatry, 137*, 103.

Patton, G.C., Wood, K., & Johnson-Sabine, E. (1986). Physical illness: A risk factor in anorexia nervosa. *British Journal of Psychiatry, 149*, 756–759.

Pitts, F.N., & Guze, S.B. (1963). Anorexia nervosa and gonadal dysgenesis (Turner's syndrome). *American Journal of Psychiatry, 119*, 1100–1102.

Powers, P.S., Malone, J.I., & Duncan, J.A. (1983). Anorexia nervosa and diabetes mellitus. *Journal of Clinical Psychiatry, 44*, 133–135.

Rodin, G.M., Johnson, L.E., Garfinkel, P.E., Daneman, D., & Kenshole, A.B. (1986). Eating disorders in female adolescents with insulin dependent diabetes mellitus. *International Journal of Psychiatry in Medicine, 161*, 49–57.

Roland, J.M., & Bhanji, S. (1982). Anorexia nervosa occurring in patients with diabetes mellitus. *Postgraduate Medical Journal, 58*, 354–356.

Rosmark, B., Berne, C., Holmgren, S., Lago, C., Renholm, G., & Sohlberg, S. (1986). Eating disorders in patients with insulin-dependent diabetes mellitus. *Journal of Clinical Psychiatry, 47*, 547–550.

Rovet, J., Ehrlich, R., & Hoppe, M. (1987). Behavior problems in children with diabetes as a function of sex and age of onset of disease. *Journal of Child Psychology and Psychiatry, 28*, 477–491.

Ryan, C.M., & Morrow, L.A. (1986). Self-esteem in diabetic adolescents: Relationship between age at onset and gender. *Journal of Consulting and Clinical Psychology, 54*, 730–731.

Schechter, N.L. (1985). Self-starvation in a diabetic adolescent. *Journal of Adolescent Health Care, 6*, 43–45.

Schotte, D.E., & Stunkard, A.J. (1987). Bulimia vs. bulimic behaviors on a college campus. *Journal of the American Medical Association, 258*, 1213–1215.

Schriock, E.A., Winter, R.J., & Traisman, H.S. (1984). Diabetes mellitus and its effects on menarche. *Journal of Adolescent Health Care, 5*, 101–104.

Schwarz, L.T., & Citrin, W. (1986). Relationship of eating patterns to glycemic control in young adult women with IDDM. *Diabetes, 35*, 224A.

Sreenivasan, U. (1984). Anorexia nervosa associated with energy-wasting disorders. *Canadian Medical Association Journal, 130*, 45–46.

Stancin, R., & Reuter, J.M. (1987, March). *Descriptive analysis of eating pathology in young women with diabetes mellitus*. Paper presented at the 8th Annual Scientific Sessions of the Society of Behavioral Medicine, Washington, D.C.

Steel, J.M., Young, R.J., Lloyd, G.G., & Clarke, B.F. (1987). Clinically apparent eating disorders in young diabetic women: Associations with painful neuropathy and other complications. *British Medical Journal, 294*, 859–861.

Szmukler, G.I. (1984). Anorexia nervosa and bulimia in diabetics. *Journal of Psychosomatic Research, 28*, 365–369.

Szmukler, G.I., & Russell, G.F.M. (1983). Diabetes mellitus, anorexia nervosa and bulimia. *British Journal of Psychiatry, 142*, 305–308.

Tattersall, R.B., & Lowe, J. (1981). Diabetes in adolescence. *Diabetologia, 20*, 577–583.

Wing, R.R., Nowalk, M.P., Marcus, M.D., Koeske, R., & Finegold, D. (1986). Subclinical eating disorders and glycemic control in adolescents in Type I diabetes. *Diabetes Care, 9*, 162–167.

Wooley, S.C., & Wooley, O.W. (1981). Overeating as substance abuse. In N. K. Mello (Ed.). *Advances in substance abuse: Behavioral and biological research*, Vol. 2 (pp. 41–67). Greenwich, CT: JAI Press, Inc.

7

Neuropsychological Sequelae of Acute and Chronic Blood Glucose Disruption in Adults with Insulin-Dependent Diabetes

Clarissa S. Holmes

Insulin-dependent diabetes is a metabolic disease which requires a high degree of patient knowledge and motivation for successful management due to the relatively complex demands of the typical medical regimen. Initially, medical and health psychologists have studied behavioral and personality factors as important variables which affect patient adherence to medical treatment. Although these variables continue to be important, it is now recognized that the complexity of the regimen also requires sufficient cognitive skills to calculate, adjust and mix insulin doses, to recall and correctly sequence a timed multistepped blood glucose monitoring procedure, and to measure and calculate caloric, cholesterol, and fat intake based upon anticipated exercise needs. These demands are sufficiently complex such that in one diabetic sample studied, up to 20% of poorly controlled ("brittle") patients, had language or other neuropsychological difficulties (e.g., memory problems) that deleteriously inhibited their understanding of and compliance with their prescribed medical regimen (Schade, Drumm, Duckworth, & Eaton, 1985). Often these neuropsychological deficits are well compensated such that it may not be immediately apparent to an untrained professional that a problem exists.

Not only does diabetes require fairly complex management skills, but research in the last 10 years indicates that glucose aberration itself is differentially associated with some neuropsychological dysfunction (Holmes, 1987a). Both acute and chronic glucose disruption, characteristic of the disease even relatively "well controlled," have been related to neuropsychologic changes. That evidence will be reviewed, along with a discussion of relevant neurologic changes that also occur and possible mechanisms of action. Comments will be limited to studies with adults, since studies of children are reviewed elsewhere (see chapter 4). Insulin-dependent diabetes will be the focus of this chapter, since it differs appreciably from non-insulin-dependent diabetes and it is more frequently associated with acute and chronic complications. See chapter 12 for a discussion of the neuropsychological sequelae of non-insulin-dependent diabetes.

Transient Changes in Neuropsychologic Function During Acute Blood Glucose Alterations

One of the more intriguing questions in the neuropsychological study of diabetes is the effect of glucose fluctuations upon mental functioning. Anecdotally, many diabetic patients report feeling slower, more lethargic, or more easily confused when their blood glucose levels are low. The brain does not have compensatory mechanisms to adapt to acute drops in blood glucose levels, which can occur from unanticipated exercise, too much insulin, or too little food, since cerebral cells can store only enough glycogen for a few minutes' use (Lund-Andersen, 1979). The brain is critically dependent upon a reservoir of continuously circulating blood sugar to maintain normal functioning.

Diabetics experience reduced cerebral reactivity in response to CO_2 challenge and relative hypoprofusion of cerebral blood flow (Dandona, James, Newbury, Woollard, & Beckett, 1978), and consequently reduced glucose metabolism. The degree to which different areas of the brain are affected by diminished glucose and neurologic symptoms (glucopenia) depends upon the order of phylogenetic evolution. The areas which evolved latest require the greatest oxygen and glucose consumption, specifically the neocortex and frontal lobes. Primitive brain structures in the myencephalic and premyencephalic regions regulate cardiorespiratory activities and are the least dependent on ambient glucose and the best preserved in its relative absence (Ensinck & Williams, 1974).

Because glucose and oxygen transport are closely related, the neurologic symptoms of deprivation of each are similar. The primary difference between the two is increased electrolytes (Na^+, K^+) and edema associated with hypoglycemia. Electrolyte disruption results in increased neural postsynaptic potentials and decreased inhibitory thresholds. The brain can survive relative loss of glucose better than loss of oxygen, but during very severe hypoglycemia both can occur. There is also some evidence of disrupted cellular energy stores of ATP during severe glucose deprivation associated with either seizure activity or coma (Ensinck & William, 1974; Lewis, Ljunggren, Ratcheson, & Siesjo, 1974).

There is no absolute correlation between different blood glucose levels and the presence of neurologic symptoms in different diabetic individuals. Older patients or those with longer disease duration, who are more likely to have atherosclerosis and compromised cerebral circulation, are also more likely to experience symptoms of glycopenia at higher blood glucose levels than younger patients or those unaffected by cardiovascular changes (Ensinck & Williams, 1974). Further, differences in insulin sensitivity and degree of previous metabolic control can also produce individual differences in hypoglycemic reactivity (Amiel, Sherwin, Simonson, & Tamborlane, 1988).

With these caveats in mind, a general guideline is presented for those who may be less familiar with glucose homeostasis. Arky (1979) reports that speech becomes slurred around 40 mg/dl, and increasing cerebral dysfunction, including convulsions and coma, can occur as blood glucose levels approach concentrations of 10–15 mg/dl. Normoglycemia occurs in the range 80–120 mg/dl and hyperglycemia, or glucose excess, is characterized by blood concentrations above 200 mg/dl. Severe hyperglycemia, which may result in neurologic disruption, occurs at much higher levels (@ 600 mg/dl). Thus, there is a much greater zone of safety in the hyperglycemic range than in the range of hypoglycemia. Diabetics often experience very labile swings in glucose levels during the course of a day since it is difficult for insulin injections to mimic the normal physiologic regulation produced by minute insulin secretions of an intact pancreas. Blood glucose levels may vary frequently and dramatically within 24 hr despite efforts to maintain adequate control. Figure 7.1 depicts the relatively stable blood glucose levels of a nondiabetic individual over the course of a day. In comparison, the more labile glucose profiles of a person with non-insulin-dependent diabetes (NIIDM) and another with insulin-dependent diabetes (IDDM) are presented. The profiles of both diabetic individuals fluctuate more than that of the nondiabetic, and the profile of the NIIDM patient has less intense fluctuations and fewer episodes of hypoglycemia than that of the IDDM patient. This is one of the factors that makes IDDM a different disease from NIDDM.

During a state of recurrent hypoglycemia cerebral metabolic adaptation occurs in response to reduced glucose availability. Studies with rats

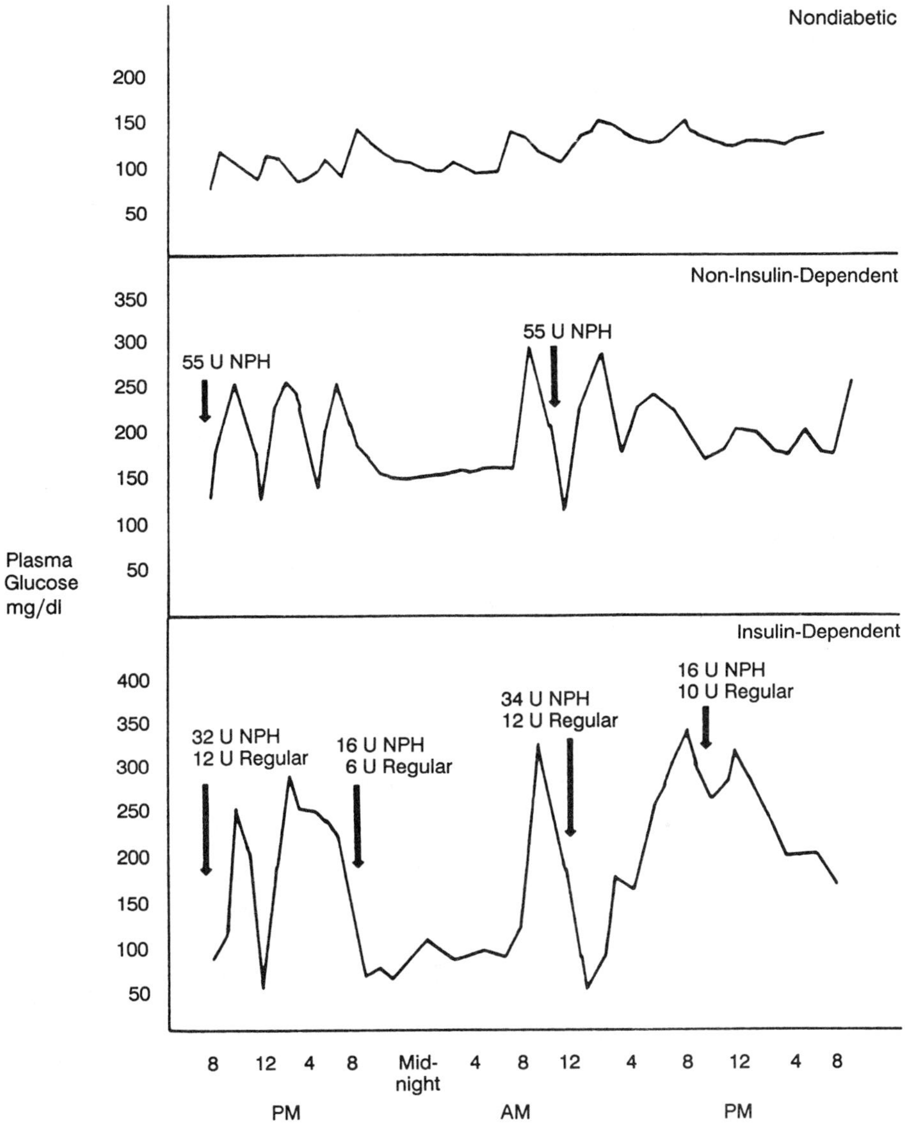

Figure 7.1. Results of hourly plasma glucose monitoring in a nondiabetic, a non-insulin-dependent diabetic, and an insulin-dependent diabetic patient during inpatient monitoring. The frequent fluctuations in plasma glucose in the diabetic compared to the nondiabetic patients are apparent. Insulin doses are indicated. Figure reprinted from DM Nathan (1983) Glycosylated hemoglobin: what is it and how to use it. *Clinical Diabetes*, 1(1), p. 3. From American Diabetes Association, Inc. Reprinted with permission.

indicate that chronic glucose depletion results in increased glucose transport across the blood brain barrier to compensate for diminished glucose availability (McCall et al., 1986). However, this adaptation takes time as demonstrated by Fourest-Fontecave et al. (1987). Using nondiabetic human subjects, they showed that fasting-induced hypoglycemia of short duration (12 hr) was associated with reduced mental clearness, while fasting of longer duration (72 hr) revealed intact mental alertness despite similar levels of stabilized hypoglycemia (40 mg/dl) during each testing period. They speculate that by 72 hr, the central nervous system had adapted to other enrgy sources such as fatty acids and recovered most functioning, although some mild neuropsychological impairments were still present.

Early Studies of Hypoglycemic Cognitive Effects

Perhaps because hypoglycemia is such a dramatic physiologic event, and it is relatively common in insulin-dependent diabetes, its effect upon cognitive performance has long been of interest to investigators. Davis (1943) studied 40 college students with electroencephalographic recordings during hypoglycemia induced via an insulin injection. While blood glucose levels ranged from 53 to 85 mg/dl, subjects showed irregular alpha activity and slower wave activity of 2–5 -s duration, suggestive of decreased vigilance. Russell and Rix-Trott (1975) first investigated the neuropsychological consequences of blood glucose alteration. In a study of 13 patients hospitalized because of obesity or suspected pituitary disorder, they found motor coordination and immediate recall were significantly impaired at glucose levels which fluctuated between 25 and 55 mg/dl. Clayson (1971) found speed of maze running and rate of learning was reduced in rats during hypoglycemia compared to normoglycemia.

Until very recently it has been difficult to unambiguously assess the effects of hypoglycemia upon cognitive performance due to the great variability that occurs between and within individuals in response to insulin injections. The advent of an automated glucose-controlled insulin infusion system (GCIIS), developed in the mid 1970s, for the first time allows glucose levels to be stabilized while cognitive functioning is assessed. The procedure consists of inserting an intravenous catheter into an arm vein in which either insulin or glucose is infused until a desired blood glucose level is achieved. Then a targeted glucose level is maintained through minute infusions of insulin or glucose as indicated for homeostasis. A second catheter is inserted into a hand vein to monitor blood glucose levels via continuous blood sampling every minute. This system best approximates normal physiologic regulation with its features of a feedback loop and the dispersion of minute quantities of insulin/glucose. Typically, catheters are placed in the nondominant hand to enable participation with the other hand in neuropsychological testing. A variation of this system is a clamp technique which relies upon manual monitoring and adjustment of glucose levels. Although intravenous access is also used, typically glucose monitoring and regulation occurs at less frequent intervals, usually every 5 to 15 min; and insulin infusion may be semiautomated via an insulin pump rather than an intravenous drip.

Acute, Transitory Neuropsychological Effects of Hypoglycemia

A group at the University of Iowa first utilized an automated glucose-controlled insulin infusion system (GCIIS; later called Biostator when it became commercially available; Ames Co., Elkhart, IN) in a series of studies designed to evaluate neuropsychological functioning during glucose alterations in diabetics (Holmes, Hayford, Gonzalez, & Weydert, 1983). In this study, we demonstrated that glucose levels could be uniformly set and maintained within and between individuals with a reasonable degree of stability (+/−4% variation). With a double-blind balanced crossover design, each subjects' neuropsychological performance during hypoglyemia (60 mg/dl) was compared to their performance during normoglycemia/control (110 mg/dl). Diminished attention was found on a simple visual reaction time (RT) task and speed of recall was slowed on a simple calculation test during hypoglycemia. On both tests, response accuracy remained intact, but performance was slower. More complex reading skills remained unaffected by glucose changes. See Table 7.1 for a detailed description of the tests administered and the method in this and all other glucose alteration studies.

This result of diminished attention on a nonverbal task was then extended to verbal measures of attention. Using the same method and design, with a slightly lower hypoglycemic level (55 mg/dl), we obtained a similar pattern of slowed responding and preserved accuracy on tasks of verbal attention and fluency (Holmes, Koepke, Thompson, Gyves, & Weydert, 1984). Verbal fluency was reduced by 18% during hypoglycemia (compared to normoglycemia), and naming performance was slowed on the Stroop test from 16 to 6% depending on whether interference was present or not, respectively. Performance decrements of 6 to 18% occurred on these brief tasks of less than 1-min duration each. When attention is required over a longer interval, and fatigue may also intervene, performance may further decline. Diminished verbal fluency has been related to lower glucose metabolism in the bilateral temporal and frontal lobes on PET scans in nondiabetics (Parks et al., 1988). Damage to the left frontal lobe has been shown to maximally affect verbal fluency scores. Our results of reduced verbal and nonverbal attention during hypoglycemia are consistent with transient compromise of the bilateral frontal lobes.

Table 7.1. Studies of Acute Glucose Disruption

Study Authors	Age Range (years) (mean)	HbA_1%	Measures	Induction Technique	Glucose Levels mg/dl	Control Condition	Control Group Nondiabetic	Glucose Level Duration (min)	Interval Between Levels (min)	Physiologic Measures
				Diabetic Subjects						
Holmes et al. (1983) $N = 12$ (6 M, 6 F)	College students	—	Visual RT[a] Rey Auditory Learning Test Mathematic Computation Reading Compreh Benton Visual Retention Test	Glucose-Controlled Insulin Infusion System (GCIIS)	(1) 300 (2) 110 (3) 60	Balanced crossover	—	30	90	—
Holmes et al. (1984) $N = 12$ M	18–35	—	Stroop Word Fluency	GCIIS	(1) 300 (2) 110 (3) 55	Balanced crossover	—	30	180	—
Herold et al. (1985) $N = 12$ (6 M, 6 F)	21–33 (31.3)	10.8	Visual RT	Bolus insulin followed by continuous infusion	(1) 85–110 (2) < 50 for 30 min otherwise fluctuating	Balanced crossover	Nondiabetics $N = 14$ (9 M, 5 F) 20–35 years	120	3–7 days	Glucagon Catecholamines Growth hormone Cortisol
Holmes et al. (1986) $N = 24$ M	18–35 (21.3)	9.6 (c)	Multichoice Visual Reaction Time Finger Tapping Visual Perception	GCIIS	(1) 300 (2) 110 (3) 55	Balanced crossover	—			—
Pramming et al. (1986) $N = 16$ M	20–46 (28)	8.7 study 8.5 sham study	Serial Sevens Tapping Digit Span Category Test Trail making	Insulin clamp	(1) 105 (2) 54 (3) 36 (4) 108	Sham study	Diabetics $N = 6$ M 20–40 years	30	50	—

			Story recall System checklist							
Heller et al. (1987) $N = 15$ (12 M, 3 F)	28–66 (36)	9.0 (N = 11) Nonreactive 9.9 (N = 4) Reactive 5–8.5 Normal	Serial 4-choice RT System Questionnaire	Glucose clamp	(1) 81 (2) 57.6 (3) 45 (4) 81	Test–Retest ABA Design	Unmatched nondiabetics $N = 10$ (8 M, 2 F) (22 yrs)	30	20	Finger tremor Heart rate Blood pressure Sweating Adrenalin
Holmes et al. (1987)[b] $N = 16$ M diabetics	18–35 (23.3)	8.8 (c) Convergent 6.9 (c) Divergent	Multichoice Auditory RT Visual Simple RT Finger Tap	GCIIS	(1) 300 (2) 110 (3) 62	Balanced crossover	—	60	120	Continuous EEG
Hoffman et al. (1989) $N = 17$ M	22–35 (28.2)	8.5 (c)	Visual/Auditory RT Pursuit Rotor Trail Making Automobile Driving Simulator	GCIIS	(1) 300 (2) 100 (3) 50	Balanced crossover	—	30	60–120	—
				Nondiabetic Subjects						
Russell & Rix-Trott (1975) $N = 10$ (5 M, 8 F) Obese or suspected pituitary disease	16–65	N/A	Pegboard Memory Problem Solving Visual Perception	Bolus-intravenous insulin	Fluctuated 25–90 during testing	—	—	30	3 days	—
Fourest-Fontecave et al. (1987) $N = 8$ M	25–34 (26.9)	N/A	Visual RT Mental Clearness & Memory Synonym Learning	(1) 12-hr fast (2) 72-hr fast with glucose/insulin clamp in each	(1) 77 40 (2) 62 40	Balanced crossover	Nondiabetic Reference Group $N = 8$ M	40–60	1 week	—

Table 7.1. (*Continued*)

Study Authors	Age Range (years) (mean)	HbA_1%	Measures	Induction Technique	Glucose Levels mg/dl	Control Condition	Control Group Nondiabetic	Glucose Level Duration (min)	Interval Between Levels (min)	Physiologic Measures
Ipp & Forster (1987) $N=7$ (6 M, 1 F)	22–41	N/A	Trail Making Test	Insulin infusion	Fluctuated 54 lowest, 64 average individually determined: (1) 1-hr before insulin (2) at time of insulin (3) 30 post-insulin (4) 90 post-insulin	No	$N=17$ (6 M, 11 F) 19–48 years Cognitive Testing only	—	—	Epinephrine
Stevens et al. (1989) $N=12$ (6 M, 6 F)	18–27 (23)	N/A	Auditory/Visual RT Finger Tapping Trail Making Test Critical Flicker Fusion Digit-Symbol Symptom Questionnaire	Glucose/insulin clamp	(1) 88.2 (2) 61.2	Balanced crossover	Nondiabetic *Ss* only $N=12$	30	60–95	Epinephrine Norepinephrine Glucagon Pancreatic polypeptide (every 15 min)

[a]Reaction Time.

We were able to further support our hypothesis of disrupted attention during low glucose levels by demonstrating a linear relationship between increasingly complex attentional demands on a visual RT task and increasing performance impairment (Holmes, Koepke & Thompson, 1986). See Figure 7.2 which illustrates that as hierarchical decision-making options increased from none, to one and two decisions, performance was more affected during hypoglycemia (7%, 10%, and 12%, respectively). Neither finger tapping nor visual perception (tachistoscopic presentation of letters) was affected by glucose alteration, providing further evidence that attention and executive function of the frontal lobes is the likely locus of cerebral dysfunctioning during mild hypoglycemia. Others have since replicated this finding indicating that finger tapping is unaffected by glucose depletion (Hoffman et al., 1989; Pramming, Thorsteinsson, Theilgaard, Pinner, & Binder, 1986), although when a planning component is added, as in the Trailmaking test, then performance decrement is likely to occur (Hoffman et al., 1989; Pramming et al., 1986). Since these first studies, both visual and auditory RT have been used frequently as a measure of attention which is sensitive to glucose depletion (Stevens, McKane, Bell, Bell, King, Hayes, 1989; Pramming et al., 1986; Heller, MacDonald, Herbert, & Tattersall 1987; Herold, Polonsky, Cohen, Levy, & Douglas, 1985).

With delayed RT demonstrated during hypoglycemia, one troubling implication of this research is the possible impact of reduced attention upon driving ability (Lasche, 1985). Recently, Hoffman and colleagues specifically addressed this question (Hoffman et al., 1989). They found impairments in visual and auditory RT at 50 mg/dl, consistent with the literature, but more complex, and overlearned, driving skills (i.e., signalling ability, braking pattern, steering, speed control) assessed by a

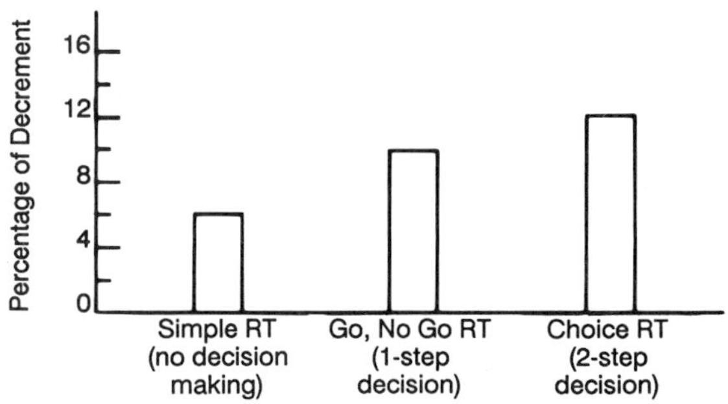

Figure 7.2. Performance decrement in RT latency at low glucose level compared to control glucose level (normoglycemia). Figure reprinted from C.S. Holmes, K.M. Koepke, and R.G. Thompson (1986). Simple versus complex performance impairments at three blood glucose levels. *Psychoneuroendocrinology, 11*, p. 356.

simulator were not impaired compared to 100 mg/dl euglycemia. Intact complex skills during relatively mild hypoglycemia is consistent with the results of others on complex tasks of categorization and reading skills (Holmes et al., 1983; Pramming et al., 1986). A word of caution is sounded by Hoffman et al. who note that a driving simulator may not sufficiently capture all the vital aspects of driving under more naturalistic conditions. Driving safety is a controversial issue since among diabetic drivers hypoglycemia may be a causative factor in 5 to 6% of all accidents (Ratner & Whitehouse, 1989; Songer et al., 1988). However, it is argued that many diabetics voluntarily limit their driving, and those individuals without a history of severe hypoglycemic episodes are less likely to have problems while driving. Most saliently, if other driving risk factors are considered, such as young age, male gender, alcohol use, previous infractions, martial status, and so on, then diabetic status does not appear to be a significant risk factor (Songer, 1989).

Counterregulatory Responses During Hypoglycemia

As part of the body's protective mechanism, when hypoglycemia occurs a number of hormones are released to counterregulate the state of deficiency. Specifically, epinephrine, cortisol, growth hormone, and glucagon are released in an effort to restore normoglycemia. The release of these hormones triggers a set of physical sensations which can include tremulousness, fatigue, sweating, and heart palpitations. These symptoms occur in response to activation of the adrenergic arm of the sympathic nervous system, primarily epinephrine discharge. Another by-product of hypoglycemia are neuroglycopenic symptoms which include difficulty concentrating, light-headedness, and disorientation; these neuropsychological effects are thought to be related to glucose depletion. The release of growth hormone and cortisol is relatively slow compared to faster acting adrenergic responses, and as a result they are less likely to play a direct role in acute neuroglycopenia.

Since both adrenergic and neuroglycopenic symptoms co-occur during hypoglycemia, an important question is posed by their association. Are neuropsychological impairments during hypoglycemia simply a reaction to the physical symptoms of feeling weak, listless, or ill? Although subjects are always blinded to study conditions in studies of glucose manipulation, if some were able to detect physical sensations, then perhaps such feedback tempered their performance, perhaps unwittingly distorting their responding through adoption of a more cautious or guarded response style. Another concern is individual variability in the onset of hypoglycemic responses since individual performance differences may be obscured by group resuls. For example, longer disease duration and poorer disease control both have been associated with diminished counterregulatory epinephrine response (Bolli et al., 1984), resulting in patients who may be severely hypoglycemic without experiencing any physical cues to warn them of their metabolic status. Patients with autonomic neuropathy (i.e., reduced blood pressure, increased heart rate), which is frequently associated with longer disease duration and poorer metabolic control, also experience reduced epinephrine counterregulation (Hoeldtke, Boden, Shuman, & Owen, 1982; Hilsted et al., 1981).

Individual Neuropsychological Patterns

Several studies have recently examined individual patterns of responding to hypoglycemia, and the relation between neuropsychological performance and adrenergic symptoms. Patterns of individual responding were first described by Herold et al. (1985) on a visual RT task given to diabetics. They found variable performance deterioration, with some subjects' RT slowing during hypoglycemia while others' RT did not. The performance of neither group could be explained by the severity or duration of hypoglycemia. In an important design refinement, these researchers evaluated the amount of counterregulatory hormones present during testing, but found it to be unrelated to performance. However, since a clamp technique was not used, glucose levels varied widely in both the euglycemic and hypoglycemic conditions, making it difficult to rule out variable glucose levels as an explanation for intersubject differences. Subjects in the study were in moderate-to-poor disease control (X $HbA_{1c} = 10.8\%$); the authors did not report the level of metabolic control for those who experienced performance deterioration versus those who did not.

Degree of metabolic control may be a significant variable to study based on a study by Holmes (1987b). Using the Biostator, with blood glucose stabilized at a very mild hypoglycemic level (62 mg/dl), two patterns of subject performance were identified on a serial auditory RT task. The auditory RT performance of some subjects (Convergent group) conformed to the visual RT pattern of increased slowness found earlier (Holmes et al., 1986), while another group of subjects displayed Divergent results and showed equivalent or slightly better performance at low compared to normal glucose levels. Both groups were similar in age, age of disease onset, and years of education, and each had high average intelligence (X IQ = 114). The only difference between groups was moderate versus rigorous metabolic control over the previous 2 months (Convergent $HbA_{1c} = 8.8\%$; Divergent $HbA_{1c} = 6.9\%$; norman range = 4.7 to 7.0%). Since Divergent subjects maintained daily glucose levels which were on average 65 mg/dl lower than the Convergent group (Goldstein, 1984), a type of state-dependent performance might have been evidenced, in that mild hypoglycemia would be a more common experience in the Divergent group. However, groups also differed in the number of episodes of hypoglycemic unconsciousness they experienced. As frequently happens to patients in more rigorous control (Arias, Kerner, Zier, Navascues, & Pfeiffer, 1985), the Divergent subjects tended to experience more episodes of hypoglycemic unconsciousness (3.6) than those in moderate disease control (0.6); a factor which has been related to poorer neuropsychological performance in children (Ryan, Vega, & Drash, 1985) and adults (Bale, 1973; Skenazy & Bigler, 1984). Episodes of unconsciousness may be the more salient explanation since, on average, the Divergent group displayed longer RT latencies on 10 out of 12 measures than did the Convergent group.

Degree of Hypoglycemia and Individual Reactivity

Heller et al. (1987) were the first investigators to thoroughly examine individual differences in physiologic responding to different levels of hypoglycemia and its association with cognitive functioning. Based on a symptom self-report checklist, only 1/15 diabetic and 2/10 nondiabetic subjects detected mild hypoglycemia ($X = 57.6$ mg/dl), yet all experienced significant neuropsychological slowing on an RT task. Epinephrine was the only counterregulatory hormone that significantly increased in all the nondiabetics and the "aware" diabetics. Heart rate, blood pressure, sweating, and tremor did not change in any subjects. These results provided initial evidence that neuropsychological disruption precedes epinephrine release in diabetics, and poorer performance is not a consequence of feeling ill. More disturbingly, mild cognitive deterioration begins before a patient is consciously or physically aware that blood glucose levels are lowered. It is unknown to what extent this diminished attention might influence a diabetic's ability to respond to an impending energy crisis; although it is known that more errors in blood glucose management occur during very high and very low glucose levels.

During moderate hypoglycemia of 45 mg/dl, all nondiabetic and 4/15 diabetic subjects experienced epinephrine response, sweating, and tremor. Subjectively "aware" diabetic and nondiabetic subjects, all of whom also experienced counterregulation, almost doubled their RT's when glucose levels were decreased from mild to moderate hypoglycemia. In contrast, "unaware" diabetics showed no additional RT slowing during moderate hypoglycemia and no counterregulatory responses. These additional findings indicate that subjective awareness of low blood glucose, as measured by self-report adjective checklist, is highly associated with the presence of counterregulatory hormones. They also demonstrate the widely recognized clinical problem that diabetic individuals with impaired counterregulatory responses are particularly vulnerable to severe hypoglycemia with little or no symptomatic cues about their glucose status. In this study, release of counterregulatory hormones in diabetic subjects occurred independently of disease duration.

Pramming et al. (1986 evaluated RT performance during mild and severe hypoglycemia (54 and 36 mg/dl, respectively). With a more striking difference between glucose levels, more distinct performance differences were obtained for diabetic subjects, indicating statistically and clinically impaired neuropsychological performance during severe compared to mild hypoglycemia. Similar to the Heller et al. study, some (2/16) of the diabetic subjects remained unaware of hypoglycemia even during severe hypoglycemia. Counterregulation was anecdotally determined by the observations of a trained experimenter. Nevertheless, the authors concluded, consistent with Heller et al., that "neuropsychological performance deteriorated at a blood glucose concentration just below 54 mg/dl in 12 of the 16 patients, though none perceived this state as hypoglycaemia" (p. 650). These were the first two studies to demonstrate that neuroglypenia appears to precede adrenergia during hypoglycemia in diabetic patients. Thus, neuropsychological changes are not a function of "feeling ill" from counterregulation.

Pramming et al. (1986) noted performance deterioration on all measures of neuropsychological functioning, including Trailmaking, Digit Span, categorization, and subtraction, unlike other studies which have found inferential skills to remain intact despite glucose alteration. This may have been a function of the statistical treatment of their data, via a paired rank sum test; raw scores were not utilized, thereby greatly reducing intraindividual and interindividual variability on performance measures. This possibility is strengthened by reviewing the means and ranges of the raw scores reported for each glucose level. Interestingly, the authors included a unique assessment device by requiring subjects to estimate the passage of 1 min at each glucose level. Although the score ranges were wide, the means (number of seconds elapsed while estimating 60 s) were within 1–2 s of 60 at all glucose levels except 36 mg/dl, during which 80 s elapsed before subjects perceived the passage of 1 min. Subjects also required much prompting to fully execute tasks, despite awareness of task demands. Difficulty with time estimation and task execution may explain why errors are so common when diabetics monitor their blood glucose at extreme levels, since a timed multistep sequence is required for accurate results.

Effects of Hypoglycemia in Nondiabetics

In nondiabetics, the relation between neuropsychological performance and adrenergic symptoms may be less clear. Heller et al. indicated that only 2/10 nondiabetics reported significant awareness of adrenergic symptoms via a checklist, yet they all experienced an increase in epinephrine levels. Even though they evidenced neuropsychological impairment during mild hypoglycemia then, this could have been related to the presence of epinephrine or some related factor and not to glucose depletion itself. Stevens et al. (1989) replicated this result with nondiabetics and showed impaired planning (Trailmaking) and slowed visual/motor memory (Digit Symbol) during mild hypoglycemia (X = 61.2 mg/dl), but again, in the presence of counterregulatory hormones (glucagon, epinephrine, pancreatic polypeptide). In contrast, Ipp and Forster (1987) attained a similar level of mild hypoglycemia ($X = 64$ mg/dl) in their nondiabetic subjects, but did *not* find neuropsychological impairment on the Trailmaking test, although they found a rise in epinephrine levels. However, glucose levels were individually determined and fluctuated in the Ipp and Forster study which may have allowed sufficient recovery time for their nondiabetic subjects to recoup from adverse hypoglycemic effects. In sum, while the precise physiologic factors underlying neuropsychological impairment during hypoglycemia remains to be determined in nondiabetics, it is known that nondiabetic counterregulatory responding is quantitatively different than that of diabetics and that different mechanisms may underlie grossly similar neuropsychological impairments in each population.

Effects of Hyperglycemia

There have been relatively few investigations of the cognitive effects of hyperglycemia. Holmes and colleagues in a series of studies (Holmes, et al., 1984; Holmes et al., 1986; Holmes, 1987b) and Hoffman et al. (1989) have shown neuropsychological functioning to be unaffected by moderate glucose excess (300 mg/dl). Based on gross physical findings, such as hyperosmolar coma when glucose levels are extremely elevated (i.e., often over 600 mg/dl), it is unlikely that moderate glucose concentrations of 300 mg/dl are sufficient to produce significant cognitive impairment. Further, moderate hyperglycemia does not have the acute life-threatening potential of hypoglycemia since there is a much larger range of short-term safety (i.e., 150–400 mg/dl) before acute physical symptoms may be evidenced. It is thought that chronic hyperglycemia is responsible for most of the long-term complications associated with diabetes, such as cardiovascular disease, blindness, and renal failure, such that it cannot be considered "safer" to diabetics than hypoglycemia in an absolute sense. An NIH multicenter national study (Diabetes Clinical Complications Trial; DCCT) is presently studying whether degree of metabolic control might be related to long-term outcome. Nevertheless, based on preliminary negative results, evaluation of the neuropsychological effects of moderate hyperglycemia in diabetics does not appear to warrant additional study at this time.

In contrast to these findings with Type I diabetics, animal studies suggest that posttraining injections of glucose can facilitate 24-hr delayed recall of an avoidance task in rats (Gold, Vogt, & Hall, 1986). Recently, Gonder-Frederick et al. (1987) provided evidence that memory may be improved in normal elderly subjects (*X* age = 67 years) during mild levels of hyperglycemia (*X* = 171 mg/dl) relative to euglycemia (*X* = 112 mg/dl). In a crossover design, subjects drank either a beverage with saccharin or glucose; order of beverage ingestion was counterbalanced across subjects. Total memory scores on the Wechsler Memory Scale were significantly better during glucose supplementation. However, a negative association was found between extremely elevated blood glucose levels and poorer memory, although maximum glucose concentrations were not reported.

Neuroelectric Correlates of Glucose Alteration

Holmes and colleagues (1987) utilized continuous EEG monitoring during neuropsychological testing at glucose levels of 55, 110, and 300 mg/dl, regulated via GCIIS. Each test period was preceded by a ½-hr interval while glucose levels were stabilized and subjects rested in a quiet room to avoid "background noise" (i.e., ocular and hand movements, etc.) in the EEG readings. No changes were found in the EEGs of 11/12 subjects, although 1 subject displayed large amplitude slow wave activity suggestive of diffuse insult. The subject's performance on neuropsychological measures did not appear more impaired than that of the others whose recordings remained intact. We concluded from these results that the neuropsychological impairments which can accompany mild hypoglycemia are not a result of changes in gross neuroelectric activity.

Pramming, Thorsteinsson, Stigsby, and Binder (1988) evaluated EEG recordings at lower glucose concentrations via bolus insulin injection followed by intravenous infusion, with blood sampling every 10 min. At a median glucose level of 36 mg/dl, alpha activity level decreased in 12/13 diabetics with a concurrent increase in theta activity, reflecting neuronal dysfunction in all leads to the cortex. The authors note that at a blood glucose level of 36 mg/dl (2 mmol/l) rabbits have an intracellular glucose concentration in the brain of close to zero. One subject who did not display EEG disruption had a slightly higher glucose level at 40 mg/dl. There was no correlation between actual blood glucose levels and EEG changes, nor age, duration of diabetes, insulin dose, HbA_{1c}, rate of glucose decline, nor anecdotal observation of hypoglycemic symptoms and patient report of symptoms. With glucose infusion, EEG abnormalities quickly reverted to normal. EEG changes appear to occur at a relatively low glucose concentration (@ 36 mg/dl) and to disappear within a very narrow blood glucose range. More of a threshold effect takes place rather than graduated onset and cessation.

Summary

Substantial evidence from a number of different research groups, using a variety of research techniques and test measures, has demonstrated that reaction time, and presumably attention, is disrupted during acute episodes of mild hypoglycemia (55–60 mg/dl) in IDDM. This effect is further exacerbated, and performance speed almost doubles, at more severe levels of hypoglycemia (45 mg/dl; Heller et al., 1987) during which transient EEG abnormalities also appear (36 mg/dl; Pramming et al., 1988). These neuropsychological effects seem to be transitory and reversible, although recent evidence in children suggests that a history of mild asymptomatic hypoglycemia in the 50 mg/dl range, is related to poorer abstraction and copying skills on the Stanford-Binet Intelligence Test (Golden et al. 1989). In addition to reaction time, diminished planning on the Trailmaking test is found, another indice indicative of frontal lobe dysfunction.

Are changes in neuropsychological functioning during hypoglycemia a result of feeling sick? Apparently not. Even before diabetic individuals begin to experience adrenergic counterregulatory hormones, which can produce uncomfortable physical sensations, attention has already begun to deteriorate (Pramming et al., 1986; Heller et al., 1987). Neuropsychological or neuroglycopenic effects of hypoglycemia seem to *precede* adrenergic or physical symptoms in IDDM. However, in nondiabetics, it has yet to be demonstrated that diminished attention precedes epinephrine counterregulation. Even though nondiabetics display the same pattern of disrupted attention at similar glucose levels as diabetics, the differences between groups in counterregulatory response may indicate that different factors underlie performance diminution.

Finally, there does not appear to be any evidence of neuropsychological disruption during acute hyperglycemia, at least not in the 300-mg/dl range which has been studied to date (Holmes et al., 1984; Holmes et al., 1986; Holmes, 1987b; Hoffman et al., 1989).

Neuropsychological Effects of Chronic Glucose Alteration

In addition to acute fluctuations in blood glucose levels, chronic glucose derangement might also disrupt optimal neuropsychological performance. Neuroimaging studies have shown that proficiency (Cerami, 1985) and site (Riege, Metter, Kuhl, & Phelps, 1985) of glucose utilization is directly related to task performance and, in some instances, to age. With increasing age, there is less overall glucose utilization by the brain (Kuhl, Metter, Riege, & Phelps, 1982), although cerebral oxygen consumption is not significantly lowered (Lammertsma et al., 1981).

It has been suggested that diabetes is a model of "premature aging" (Kent, 1976) because of the accelerated microvascular changes which occur and lead to atherosclerosis of the blood vessels. This process results in an increased incidence of cardiovascular disease and insult in the form of blood vessel infarction. Decreased blood flow to peripheral arteries is particularly common, and peripheral nerve damage secondary to ischemia results in well-known diabetic foot disease, among other neuropathic conditions. Newrick et al. (1987) demonstrated that diabetic patients with peripheral neuropathy had a reversed nerve-vein oxygen gradient (NVOG) which correlated with disease duration. There was also suggestion of reduced blood flow since reversed NVOGs were correlated with capillary diffusing distance and basal cell membrane thickening. All of these physiologic indicators were significantly correlated with measures of clinical pathology on vibratory and thermal thresholds.

Atherosclerotic changes occur in a slow cumulative progression, and a similar gradual occlusion can take place in the cerebral arteries either through the natural aging process or precociously through a disease process. PET scans conducted with patients who were hypertensive, with or without arteriosclerosis, revealed reduced cerebral blood flow and both lowered oxygen and glucose delivery to the brain (Dastur et al., 1963). Among nondiabetic patients, PET scan changes have been correlated with age-related performance decline on some tasks. Riege et al. (1985), who studied nondiabetic subjects aged 27 to 78 years, found better regional glucose utilization to the frontal-subcortical brain area was associated wtih younger age and better memory for verbal and nonverbal information. Although age-related differences in regional cerebral metabolism were few, evidence was found of an overall reduction in mean glucose metabolism and reduced metabolism in Broca's area. Older subjects (above age 48) with lowered Broca's area glucose consumption displayed a concomitant decrease in verbal and verbally mediated memory. Similarly, organizational memory encoding, which declines with age, was related to superior-frontal metabolic ratios. These age-associated differences in site and degree of glucose utilization in the brain may explain why elderly nondiabetic patients (X age = 67 years) in the Gonder-Frederick et al. study (1987) improved their memory during mild hyperglycemia (X = 171 mg/dl) following glucose ingestion, compared to a euglycemia condition (X = 112 mg/dl).

Although PET scans and other sophisticated neuroimaging studies have yet to be conducted with diabetic subjects, a high percentage of even newly diagnosed diabetic patients have been shown to have a relative hypoprofusion (44%) or no increase (17%) in blood flow to the frontal lobes following CO_2 challenge (Dandona et al., 1978). These patients had an impaired reactivity to CO_2 and reduced dilation of the cerebral vessels. Should subtle vascular changes occur, blood flow to the peripheral projections of the brain (i.e., the frontal lobes) would likely be first and most affected. If such changes occur, then initially one might expect subtle neuropsychological effects prior to any ultimate event that might occur such as severe cerebrovascular accident or stroke.

Although evidence of disrupted attentional performance and other neuropsychological skills will be presented, which may be indicative of atypical brain functioning, it is important to remember that these skills are also highly sensitive measures and vulnerable to almost any disruption including fatigue, anxiety, or mild depression which might accompany a chronic disease, in addition to low task motivation. Thus, underlying mechanisms discussed must remain speculative until definitive neuroimaging studies are available to confirm or disconfirm hypotheses of disrupted cerebral glucose utilization. Further, just as individuals differ in their predilection toward heart disease based on family history, diet, and diabetic disease factors, one would anticipate differences in cerebral susceptibility and recovery as well. In short, diabetic individuals are not a homogeneous population and careful study of disease correlates or other risk factors will be necessary to identify those who might be at greater risk for neuropsychological disruption.

Evoked Potential Studies

Aside from neurologic changes associated with long-term, possibly degenerative, disease factors, it appears that glucose disruption may be associated with immediate, but mild, neurologic sequelae. Several studies have examined auditory and visual cortical evoked potentials in patients who were newly diagnosed and/or who were without clinical neuropathies. Pozzessere et al. (1988) found that 36% of their IDDM subject group aged 18–32 years ($\bar{X}$ age = 23.0), all of whom had been diagnosed with diabetes for less than 4 years, evidenced clinically significant (>3 SDs) reductions in cortical transmission times on at least one of four measures of visual, auditory, or either of two somatosensory evoked potentials (after stimulation of median and tibial nerves). This evidence of so-called "central encephalopathy," a term coined by Reske-Nielsen & Lundbaek (1963), occurred in the absence of peripheral neuropathy to median, tibial, or optic nerves. The P100 latency, which represents the response of the visual cortex to retinal stimulation, was unrelated to indices of metabolic control. In contrast, brainstem auditory evoked responses (BAERs) and somatosensory evoked potentials (EPs) were positively correlated with metabolic control (HbA_{1c}), indicating that poorer metabolic control was related to longer latencies.

The findings of Pozzessere et al. differ from those of other research groups who have not found an association between degree of metabolic control and reduced BAERs. However, others (Donald et al., 1984; Fedele et al., 1984; Fedele et al., 1984) have employed more heterogeneous groups which have varied widely in age (i.e., 16–60 years and 15–40 years, respectively) and disease duration (i.e., 1 month–45 years and 2 months–32 years, respectively), such that subject diversity on these variables may have interacted with or "washed out" effects of metabolic control. Nevertheless, despite sampling and measurement differences, all studies have demonstrated that diabetic subjects, even those who are newly diagnosed, evidence reduced cortical evoked potentials compared to nondiabetic controls. Further, these effects were found even though there was no evidence of peripheral or autonomic neuropathy.

What is the impact of EP changes upon performance? Only one research group has examined the functional correlates of reduced central conduction velocities in diabetic subjects and found no association between articulatory reaction times or IQ, and BAERs (Donald et al., 1984). It is difficult to evaluate this finding in depth, since the focus of the study was BAERs and no specific data were reported from the psychological measures to allow determination of response levels or variability. An earlier pilot study, with a smaller sample of the same subjects (N = 10; Donald et al., 1980) found diabetics had slower decision-making times on a choice reaction time task compared to a control group (Donald et al., 1980), which also was unrelated to EP latencies. See Table 7.2. Despite their failure to find neuropsychological correlates of BAERs, Donald et al. (1984) nevertheless demonstrated significantly longer BAERs in diabetics at an earlier age than nondiabetics. Diabetic subjects showed an increase in Wave I-V interpeak latencies between ages 20 and 45 while nondiabetic controls showed no significant increase in latencies until after age 50. The slowed responding of diabetic subjects occurred 10–15 years before an age-related decline would be expected as part of the natural aging process.

There also is evidence that subtle visual alterations occur earlier in the disease process than previously realized. Trick, Burde, Kilo, Gordon, and Santiago (1987) found a high incidence of abnormal visual responses in diabetic patients who were without overt retinopathy. They found that 50–60% of diabetics they studied (n = 30) still presented some form of visual dysfunction in one or more of the following: hue discrimination, spatial/contrast resolution, and neural processing in the retina or visual cortex (i.e. evoked potentials). However, the degree of association between one or more of these conditions was not reported. It is not known if reduced EPs were correlated with functional decrements in color discrimination and contrast resolution.

In sum, there is accumulating evidence that mild, subclinical central neuropathic alterations may occur in diabetics, even those who are re-

Table 7.2. Studies of Chronic Glucose Disruption

Study Authors	Age Range (years) (mean)	Range of Disease Duration (years) (mean)	HbA_1c[a] (%)	Range of Age/Onset (years) (mean)	Neuropsychology Measures	Control Group	Physiologic Measures
Miles & Root (1922)	15–55 (46) N=40	—	—	—	Digit Cancellation Memory Span for Digits & Words Simple Addition	Friends Relatives	—
Bale (1973)	20–64 (47) N=100	24 (15–45)	—	3–48 (25)	Walton–Black Word Learning Test	—	—
Donald et al. (1980)	16–55 (38) N=10	20 (5–37)	—	—	WAIS subtests Auditory RT[a]	Age and sex-matched controls	Sural MCV Evoked Potentials Auditory/ Articulatory RT
Donald et al. (1984)	16–60 (38.1) N=50	13 (1–45)	9.1	5–60	WAIS[b] subtests Memory scale	Age-matched controls	Brainstem Auditory-evoked Potential late Auditory Evoked Potential Nerve conduction Velocity (NCV)
Franceschi et al. (1984)	18–35 (25.8) N=37	7.6	12.7 Patients admitted to hospital in poor control		Raven's Progressive Matrices Wechsler Memory Scales	Age, sex & SES matched controls selected from	—

					WAIS subtests Attn-Concentration	Orthopedic inpatient ward	
Lawson et al. (1984)	16–60 N = 48	13 (0.1–45)	—	5–60	Wechsler Memory Scale WAIS subtests Figure Drawing Word Repetition	Age-matched controls had more education	Median NCV
Skenazy & Bigher (1984)	18–47 (28.0) N = 39	1–31 (17)	—	1–36 (13)	Halstead–Reitan WAIS	Chronically ill group & Healthy control	—
Holmes (1986)	18–35 (22.5)	(8.0)	Moderate 8.2 Poor 12.4(c)	(13)	WAIS	—	Median NCV
Baade (1988)	20–49 (30.3) N = 35	2–26 (13)	Good < 7.9 Fair 8.0–9.2 Poor > 9.2	13 (0.2–47)	Halsted–Reitan WAIS WRAT-R[c] Grooved Pegboard	Age, sex, and SES matched controls	—
Holmes, Tsalikian, & Yamada (1988)	18–35 (23.3) N = 16	(7.1)	Moderate 10.1 Near-normal 6.9	(16.6)	Visual & Auditory RT[a] WAIS subtests Pegboard Tasks	—	Continuous EGG

[a]RT = Reaction Time measure of attention.
[b]WAIS = Wechsler Adult Intelligence Scale.
[c]WRAT-R = Wide Range Achievement Test-Revised.

cently diagnosed and/or without overt peripheral, retinal, or autonomic neuropathy. It is not known why such changes may occur. It has been suggested that increased reservoirs of glucose, related to insulin insufficiency, may increase aldose reductase activity and lead to neuronal demyelinization or axonal degeneration (Pozzessere et al., 1988). Because it is known that axonal dysfunction may precede demyelinating lesions, if poor metabolic control is a significant factor, it could be beneficial to reexamine poorly controlled patients once better metabolic control is achieved to determine if EP slowing is reversible (Algan et al., 1989).

It is important to note that there is individual variability on these cortical measures. Despite the fact that groups of diabetic subjects generally have slower EPs than groups of nondiabetic controls, often a few subjects with clinically deviant responses can skew the group mean and produce unrepresentative results. Even within individuals, when bilateral conduction times are assessed, unilateral disruption often occurs, suggesting that differential nerve vulnerabilities can occur idiosyncratically within the same person (Pozzessere, 1988). Ideally, in the future, such data could be reported both as group means and as the percentage of individuals who significantly differ from normative expectation. A final, and more important, caution is warranted. The functional impact of these difficulties may be small or undetectable since throughout the lifespan, including senescence, the healthy brain demonstrates plasticity and redundancy in function (Creasey & Rapoport, 1985). Approximately 10 to 100 billion neurons are present in the healthy young adult brain, with about 10,000 connections per neuron (Vijayashankar & Brody, 1979). The brain may well tolerate minor neural slowing or cellular disruption and loss with no concomitant loss of function.

Neuropsychological Studies of Chronic Glucose Alteration

Historically, Miles and Root (1922) were among the first to examine the overall cognitive status of diabetic patients, and compare their performance to a control group consisting of friends and relatives. They found diabetic performance was slowed approximately 20% on tests of attention and memory, but accuracy remained intact. Overlearned, highly familiar tasks were less affected than novel retention tasks. Performance scores were not compared to disease variables. See Table 7.2 for the details of this and other neuropsychological studies reported here.

Bale (1973) was among the first contemporaneous investigators to evaluate a group of diabetics that varied widely in age (ages 20–64), with relatively late disease onset ($X = 25$ years) and long disease duration ($X = 24$ years). He used the Walton-Black Word Learning Test and found 17% of his diabetic sample and none of the controls scored in the dysfunctioning range. Neither age of disease onset nor length of disease duration was related to performance but episodes and severity of hypoglycemic reactions were related to poorer performance. Interestingly, six of the diabetic patients and none of the controls had a history of cerebrovascular accident, but only one of the six with a history of stroke scored in the dysfunctional range on the Walton-Black. These findings suggest that hypoglycemic episodes and not cerebrovascular disease were more of a factor related to poor performance.

Skenazy and Bigler (1984) and Baade (1988) each administered the Wechsler Adult Intelligence Scale (WAIS) and a traditional neuropsychological battery, the Halsted-Reitan, to a group of diabetics and nondiabetic controls matched for age, gender, and educational level. Both research groups had demographically similar diabetic samples with age restricted to early and middle adulthood (@ 20–50 years) and a similar length of disease duration (X years = 17 and 13, respectively). Baade found that diabetics performed more poorly than controls in four broad categories of tests: sensory/motor, fund of knowledge, problem solving, and attention/memory. Diabetic subjects also were less verbally fluent, although motor speed was intact. Greatest differences were seen in lower fund of knowledge, despite similar educational backgrounds. Specifically, diabetic Verbal IQs were lower than control IQs, directly related to lower Information and Vocabulary subtests; Spelling and Reading scores from the Wide Range Achievement Test-Revised were also lower. Diabetics had scores that were mildly deflated (@ 7 points) compared to controls; however, the standard deviations indicated more variability among the performance of diabetics, suggesting that some individuals might be more clinically different than others. Skenazy and Bigler (1984) also found their diabetic sample performed more poorly than controls, but primarily on somatosensory tests and the Performance IQ. Poorer performance was linked to severity of hypoglycemic episodes in their study. Results of this study more closely parallel those of studies with children, which implicate episodes of unconsciousness to be associated with poorer spatial and nonverbal abilities (Ryan, Vega, and Longstreet, 1984). In contrast, episodes of severe hypoglycemia were not reported in Baade's study.

Franceschi et al. (1984) examined diabetic subjects admitted to the hospital because of poor metabolic control (X $HbA_{1c} = 12.7\%$). Their performance on selected WAIS subtests, the Wechsler Memory Scale, and tests of attention was compared to that of a control group from an orthopedic inpatient ward matched for age, gender, and SES. Diabetic patients were relatively young ($X = 26$ years), with relatively short disease duration ($X = 7.6$ years). Age of disease onset was not evaluated as a variable. Results revealed that these younger diabetic patients, with relatively short disease duration and poor metabolic control, evidenced intact global intellectual functioning (although only selected WAIS subtests were administered), but poorer memory and conceptual (Block Design and Similarities) abilities.

Holmes and colleagues (1986) administered a hierarchical visual reaction time (RT) measure to diabetic subjects following blood glucose monitoring done for descriptive purposes. Blood glucose levels varied widely across individuals during testing (X = 275 mg/dl; range 60–400 mg/dl). In addition to the RT measures, intelligence (WAIS) and academic achievement tests were administered to diabetic men between the ages of 18 and 35 (X age = 22 years). A stepwise regression indicated that metabolic control and age of diabetes onset were the two best predictors of intellectual performance. Ambient blood glucose was unrelated to performance, probably because it varied so widely. Men in poorer metabolic control ($HbA_{1c} > 11\%$; $X = 12.4\%$) had lower verbal IQs (8 points) than those in moderate control (X $HbA_{1c} = 8.2\%$). Specifically, the Vocabulary and Information subtests were lower. indicative of a reduced fund of acquired information, even though subjects in poorer control were demographically similar in amount of education, age, full-scale IQ, and had similar math computation and reading skills with which to acquire new information. Scores were statistically lower, but were still within the average range. When early onset (< 13 years) and poor control were examined together, Similarities scores, an index of conceptual ability, were lowered. Attention was diminished on a simple RT task and was unrelated to motor nerve conduction velocity, motor speed, or visual perception, suggesting that cognitively based attention was diminished rather than other subcomponent skills.

Diminished attention was also found in association with metabolic control in another study which examined auditory and visual reaction times in a different sample of young diabetic men (Holmes, Tsalikian, & Yamada, 1988). Patients were again between 18 and 35 years (X = 23.3) and without any secondary disease complications. During testing, blood glucose levels again varied widely (X = 197 mg/dl), regardless of previous metabolic control that was either near-normal (HbA_{1c} nondiabetic range = 4.7 to 7.0%; $X = 6.9\%$) or moderate ($X = 10.1\%$). Subjects in near-normal control displayed poorer auditory and visual attention than subjects in moderate disease control. Groups did not differ in age, education, IQ (X=115), age of disease onset (X=16.5 years) or disease duration (X=7 years). Subjects in near-normal control, who maintained HbA_{1c} values in the nondiabetic range, showed a trend toward more episodes of hypoglycemic unconsciousness than those in moderate control (3.6 vs. 0.3, respectively). More rigorous metabolic control, in the nondiabetic range, has been associated with more episodes of severe hypoglycemia (Goldstein, 1984), which in turn has been related to poorer neurologic and neuropsychological outcome (Ingram, Stark, & Blackburn, 1967; Ryan, Vega, & Drash, 1985; Bale, 1973; Baade, 1988). When results from the visual RT in this study are combined with those from the Holmes' (1986) study, degree of attention appears associated with degree of metabolic control in a possible U-shaped rela-

Figure 7.3. Mean response time (+/− SD) to a simple visual reaction time task by degree of prevailing blood glucose control. Data at HbA_1c of 8.2 and 12.4% are from insulin-dependent patients reported in CS Holmes (1986) Neuropsychological profiles in men with insulin-dependent diabetes. *Journal of Consulting and Clinical Psychology, 54*, pp 386–389. Figure reprinted from CS Holmes (1988) Blood glucose control and visual and auditory attention in men with insulin-dependent diabetes. *Diabetic Medicine, 5*, p. 638.

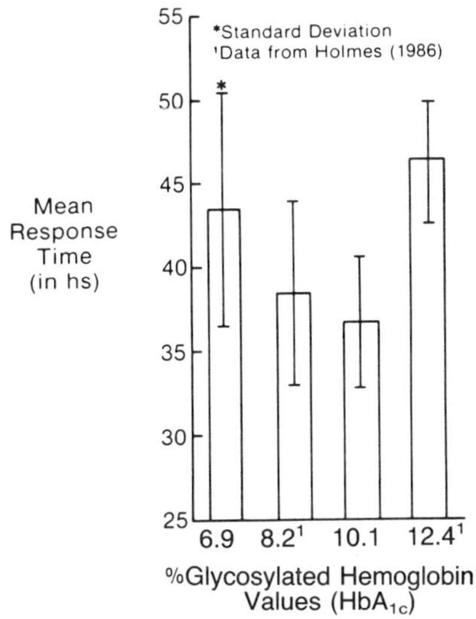

tion. Figure 7.3 presents the combined visual RT findings. Very rigorous and very poor control each are associated with longer response latencies, than is relatively moderate disease control (X $HbA_{1c} = 8.2\%$ and 10.1%).

Summary

Early studies have compared diabetic patients to nondiabetic controls and generally have found intact global intelligence, but poorer performance on specific measures of memory and attention (Donald et al., 1980; Lawson et al., 1984; Franceschi et al., 1984; Baade, 1988), and poorer word learning ability (Bale, 1973). Although overall intelligence has been intact, Baade (1988) found poorer Verbal IQ, related to lower fund of general information (Information and Vocabulary subtests) and poorer nonverbal problem solving and visual/motor skills. Skenazy and Bigler (1984) showed their diabetic sample to have poorer Performance IQ and motor strength, which was related to number of episodes of hypoglycemic unconsciousness. Bale (1973) also found hypoglycemic blackouts to relate to significantly poorer performance in 17% of his diabetic sample who had test scores in the clinically dysfunctional range. Because of the high incidence of cerebrovascular insult and hypoglycemic unconsciousness in his study patients, Bale's results provide a unique perspective about possible underlying atherosclerotic factors versus hypoglycemic insult as correlates of neuropsychological functioning. Hypoglycemic blackouts were more frequently associated with poorer performance than was history of stroke on a word learning task. This finding awaits further replication with a more diverse array of neuropsychological tasks.

Since diabetes has an incipient onset, even newly diagnosed individuals appear to have an increased incidence of reduced cortical evoked potentials, both visual and auditory. This occurs before there is any other overt sign of disease complications. In addition, to this "central neuropathy" as it has been termed, there is evidence that peripheral neuropathy, often characteristic of longer disease duration and/or poorer control, may also be associated with slowed responding or selective impairments.

From a series of studies on the effects of acute versus chronic glucose disruption by Holmes and colleagues, some tentative descriptions emerge of the neuropsychological correlates of different disease parameters. It appears that acute mild hypoglycemia relates to transient impairments in auditory and visual attention *and* decision-making skills (Holmes, Koepke, & Thompson, 1986; Holmes, 1987b) while extremes in chronic glucose control (measured by glycosylated hemoglobin) are related to decreased auditory and visual attention, but *intact* decision-making (Holmes, 1986; Holmes, Tsalikian, & Yamada, 1988). Further, when wide differences occurred in unregulated blood glucose levels across subjects at the time of testing, as typically happens in these descriptive studies, then interindividual variability was so great that subtle differences in attention were masked. Instead, chronic metabolic control (HbA_{1c}) and age of diabetes onset were more salient predictors of performance in very homogeneous samples of diabetics. However, different disease mechanisms may underlie the performances of patients in very rigorous and very poor control; those in very good control had an increased incidence of hypoglycemic unconsciousness, which appears to be consistently related to poorer performance, while those in very poor control did not.

Implications and Directions for Further Research

There appears to be a growing preponderance of evidence that insulin-dependent diabetes is associated with a variety of usually mild neuropsychological impairments. Initial studies have focused upon demonstrating that diabetic patients differ from nondiabetic controls on a variety of measures. Often these studies have involved large surveys of heterogeneous diabetic patients such that specific disease factors which might predispose patients to neuropsychological difficulties were obscured. Broad age ranges in subject samples are particularly troublesome, since most neuropsychological tests are sensitive to age effects. Even with a suitably matched control group, interesting results may "wash-out" against such wide variations in age, and resultant intertwined variables of age of disease onset and length of disease. Gender can also differentially affect some neuropsychological tasks and should be considered as a factor in study design. Perhaps at this juncture, more information is to be gained by determining which disease factors are implicated in poorer performance through more careful patient description and selection.

Based on work thus far, there is a preliminary indication of salient disease factors which deserve more careful study. None is likely to be more controversial than hypoglycemic unconsciousness because of its close association with more rigorous metabolic control (Goldstein, 1984). Indeed, as preliminary resuls from the multicenter Diabetes Clinical Complications Trial (DCCT) have indicated, near-normal metabolic control is possible with multiple daily blood glucose checks and multiple insulin injections. However, along with achieving blood glucose values in the nondiabetic range of 80 to 120 mg/dl, comes an increased incidence of severe hypoglycemic reaction and unconsciousness. Near-normal control leaves little margin for error in adjusting insulin levels, anticipating exercise needs, or calculating dietary intake. Hypoglycemic unconsciousness appears to be one of the most serious disease variables, in that Reske-Nielsen and Lundbaek (1963) in a multiple-case study found protracted episodes of unconsciousness appeared related to pathohistologic changes in diabetic brains at autopsy. It is unknown what impact, if any, less severe episodes may have. Recently, however, there has been evidence that multiple episodes of even mild asymptomatic hypoglycemia (i.e., in the 50-mg/dl range) are associated with neuropsychological differences in children (Golden et al., 1989). With the advent of memory glucometers to more reliably assess daily blood glucose fluctuations among diabetic patients, it should be possible to better describe this phenomenon.

The selective deficits which have been found in diabetic performance on verbal and nonverbal attentional tasks during hypoglycemia are consistent with diminished attentional deployment and decision-making characteristic of the frontal lobes. However, this possible site of neural action in diabetes, and the precise underlying mechanism of action, remains to be determined. Answers should be available before long since the necessary technologies exist to determine what, if any, association might exist between diabetic performance decrements and cerebral glucose utilization. The sizable degree of performance impairment found during hypoglycemia in some studies, of up to an 18% decrement, on brief measures of 1 min or less each, cause one to speculate about possible performance decrements in a school or work setting when performance must be sustained over a longer interval and the effects of fatigue may further compromise performance. To date, no one knows what might happen to performance under more naturalistic conditions. Prediction of "real-life" functioning could be especially important to children who must acquire novel information in school, and who are particularly prone to wider fluctuations in glucose level due to more brisk epinephrine counterregulation (Amiel, Simonson, Sherwin, Lauritano, & Tamborlane, 1987) and greater sensitivity to insulin (Ternand et al., 1982). We are presently conducting a longitudinal evaluation of diabetic children to determine the effect of acute and chronic glucose deviations upon school performance.

Acknowledgments. This work was supported in part by the National Institute of Diabetes, Digestive and Kidney Diseases Grants 1 R23 AM 31464 and 1R01 DK37545 and RR 59 from the General Clinical Research Centers Branch. Drs. Eva Tsalikian and James Hansen provided helpful comments on earlier drafts of this chapter.

References

Algan, M., et al. (1989). Visual evoked potentials in diabetic patients. *Diabetes Care, 12*, 227–229.

Amiel, S.A., Sherwin, R.S., Simonson, D.C., & Tamborlane, W.V. (1988). Effect of intensive insulin therapy on glycemic thresholds for counterregulatory hormone release. *Diabetes, 37*, 901–907.

Amiel, S.A., Simonson, D.C., Sherwin, R.S., Lauritano, A.A., & Tamborlane, W.V. (1987). Exaggerated epinephrine responses to hypoglycemai in normal and insulin-dependent diabetic children. *Journal of Pediatrics, 110*, 832–837.

Arias, P., Kerner, W., Zier, H., Navascues, I., & Pfeiffer, E.F. (1985). Incidence of hypoglycemic episodes in diabetic patients under continuous subcutaneous insulin infusion and intensified conventional insulin treatment: assessment by means of semiambulatory 24-hour continuous blood glucose monitoring. *Diabetes Care, 8*, 134–139.

Arky, R.A. (1979). Hypoglycemia. In G. F. Cahill, W.D. Odell, L. Martini, J.T. Potts, D.H. Nelson, E. Steinberger, & A.I. Winegrad (Eds.). *Endocrinology, Vol. 2* (pp. 1099–1120). New York: Grune & Stratton.

Baade, L.E. (1988). *Neuropsychological test differences between insulin-dependent diabetic adults and matched controls.* Paper presented at The International Neuropsychological Society, New Orleans, LA.

Bale, R.N. (1973). Brain damage in diabetes mellitus. *British Journal of Psychiatry, 122*, 337–341.

Bolli, G., DeFeo, P.D., Cosmo, S.D., Perriello, G., Angeletii, G., Ventura, M.R., Santeusanio, F., Brunetti, P., & Gerich, J.E. (1984). Effects of long-term optimization and short-term deterioration of glycemic control on glucose counterregulation in type I diabetes mellitus. *Diabetes, 33*, 394–400.

Cerami, A. (1985). Glucose as a mediator of aging. *Journal of American Geriatric Society, 33*, 626–634.

Clayson, S.J. (1971). Effect of hypoglycemia on T-maze learning in rats. *Physical Therapy 51*, 991–999.

Creasey, H., & Rapoport, S.I. (1985). The aging human brain. *Annals of Neurology, 17*, 2–10.

Dandona, P., James, I.M., Newbury, P.A., Woollard, M.L., & Beckett, A.G. (1978). Cerebral blood flow in diabetes mellitus: Evidence of abnormal cerebrovascular reactivity. *British Medical Journal, 2*, 325–326.

Dastur, D.K., Lane, M.H., Hansen, B.D., et al. (1963). Effects of aging on cerebral circulation and metabolism in man. In J.E. Birren, R.N. Butler, S.W.

Greenhouse, et al. (Eds.). *Human aging, a biological and behavioral study* (USPHS Publication 986, pp. 59–76). Washington, DC: U.S. Government Printing Office.

Davis, P.A. (1943). Effect on the electroencephalogram of changing the blood sugar level. *Archives of Neurology and Psychiatry, 49*, 186–194.

Donald, M.W., Bird, C.E., El-sawy, R., Hart, R., Lawson, S., Letemendia, F.J.J., Surridge, D.H.C., & Wilson, D.L. (1980). Cortical evoked potentials and auditory decision times of diabetics. *Progress in Brain Research, 54*, 516–521.

Donald, M.W., Erdahl, D.L.W., Surridge, D.H.C., Monga, T.N., Lawson, J.S., Bird, C.E., & Letemendia, F.J.J. (1984). Functioning correlates of reduced central conduction velocity in diabetic subjects. *Diabetes, 33*, 627–633.

Ensinck, J.W., & Williams R.H. (1974). Disorders causing hypoglycemia. In R.H. Williams (Ed.). *Textbook of endocrinology* (5th ed.) (pp. 627–659). Philadelphia: W.B. Saunders Co.

Fedele, D., Martini, A., Cardone, C., Comacchio, F., Bellavere, F., Molinari, G., Negrin, P., & Crepaldi, G. (1984). Impaired auditory brainstem-evoked responses in insulin-dependent diabetic subjects. *Diabetes, 33*, 1085–1089.

Fourest-Fontecave, S., Adamson, U., Lins, P.E., Ekblom, B., Sandahl, C., & Strand, L. (1987). Mental alertness in response to hypoglycaemia in normal man: The effect of 12 hours and 72 hours of fasting. *Diabete and Metabolisme, 13*, 405–410.

Franceschi, M., Cecchetto, R., Minicucci, F., Smizne, S., Baio, G., & Canal, N. (1984). Cognitive processes in insulin-dependent diabetes. *Diabetes Care, 7*, 229–231.

Gold, P.E., Vogt, J., & Hall, J.L. (1986). Posttraining glucose effects on memory: Behavioral and pharmacological characteristics. *Behavioral and Neural Biology, 46*, 145–155.

Golden, M.P., Ingersoll, G.M., Brack, C.J., Russell, B.A., Wright, J.C. & Huberty, T.J. (1989). Longitudinal relationship of asympotomatic hypoglycemia to cognitive function in IDDM. *Diabetes Care, 12*, 89–93.

Goldstein, D.E. (1984). Is glycosylated hemoglobin clinically useful? *New England Journal of Medicine, 318*, 384–385.

Gonder-Frederick, L., Hall, J.L., Vogt, J., Cox, D.J., Green, J., & Gold, P.E. (1987). Memory enchancement in elderly humans: Effects of glucose ingestion. *Physiology & Behavior, 41*, 503–504.

Heller, S.R., MacDonald, I.A., Herbert, M., & Tattersall, R.B. (1987). Influence of sympathetic nervous system on hypoglycaemic warning symptoms. *Lancet, 2*, 359–363.

Herold, K.C., Polonsky, K.S., Cohen, R.M., Levy, J., & Douglas, F. (1985). Variable deterioration in cortical function during insulin-induced hypoglycemia. *Diabetes, 34*, 677–685.

Hilsted, J., Madsbad, S., Krarup, T., Sestoft, L., Christensen, N.J., Tronier, B., & Galbo, H. (1981). Hormonal, metabolic, and cardiovascular responses to hypoglycemia in diabetic autonomic neuropathy. *Diabetes, 30*, 626–633.

Hoeldtke, R.D., Boden, G., Shuman, C.R., & Owen O.E. (1982). Reduced epinephrine secretion and hypoglycemia unawareness in diabetic autonomic neuropathy. *Annals of Internal Medicine, 96*, 459–462.

Hoffman, R.G., Speelman, D.J., Hinnen, D.A., Conley, K.L., Guthrie, R.A., & Knapp, R.K. (1989). Changes in cortical functioning with acute hypoglycemia and hyperglycemia in type I diabetes. *Diabetes Care, 12*, 193–197.

Holmes, C.S. (1986). Neuropsychological profiles in men with insulin dependent diabetes. *Journal of Consulting and Clinical Psychology, 54*, 386–389.

Holmes, C.S. (1987a). Cognitive functioning and diabetes: Broadening the paradigm for behavioral and health psychology? *Diabetes Care, 10*, 273–290.

Holmes, C.S. (1987b). Metabolic control and auditory information processing at altered glucose levels in insulin-dependent diabetes. *Brain and Cognition, 6*, 161–174.

Holmes, C.S., Hayford, J.T., Gonzalez, J.L., & Weydert, J.A. (1983). A survey of cognitive functioning at different glucose levels in diabetic persons. *Diabetes Care, 6*, 180–185.

Holmes, C.S., Koepke, K.M., & Thompson, R.G. (1986). Simple versus complex neuropsychological impairments during three blood glucose levels. *Psychoneuroendocrinology, 11*, 353–357.

Holmes, C.S., Koepke, K.M., Thompson, R.G., Gyves, P., & Weydert, J.A. (1984). Verbal fluency and naming skills in type I diabetes at different glucose levels. *Diabetes Care, 7*, 454–459.

Holmes, C.S., Tsalikian, E., & Yamada, T. (1988). Blood glucose control and visual and auditory attention in men with insulin-dependent diabetes. *Diabetic Medicine, 5*, 634–639.

Ingram, T.T.S., Stark, G.D., & Blackburn, I. (1967). Ataxia and other neurological disorders as sequels of severe hypoglycemia in childhood. *Brain, 90*, 851–862.

Ipp, E., & Forster, B. (1987). Sparing of cognitive function in mild hypoglycemia: Dissociation from the neuroendocrine response. *Journal of Clinical Endocrinology and Metabolism, 65*, 806–810.

Kent, S. (1976). Is diabetes a form of accelerated ageing? *Geriatrics, 31*, 141–151.

Kuhl, D.E., Metter, E.J., Riege, W.H., & Phelps, M.E. (1982). Effects of human aging on patterns of local cerebral glucose utilization determined by the F-18 Fluoro-deoxyglucose method. *Journal of Cerebral Blood Flow & Metabolism, 2*, 163–171.

Lammertsma, A.A., Frackowiak, R.S., Lenzi, G.L., Heather, J.D., Pozzili, C., & Jones, T. (1981). Accuracy of the oxygen-15 steady state technique in measuring CBF and CMRO2. *Journal of Cerebral Blood Flow & Metabolism, 1*, S3–4.

Lasche, E. M. (1985). The diabetic driver. *Diabetes Care, 8*, 189–191.

Lawson, J.S., Erdahl, D.L.W., Monga, T.N., Bird, C.E., Donald, M.W., Surridge, D.H.C., & Letemendia, F.J.J. (1984). Neuropsychological function in diabetic patients with neuropathy. *British Journal of Psychiatry, 145*, 263– 268.

Lewis, L.D., Ljunggren B., Ratcheson, R.A., & Siesjo, B.K. (1974). Cerebral energy state insulin-induced hypoglycemia, related to blood glucose and to eeg. *Journal of Neurochemistry, 23*, 673–679.

Lund-Andersen, H. (1979). Transport of glucose from blood to brain. *Physiology Review, 59*, 305.

McCall, A.L., Fixman, L.B., Fleming, N., Thornheim, K., Chick, W., & Ruderman, N.B. (1986). Chronic hypoglycemia increases brain glucose transport. *American Journal of Physiology, 251*, 442–447.

Miles, P., & Root, H.F. (1992). Psychologic tests applied to diabetic patients. *Archives of Internal Medicine, 30*, 767–777.

Newrick, P.G., Ford, I., Greaves, M., Malik, R., Sharma, A.K., Willars, G., Tomlinson, D.R., Bouton, A.J., & Ward, J.D. (1987). Clinicopathological correlates of human diabetic neuropathy. *Diabetes 36*, Supplement 1, 86A.

Parks, R.W., Lowenstein, D.A., Dodrill, K.L., Barker, W.W., Yoshii, F., Chang, J.Y., Emran, A., Apicella, A., Sheramata, W.A., & Duara, R. (1988). Cerebral metabolic effects of a verbal fluency test: A PET scan study. *Journal of Clinical and Experimental Neuropsychology, 10*, 565–575.

Pozzessere, G., Rizzo, P.A., Valle, E., Mollica, M.A., Meccia, A., Morano, S., Di Mario, U., Andreani, D., & Morocutti, C. (1988). Early detection of neurological involvement in IDDM and NIDDM: Multimodal evoked potentials versus metabolic control. *Diabetes Care, 11*, 473–480.

Pramming, S., Thorsteinsson, B., Stigsby, B., Binder, C. (1988). Glycaemic threshold for changes in electroencephalograms during hypoglycaemia in patients with insulin dependent diabetes. *British Medical Journal, 296*, 665–667.

Pramming, S., Thorsteinsson, B., Theilgaard, A., Pinner, E.M., Binder, C. (1986). Cognitive function during hypoglycaemia in type I diabetes mellitus. *British Medical Journal, 292*, 647–650.

Ratner, R.E., & Whitehouse, F.W. (1989). Motor vehicles, hypoglycemia, and diabetic drivers. *Diabetes Care, 12*, 217–222.

Reske-Nielsen, E., & Lundbaek, K. (1963). Diabetic encephalopathy: Diffuse and focal lesions of the brain in long-term diabetics. *Acta Neurologica Scandinavica, 39*(Suppl. 4), 273–290.

Riege, W.H., Metter, E.J., Kuhl, D.E., & Phelps, M.E. (1985). Brain glucose metabolism and memory functions: Age decrease in factor scores. *Journal of Gerontology, 40*, 459–467.

Russell, P.N., & Rix-Trott, H.M. (1975). An exploratory study of some behavioural consequences of insulin induced hypoglycaemai. *New Zealand Medical Journal, 81*, 337–340.

Ryan, C., Vega, A., & Drash, A. (1985). Cognitive deficits in adolescents who developed diabetes early in life. *Pediatrics, 5*, 921–927.

Ryan, C., Vega, A., Longstreet, C. (1984). Neuropsychological changes in adolescents with insulin-dependent diabetes. *Journal of Consulting Clinical Psychology, 52*, 335–342.

Schade, D.S., Drumm, D.A., Duckworth, W.C., & Eaton, P. (1985). The etiology of incapacitating brittle diabetes. *Diabetes Care, 8*, 12–20.

Skenazy, J.A., & Bigler, E.D. (1984). Neuropsychological findings in diabetes mellitus. *Journal of Clinical Psychology, 40*, 246–258.

Songer, T.J. (1989). Drivers with diabetes: Innocent until proven guilty. *Diabetes Care, 12*, 133–134.

Songer, T.J., LaPorte, R.E., Dorman, J.S., Orchard, T.J., Cruickshanks, K.J., Becker, D.J., & Drash, A.L. (1988). Motor vehicle accidents and IDDM. *Diabetes Care, 11*, 701–707.

Stevens, A.V., McKane, W.R., Bell, P.M., Bell, P., King, D.J., & Hayes, J.R. (1989). Psychomotor performance and counterregulatory responses during mild hypoglycemia in healthy volunteers. *Diabetes Care, 12*, 12–17.

Ternand, C., Go, V.L.W., Gerich, J.E., et al. (1982). Endocrine pancreatic a response of children with onset of insulin-requiring diabetes before age 3 and after age 5. *Journal of Pediatrics, 101*, 36–39.

Trick, G.L., Burde, R.M., Kilo, C., Gordon, M.O., & Santiago, J.V. (1987). Abnormal visual function associated with diabetes mellitus. *Diabetes 36*, Supplement 1, 17A.

Vijayashankar, N., & Brody, H. (1979). A quantitative study of the pigmented neurons in the nuclei locus coeruleus and subcoeruleus in man as related to aging. *Journal of Neuropathology and Experimental Neurology, 38*, 490–497.

8

Symptom Perception and Blood Glucose Feedback in the Self-Treatment of IDDM

Linda A. Gonder-Frederick and Daniel J. Cox

Introduction

In behavioral models of health care, subjectively experienced symptoms play a critical role in medical help-seeking and self-treatment efforts (Pennebaker, 1982). Put most simply, this means that people tend to seek medical advice only when unpleasant or unusual symptoms occur, and typically follow medical recommendations only until their discomfort is alleviated. On a more complex level, symptoms help form the "common sense" mental representation of an illness that guides the process of health care decision making (Leventhal, Meyer, & Nerenz 1980; Nerenz & Leventhal, 1983). Although important in any illness model, symptoms play an even more significant role in the management of Type I, or insulin-dependent diabetes mellitus (IDDM). As discussed in previous chapters, the self-regulation of glucose metabolism involves a complex regimen that demands an enormous amount of decision making on the part of the patient. One of the factors that influences these self-treatment decisions is feedback concerning glucose levels, including subjectively perceived symptoms.

This chapter reviews findings from an ongoing 9-year investigation of blood glucose (BG) symptoms and perception in IDDM patients. Both the research program and this chapter focus on four major areas of interest. The first section examines the role of BG feedback in self-treatment, addressing questions such as: Why are symptoms and other forms of BG feedback important in diabetes management? To what extent do patients utilize perceived symptoms in making self-treatment decisions? The second section reviews research looking at the nature of subjective BG symptoms, addressing questions such as: To what extent are diabetic glucose fluctuations symptomatic and what are the symptoms associated with abnormally low (hypoglycemic) and abnormally high (hyperglycemic) BG levels?

The third section reviews studies assessing the accuracy of BG perception, focusing on questions such as: How accurately can IDDM patients detect hypoglycemia and hyperglycemia and what are the most common errors made? In addition, what are the clinical implications of errors in BG perception? Finally, the fourth section describes the development and assessment of an intervention designed to improve patients' ability to estimate BG levels, addressing the questions: Can ability to recognize BG symptoms be improved and, if so, what effects can this have on self-treatment behaviors and diabetes control? The chapter concludes with a summary of these findings and a discussion of ongoing and future research directions. We begin with an exploration into the role of glucose feedback, including perceived symptoms, in the self-treatment of IDDM.

BG Feedback and Self-Treatment

With IDDM, metabolic functions usually performed automatically by the body must be duplicated by self-treatment behaviors. These functions include: monitoring BG levels, calculating the effects of food intake and activity, determining insulin dose, and administering insulin. BG monitoring is critical to both short-term and long-term control of diabetes. Feedback about BG is necessary to: avoid hypo and hyperglycemia; adjust food intake, exercise, and insulin; monitor overall diabetes control; and evaluate the effectiveness of self-treatment decisions. For example, if BG is too low, some form of quickly metabolized carbohydrate is needed to raise glucose levels. If BG is too high, it should be lowered and ketone levels should be tested. The IDDM patient has two major sources for BG information: (1) self-measurement of glucose or urine and (2) perception of subjective symptoms that signal hypoglycemia and hyperglycemia.

Until the last decade, the only available method of self-monitoring was urine testing for hyperglycemia, indicated by the presence of glucose or ketones. Since the renal threshold for glycosuria is quite high, urine testing provides very limited information. Although helpful in avoiding severe hyperglycemia and ketoacidosis, the patient obtains no information concerning more moderate hyperglycemic episodes or hypoglycemia from urine testing. The ability to monitor BG has dramatically improved in recent years with the development of methods that allow patients to measure their own BG levels. These tests are performed by obtaining one drop of whole blood, via a finger prick, which is placed on a glucose/peroxidase reagent strip. Color change on the reagent strip can be visually interpreted, or read by a reflectance meter which provides a digital readout of BG level.

With frequent SMBG, patients can make subtle adjustments in daily treatment; for example, increasing morning insulin dose if BG is higher than usual before breakfast, or eating a snack before exercise if BG is moderately low. Numerous studies have shown that the more intensive regimens involving this type of daily "fine-tuning," including multiple daily injections and insulin pump therapy, lead to better metabolic control (e.g., Schiffrin & Belmonte, 1982). Unfortunately, numerous problems prevent this ideal utilization of SMBG. SMBG can be expensive and inconvenient, and many patients are unable or unwilling to measure BG as frequently as needed (several times each day) to improve diabetes control (see Gonder-Frederick, Cox, Pohl, & Carter, 1984).

Even if patients are willing to follow recommendations, there may be problems. In a recent adherence study, we found that patients were using SMBG as frequently as their physicians had recommended (Gonder-Frederick, Julian, Cox, Clarke, & Carter, 1988). However, the majority of their physicians had recommended only one or two daily measurements, not enough to obtain better metabolic control. Even more importantly, the majority of diabetic patients do not even use SMBG, although the American Diabetes Association has recommended it for nearly all types of patients.

The other source of BG feedback is perception of glucose-related symptoms. Patients with IDDM are taught to monitor certain symptoms as signs of hypoglycemia and hyperglycemia, and to take some corrective action when these symptoms occur. For example, almost all insulin-dependent patients are instructed to eat or drink carbohydrates when hypoglycemic symptoms such as trembling and sweating occur. Surveys have shown that the vast majority of patients experience symptoms with hypoglycemia and hyperglycemia, and most believe they can accurately recognize these symptoms (Gonder-Frederick, Cox, Pennebaker, & Bobbitt, 1986; O'Connell et al., 1984). Traditionally, the medical community has encouraged patients to consider symptoms in making self-treatment decisions, based on the assumption that the symptoms of low and high BG are well documented and easily recognized.

There is much evidence that, even when a method is available to objectively measure health status, people will continue to rely on and trust symptom feedback (Leventhal et al., 1980; Nerenz & Leventhal, 1983; Pennebaker, 1982). To see if this occurs in diabetes, we surveyed 80 IDDM patients who used home SMBG and asked them to report "the first four things you do when you feel like your blood suger is low" (Gonder-Frederick & Cox, 1986). Only one third of the respondants indicated they would check their BG level before taking some action to treat themselves for hypoglycemia. More than half never checked their BG when they felt hypoglycemic symptoms. Rather, they reported a variety of self-treatment behaviors, many of which (e.g., lying down, trying to relax) would have no effect on reversing hypoglycemia. Similar irrelevant behaviors in response to BG symptoms have been found in other studies (O'Connell et al., 1984).

Thus, for a variety of reasons, perceived symptoms and subjective estimates of BG level can have significant influence on self-treatment of diabetes, in patients who use SMBG as well as those who do not. From a clinical perspective, this means that appropriate self-treatment depends, to some extent, on a patient's ability to accurately recognize and interpret BG symptoms and other cues. This also means that errors in BG perception can lead to errors in treatment decisions. For example, the patient who "feels" weak and trembly due to physical exhaustion, misinterprets these symptoms as hypoglycemia, and then drinks a soda to raise BG might become hyperglycemic. The patient who decides to skip a bedtime snack because of "feeling" too high may become hypoglycemic during the night.

BG Symptoms

Although critical to self-management of diabetes, BG symptomatology and perception have received very little empirical attention. We began our investigation by testing some of the traditional assumptions about glucose symptomatology with the following questions: To what extent are hypoglycemia and hyperglycemia associated with perceived symptoms? What symptoms are most commonly related to BG extremes? And, are these symptoms the same for all IDDM patients? In the first study, hospitalized patients followed a repeated measures design in which they rated a symptom checklist just prior to a measurement of actual BG level, repeating this procedure seven times each day for one week (Pennebaker et al., 1981). The symptom checklist was composed of 19 symptoms commonly included in educational materials, i.e., the symptoms patients are taught to monitor as signs of hypoglycemia and hyperglycemia.

To identify symptoms related to low and high BG measurements, we first computed standard between-subject correlations between BG measurements and ratings of each symptom item. None of the 19 symptom items correlated significantly with BG, indicating that there were no standard symptoms associated with hypoglycemia or hyperglycemia across this group of patients. Within-subject correlations were then computed to identify symptoms related to glucose for individual patients. This approach to the data revealed that symptoms were related to both hypoglycemia and hyperglycemia, but that the pattern of symptoms differed greatly from person to person. This means that, for some people, trembling and sweating are the symptoms most strongly related to hypoglycemia, but for other people, these symptoms are unrelated to hypoglycemia and different symptoms, such as difficulty in thinking, occur with low BG.

The idiosyncracy of BG symptoms has been replicated in several subsequent studies (Freund, Bennett-Johnson, Rosenbloom, Alexander & Hansen, 1986; Gonder-Frederick et al., 1986; Gonder-Frederick, Cox, Bobbitt, & Pennebaker, 1989; Moses & Bradley, 1985). These idiosyncratic symptoms are fairly reliable over time (Cox, Gonder-Frederick, Pohl, & Pennebaker, 1983), but changes in metabolic control or diabetic complications, such as autonomic neuropathy, may alter physiological responses to BG fluctuations and, consequently, subjective symptoms (Bulpitt, Shaw, Clifton, & Bloom, 1981; Hoeldtke, Boden, Shuman, & Owen, 1982).

Table 8.1 summarizes the symptoms we have found to be most commonly related to hypoglycemia and hyperglycemia. In general, hypoglycemia appears to be, by far, more symptomatic than hyperglycemia. The symptoms most frequently related to low BG are trembling, sweating, heart palpitations, difficulty concentrating, and mental confusion. Most hypoglycemic symptoms appear to be either adrenergic or neuroglycopenic in nature. Adrenergic symptoms are caused by epinephrine secretion in response to hypoglycemia, which causes the liver to release and convert its stored glycogen. The neuroglycopenic symptoms reflect disruption of brain and behavioral function due to depletion of brain glucose.

The symptoms most frequently related to hyperglycemia are dryness in the mouth, eyes, or throat, increased thirst, increased need to urinate, and painful or tingling sensations in extremities. Some of these

Table 8.1. Symptoms and Moods Commonly Related to Blood Glucose in IDDM Patients

Hypoglycemia	Hyperglycemia	Hypoglycemia and Hyperglycemia
Trembling	Dryness in Mouth or Throat	Blurry Vision
Sweaty	Sweet or Funny Taste in Mouth	Fatigue
Pounding Heart	Need to Urinate	Weakness
Mental Confusion	Pain, Tingling in Extremities	Numbness
Slurred Speech	Alert, Energetic	Heavy Breathing
Anxiety/Nervousness	Relaxed	Queasy Stomach
Lightheaded		Headache
Hunger		Salivation
		Frustrated
		Irritated/Angry

symptoms reflect the body's attempts to remove excess glucose from the system through the urinary system. Pain and other sensations in the extremities may be associated with neuropathology in the peripheral nervous system, a very common diabetic complication. There is evidence that, in patients with peripheral neuropathy, hyperglycemia produces a reduction in pain threshold (Boulton, Drury, Clarke, & Ward, 1982; White, Waltman, Krupin, & Santiago, 1981).

In addition to physical symptoms, Table 8.1 shows that diabetic BF can also be associated with changes in subjective mood states (Gonder-Frederick et al., 1989; Moses & Bradley, 1985). In general, low BG is associated with negative or unpleasant emotions, most frequently anxiety-like feelings. Mood changes associated with hypoglycemia, like symptoms, are most likely related to epinephrine secretion and brain glucose depletion. High BG can be associated with either positive or negative mood changes. Some patients experience irritablity and frustration with hyperglycemia, while others feel alert, calm, or some other subjectively pleasant state with higher BG levels.

Table 8.1 also presents those symptoms that can be associated with either hypoglycemia or hyperglycemia. In other words, these symptoms are related to hypoglycemia for some people, and related to hyperglycemia for others. The fact that a symptom such as nausea can be associated with low BG for some people and high BG levels for others has obvious implications for patient education concerning glucose symptoms. Traditionally, symptom education has been based on the assumptions that the symptoms associated with hypoglycemia and hyperglycemia are quite distinct and that diabetic symptomatology is relatively consistent across individual patients. The data support neither of these assumptions. Further discussion of the implications of symptom studies for education and other aspects of diabetes treatment can be found in Cox et al., (1985).

Accuracy of Symptom Beliefs

Since BG extremes are associated with perceived symptoms and patients use these symptoms to guide treatment decisions, it is important to know the extent to which patients can accurately recognize BG symptoms. We first focused on the accuracy of patient's *beliefs* about their own BG symptoms (Gonder-Frederick et al., 1986). The method used was essentially a replication of the procedure described previously—subjects rated theri symptoms prior to SMBG, repeating this procedure several times each day over a period of approximately 10 days. At the end of this period, subjects were asked to rate the extent to which they believed each symptom item to be related to their own hypoglycemia and hyperglycemia. With these data, we were able to empirically identify symptoms related to low and high BG for each person and to compare these *actual* symptoms to *believed* symptoms.

To quantify accuracy of symptom beliefs, each symptom item was categorized into one of four cells analogous to the dependent measures used in Signal Detection research to measure accuracy of sensory perception—Hits, Misses, False Alarms, and Correct Rejections (Swets, 1973). Accurate beliefs fell into one of two categories: (1) symptoms believed to be related to low or high BG that were actually related and (2) symptoms believed to be unrelated to BG that were actually unrelated (Hits and Correct Rejections, respectively). Inaccurate beliefs also fell into one of two categories: (1) symptoms believed to be related to BG that were actually unrelated and (2) symptoms believed to be unrelated to BG that were acutally related (False Alarms and Misses).

Accurate beliefs (Hits and Correct Rejections) occurred significantly more frequently than inaccurate beliefs (False Alarms and Misses) for both hypoglycemic and hyperglycemic symptoms. Beliefs about hypoglycemic symptoms were more accurate than beliefs about hyperglycemic symptoms. Females had a higher rate of both hits and false alarms, whereas males had a higher rate of both Correct Rejections and Misses, especially missed hypoglycemic symptoms. However, symptom belief accuracy varied greatly across individual subjects, with Hit rates ranging from 0% to 100%. The most common error in symptom beliefs were False Alarm beliefs. In fact, the rate of False Alarm beliefs was higher than the rate of Hits for almost half of the subjects. On the average, subjects reported two to three False Alarm symptom beliefs. Similar results have recently been reported by O'Connell, Hamera, Schorfheide, and Guthrie (1989) who found that diabetic subjects were not aware of their most reliable symptoms.

These findings suggest that many diabetic patients are monitoring symptoms for BG information, when, in realilty, these symptoms are not even related to their own glucose changes. Such erroneous symptom beliefs may be especially common in chronic diseases that require constant monitoring of some particular physical parameter. To the IDDM person attempting to monitor and regulate BG, any change in perceived symptoms or health status may be readily interpreted as glucose or diabetes related (Taylor and Fiske, 1978). We have frequently encountered this type of symptom misattribution in clinical work with diabetic patients. For example, one woman believed that her frequent headaches were caused by high BG levels. A symptom analysis, however, found no relationships between occurrence of her headaches and episodes of hyperglycemia. Rather, the headaches appeared to relate to stress at work. Nonetheless, the young woman continued to believe that her headaches were glucose related, even when presented with objective evidence to the contrary. Once formed, symptom beliefs appear to be resistant to change, a phenomenon observed in hypertensive, as well as diabetic, patients (Leventhal, Meyer, & Nerenz, 1980).

Ability to Recognize Hypoglycemia and Hyperglycemia

In addition to symptom feedback, the IDDM patient has a number of other potential sources of information about glucose levels: time of day, type/timing/amount of last insuline dose, amount of food eaten, activity levels, and so one. Thus, both *internal* cues (changes in symptoms, moods, performance) and *external* cues, such as those listed above, will influence a person's ability to predict and recognize BG extremes. In our first study of BG detection, ability to estimate BG levels on the basis of internal and external cues was tested under two different conditions: (1) in a hospital setting where glucose levels were manipulated via a glucose/insulin infusion system and (2) in the home environment prior to daily SMBG (Cox, Clarke, et al., 1985).

In the hospital condition, subjects were connected to the Biostator (Ames Division, Miles Laboratories, Elkhart, IN), making it possible to manipulate BG levels to low, normal, and high ranges (50 to 300 mg/dl) while constantly monitoring glucose measurements. Subjects were kept blind to glucose measurements and asked to estimate their current BG every 10 min throughout the 9-hr protocol (a total of 54 trials). The purpose of this condition was to test accuracy in a setting that prohibited use of external cues to BG, such as time of day, forcing the subject to rely on symptom feedback to estimate current glucose.

After hospital testing, subjects were asked to estimate BG levels before daily SMBG at home for a 2-week period (for a total of at least 40 trials). They were instructed to use both internal and external cues when making these estimates. To ensure that home estimates provided valid data, a subgroup of subjects entered estimated and acutal BG measurements into a programmed handheld computer (Sharp 1500A, Paramus, NJ) containing an internal clock. Since development of reagent strips required at least 50 s, any actual BG entries in less than 50 s indicated that BG level was measured before estimated. Use of this procedure in this and subsequent studies has shown that such data manipulation is extremely rare.

Before reviewing the results of this study, the issue of *measurement of accuracy* must be addressed. Most studies comparing patient-generated measures of BG to reference measurements have used one of two statistical approaches: (1) correlations between patient and reference values or (2) computation of deviation from reference value. Both approaches are problematic in that they focus on statistical significance while ignoring clinical significance of errors (Clarke, Cox, Gonder-Frederick, Carter, & Pohl, 1987; Cox et al., 1985; Koschinsky, Dannehl, & Gries, 1988). For example, an estimated BG of 50 mg/dl deviates 100% from an actual BG concentration of 25 mg/dl. Clinically, however, these two values do not differ because, in both instances, estimated hypoglycemia would lead to carbohydrate intake to raise BG.

On the other hand, the 100% deviation between an estimated BG of 150 and an actual BG is 300 is clinically significant since the patient is unaware that glucose needs to be lowered.

Figure 8.1 shows the Error Grid Analysis (EGA) which was developed as an asssessment of accuracy that does take into consideration the clinical implications of errors in BG estimation (Cox et al., 1985; Clarke, et al., 1987). EGA involves plotting BG estimates against reference values such that each estimate falls above or below the diagonal line, into either the upper or lower portion of one of the five error zones. Estimates that fall above the diagonal are overestimates of BG and estimates that fall below the diagonal are underestimates.

The EGA also assigns each estimate to one of the five zones (upper or lower A through E Zones) that distinguish clinically accurate and clinically dangerous errors in estimation. These logically symmetrical zones are based on two assumptions: (1) when actual BG level is below or above certain criterion values, some action to reverse its direction is needed and (2) when a person estimates BG level to be below or above certain criterion values, some action to reverse its direction will be taken. One feature of the EGA is that these criterion values, and thus the error zones, can be altered to reflect different treatment goals. In addition, EGA can be used to compare *any* estimate of BG to *any* reference value; for example, reflectance meter values to laboratory assessments to evaluate the accuracy of different meters or patient-generated measurements (see Clarke et al., 1987; Cox, Herrman, et al., 1988;

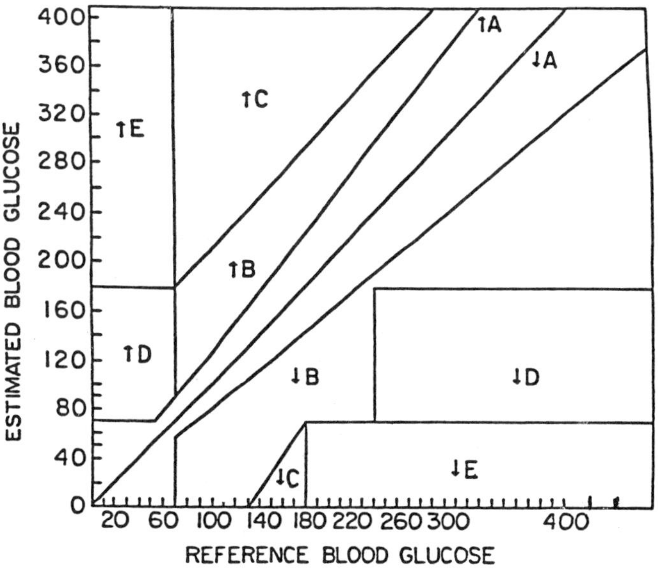

Figure 8.1. Error grid.

Cox, Moll, Gonder-Frederick, Savory, & Jones-Garrison, 1988; Pohl, Gonder-Frederick, Cox, & Evans, 1985).

Estimates that fall into upper or lower A Zones are considered *clinically accurate.* These estimates are either within 20% of a reference or "actual" BG value, or estimates of hypoglycemia when actual BG is below 70 mg/dl. Estimates that fall into B Zones are *benign errors*; that is, either no change in treatment would result, or the change would have negligible effects on self-treatment decisions or metabolic status. The remaining zones (C, D, and E) represent estimation errors that could be clinically dangerous. C Zone errors indicate that BG was believed to be in an unacceptable range when actual BG was acceptable, possibly resulting in inappropriate actions to raise or lower glucose. D Zone errors indicate that the person failed to detect an unacceptably low (upper D) or high (lower D) BG level, potentially leading to failure to provide needed treatment. Finally, E Zone errors represent instances when a person believes BG is too high when it is actually too low, or, conversely too low when it is actually too high. Such errors could result in clinically dangerous, even life-threatening mistakes in self-treatment.

Figure 8.2 shows the frequency of estimates falling into each zone of the EGA results in both the hospital and home conditions of the study described above (Cox et al., 1985). The majority of estimates were clinically accurate. A total of 46% of hospital estimates and 54% of home estimates fell into the A Zones, indicating that subjects were more accurate in the setting that provided both internal and external information about BG. A total of 18.8% of the hospital estimates and 13% of the home estimates fell into the clinically dangerous zones. The most common errors were D Zone estimates, i.e., believing BG to be in a euglycemic range when it was actually too low or too high. Only a very few Zone E errors were made and Zone C errors almost never occurred.

This same pattern in errors has been replicated in subsequent studies, with failure to detect hypoglycemia and hyperglycemia consistently being the most common type of error in BG estimation (Cox, Carter, Gonder-Frederick, Clarke, & Pohl, 1988; Cox, Gonder-Frederick et al., 1989; Gonder-Frederick, Snyder & Clarke, 1989). EGA results can be reduced to a single measure—the Accuracy Index, derived by substracting the sum of upper and lower C, D, and E zone estimates from the sum of upper and lower A zone estimates. Across subject groups from the three studies of IDDM adults, Accuracy Indexes have ranged from 35% to 51% with a mean of 41.7% (Cox, Clarke et al., 1985; Cox, Carter, et al., 1988; Cox, Gonder-Frederick, Snyder & Clarke, 1989).

Across studies, AI has not been found to be related to age, sex, duration of diabetes, or frequency of SMBG. However, accuracy may be marginally related to duration of SMBG, as well as glycosylated hemoglobin, suggesting that better BG detection contributes to improved metabolic control (Cox, Gonder-Frederick, et al., 1989). In every study,

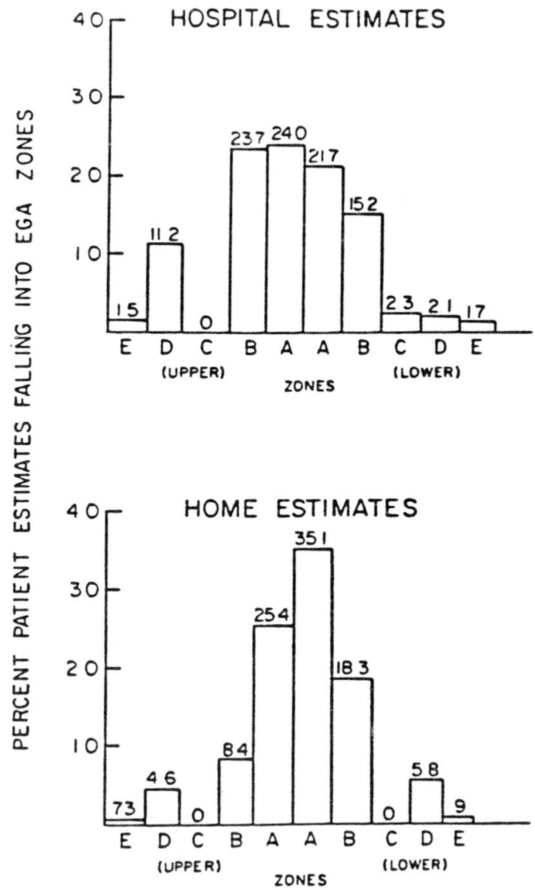

Figure 8.2. Error grid analysis of BG estimates in hospital and home tests.

the subject's confidence in ability to estimate his own BG has been found to be *unrelated* to measured accuracy, suggesting that patient's self-reports concerning symptom recognition should be viewed with some caution.

The high frequency of observed failures to detect hypoglycemia contrasts directly with the traditional assumption that low BG symptoms are easily recognized and interpreted. In fact, our results demonstrate that patients may fail to detect as many as 50% of their low BG episodes (Cox, Gonder-Frederick, Snyder & Clarke, 1989). Failure to detect hypoglycemia does not necessarily suggest that the episode was asymptomatic. During insulin infusion protocols, we have frequently observed patients become extremely symptomatic—sweating, trembling, slurring words, becoming confused—yet not detect these symptoms and continue to estimate their BG level to be in a normal or high range. However, it should also be emphasized that individual subjects differ greatly in their ability to recognize hypoglycemia and hyperglycemia. Some people are extremely accurate about their symptoms and are able to quickly detect hypoglycemia and/or hyperglycemia, while others have difficulty recognizing even extremely abnormal BG levels.

We have recently tested accuracy of BG estimation in diabetic children (ages 5 to 11 years). (Gonder-Frederick, Snyder, and Clarke, 1989). Since management of pediatric diabetes also requires the parents to monitor for BG symptoms, we also examined ability to estimate children's BG by their parents. Figure 8.3 summarizes the EGA results from this study, showing that both parents and their children made quite a high rate of serious errors (C, D, and E Zones) in BG estimation. In fact, the frequency of clinically serious estimates was as high as the frequency of clinically accurate estimates (A Zones) for both parents and children. AIs for both parents and children, with means of 5.03% and − 1.05%, respectively, were much lower than those found in the studies of adult subjects.

Like adult subjects, the most common error in BG estimation was failure to detect hypoglycemia and hyperglycemia. Both parents and children showed a significant tendency to underestimate the child's BG. Unlike adult subjects, however, children showed a tendency to report low BG levels when actual BG was above 180 mg/dl (lower E Zone errors). The increased frequency of these errors may reflect misinterpretation of physical symptoms associated with high BG levels in children. It may also reflect reinforcement contingencies since children are

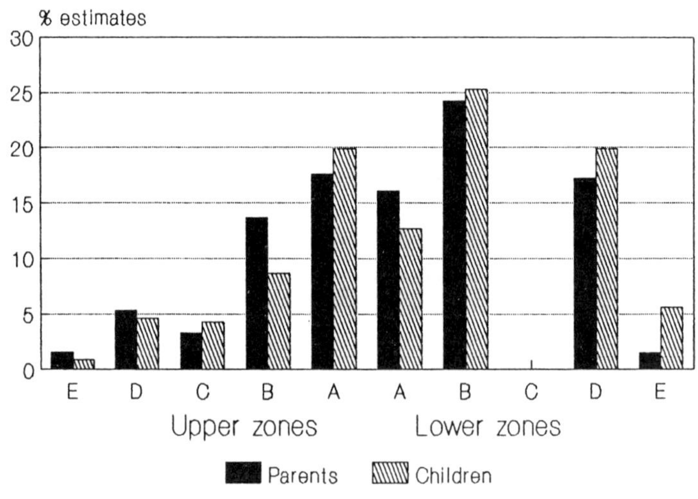

Figure 8.3. Error grid analysis. Results from pediatric study.

typically given something sweet to eat or drink when they report hypoglycemic symptoms.

The accuracy studies demonstrate that Type I patients frequently make errors when estimating their own BG levels, often misinterpreting or failing to detect symptoms and other glucose-relevant information. Many of these errors could have serious clinical implications. The ability to recognize extremes in BG appears to be especially poor in diabetic children and their parents. There is a great deal of individual variability in BG estimation, however, there is also strong evidence that individual patients are not accurate about their own ability to recognize hypoglycemia and hyperglycemia. Clinically, these results suggest that patients should not be encouraged to treat themselves on the basis of "perceived" BG levels. Rather, they should be encouraged to use SMBG or other testing methods before taking actions to adjust glucose.

Intervention to Improve BG Perception

Regardless of accuracy, however, there is reason to assume that people will continue to rely on their symptoms and perceived BG levels to guide self-treatment. For this reason, we have developed and tested a systematic training program designed to improve ability to recognize and predict hypoglycemia and hyperglycemia. This section describes that program and summarizes the evidence for its benefits.

The program is called *Blood Glucose Awareness Training* (BGAT) and is conducted in seven weekly group sessions, with daily "homework" between sessions. These sessions follow a structure provided by a BGAT manual composed of seven chapters, so that each chapter (week) focuses on some different internal or external cue to BG. (The BGAT Manual is available upon request). Three areas of skill training are involved: (1) increasing general awareness of and attention to somatic cues, (2) increasing knowledge about the effect of various factors (e.g., insulin, exercise, psychological stress) on personal BG fluctuations and (3) increasing awareness of internal cues that are reliably related to personal BG fluctuations.

But the most important learning component of BGAT is the daily BG Diary kept by each participant throughout training. Several times each day, participants complete a diary entry just prior to SMBG. This requires the individual to (1) "scan" themselves for glucose information, taking into consideration other glucose-relevant factors (e.g., food intake), (2) then estimate BG level on the basis of these cues, (3) measure and record actual glucose value and, finally, (4) plot the estimate on a graph of the EGA and evaluate its accuracy. This procedure provides the opportunity to systematically practice BG detection and receive immediate feedback concerning accuracy.

During the weekly sessions, BG Diaries are reviewed. Patterns of errors are examined, such as consistent overestimation or underestimation of actual glucose level. Since many people tend to "normalize" their BG when they estimate, one of the first adjustments often needed is *increasing the potential range* of glucose estimates. Other patterns are also common; for example, poorer accuracy at certain times of the day or inability to detect low BG measurements. By examining the types of symptoms and other information considered when each estimate was made, participants can begin to distinguish those cues that were predictive from those that were misleading and begin to identify reliable symptoms.

The utility of BGAT has now been tested in three separate studies, using a pre–post design in which accuracy of BG estimation is assessed prior to and following intervention. Figure 8.4 shows the pre-BGAT and post-BGAT Accuracy Index from each group and study. In the first study (Cox, Carter, et al., 1988), 20 subjects were randomly assigned to either BGAT or Stress Management (placebo) classes that met weekly. Since this study was conducted before the current training manual and program were developed, weekly sessions did not focus on specific content areas. Rather, BGAT subjects kept BG Diaries that were reviewed during group discussions.

EGA of pretraining and posttraining estimates showed that BGAT improved BG estimation, with increased frequency of accurate estimates (A Zones) and reduced frequency of serious errors (lower D Zone) involving failure to detect hyperglycemia. There was no improvement in the control group. As can be seen in Figure 8.4, pre-Accuracy

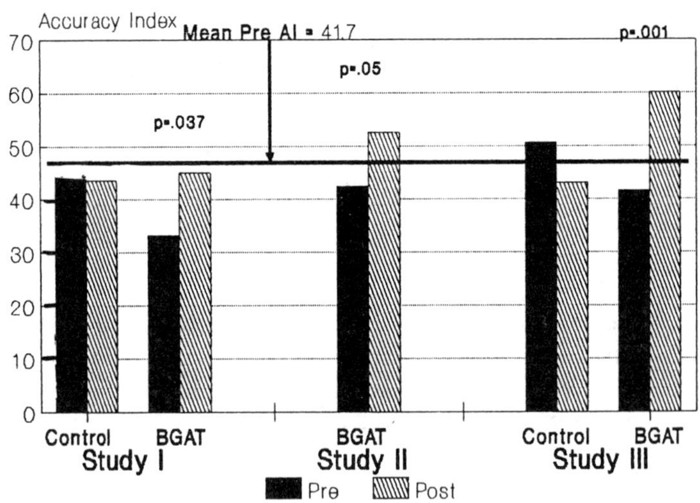

Figure 8.4. Pre-BGAT and post-BGAT results.

Indexes and post Accuracy Indexes for the BGAT and control groups were 42% and 53%, and 34% and 45%, respectively. In the BGAT group, 70% of the subjects showed improvement, whereas in the control group, only 40% of the subjects showed improvement.

Based on the experience and information obtained from Study I, an initial BGAT manual and program structure was developed. A second study (Cox, Carter, et al., 1988) tested the utility of this training program, as well as the effect of increased group size (16 individuals). Figure 8.4 shows that BG estimation was again improved. As in Study I, the frequency of accurate estimates increased after training, and the number of serious errors decreased (a 30% reduction). However, in this study, improvement in detection of hypoglycemia (reduced upper D Zone errors) rather than hyperglycemia was observed. Again, the majority (87%) of subjects showed improvement in BG estimation after training. In both studies, degree of improvement was negatively related to pre-BGAT accuracy, indicating that the intervention was most beneficial for those subjects who showed the poorest ability prior to intervention.

The last study has just been completed and replicates the pattern of results described above (Cox, Gonder-Frederick, et al., 1989). In comparison to control subjects, who showed no change in Accuracy Index, BGAT subjects showed significant improvement with pretraining to posttraining scores increasing from 41% to 60%. As in Study I, A Zone estimates increased and lower D Zone errors decreased, indicating better estimation of hyperglycemia. In addition to replicating previous results, there was also evidence that BGAT may contribute to improved metabolic control. Posttraining glycosylated hemoglobin levels (mean = 10.8%) were significantly lower than pretraining levels (mean = 12.2%) in the BGAT group, but did not change in the control group.

Taken together, these three studies provide strong evidence that a relatively simple and inexpensive intervention fan improve ability to estimate BG in Type I adults. In every study, BGAT increased the rate of clinically accurate estimates and decreased the rate of errors that could lead to potentially dangerous self-treatment decisions. BGAT may also contribute to positive changes in diabetes control, presumably an indirect effect caused by improvements in self-treatment behavior. The intervention appears to be most beneficial for those patients who have the most difficulty estimating BG, suggesting that it might be especially applicable for certain subgroups of diabetic patients.

For example, patients with autonomic neuropathy and deficient hormonal counterregulation may have difficulty recognizing hypoglycemia due to decreased adrenergic symptoms. Medications, such as beta-blockers, can also mask symptoms. BGAT may also be beneficial when there is a history of frequent or sudden-onset hypoglycemia, or history of hypoglycemia-related accidents. Patients attempting to gain better diabetes control through more intensive regimens also experience more frequent hypoglycemic episodes (Amiel, Tamborlane, Simonson, & Sherwin 1987). Finally, our data suggest that diabetic children and their parents need to improve BG estimation skills and reduce potentially serious errors. This may be especially true for parents of very young diabetic children, who may have increased need to avoid frequent or severe hypoglycemia, which appears to have negative impact on cognitive development in children under age 5 (Ryan, 1988).

Summary and Future Directions

The research reviewed in this chapter can be summarized by the following conclusions: (1) Subjective symptom perception and BG estimation play an important role in the self-treatment of IDDM; (2) abnormally low and high BG levels are associated with subjective symptoms, but the symptoms related to hypoglycemia and hyperglycemia are quite idiosyncratic; (3) IDDM patients may overattribute their physical symptoms to glucose levels, or may fail to detect signs of glucose extremes, therefore beliefs about BG symptoms are not always accurate; (4) ability to detect hypoglycemia and hyperglycemia differs greatly across individuals, but most patients appear to make clinically serious errors when estimating their BG, with some patients making an unacceptably high rate of serious errors; (5) the most common error in BG estimation is failure to detect hypoglycemia and hyperglycemia; (6) self-reported ability to detect BG (confidence) is not related to measured accuracy; (7) with systematic training, ability to recognize symptoms and predict BG fluctuations can be improved; and (8) improved accuracy in recognizing extreme BG levels may contribute to improvements in metabolic control.

Research is continuing in each of these areas—BG symptomatology, BG detection, and intervention. One area of special interest involves the mechanisms underlying idiosyncracy in glucose symptomatology. Differences in perceived symptoms may occur because of differences in physiological responses; for example, individual differences in hormonal responses, neuropathology, and chronic metabolic status. An alternative possibility is that symptom idiosyncracy reflects individual differences in psychological variables that influence symptom attention and interpretation. To test this question, several studies are using a protocol involving a 2-hr insulin infusion to manipulate BG to hypoglycemic levels. During these manipulations, a variety of measures related to glucose changes are obtained, including hormone levels (epinephrine, glucagon, cortisol), heart rate, blood pressure, skin conductance, temperature changes, and subjective symptom reports.

The results of the two completed studies suggest that both physiological and psychological differences contribute to symptom idiosyncracy. The purpose of the first study (Clarke et al., 1988) was to determine the reliability of a device designed to detect hypoglycemic episodes (Sleep Sentry, Teledyne Avionics, Charlottesville, VA). This device is worn like a wristwatch and sounds an alarm in response to skin moisture (sweat) and temperature changes associated with hypoglycemia. During hypoglycemia, both skin moisture and temperature changes varied greatly across individual subjects. Despite equivalently low BG levels (approximately 50 mg/dl), the alarm sounded in only half of the subjects. Furthermore, none of the physiological measures differentiated those cases in which the alarm sounded from those in which it did not. In addition, there was no relationship between preceived sweating and activation of the alarm.

Preliminary analysis of a second study suggests that the BG level at which physiological responses to hypoglycemia occur also varies across individual subjects (Cox, Antoun, et al., 1989). For example, hormonal counterregulation can occur at 55 mg/dl in some subjects, while others show no change in epinephrine until BG reaches 35 mg/dl. The BG threshold for subjective symptom perception also varies across individuals, as does the particular symptoms which appear first. Surprisingly, these data also indicate that adrenergic (e.g., pounding heart) and neuroglycopenic symptoms (e.g., mental confusion) appear as the first symptoms of hypoglycemia with equal frequency across subjects. This finding calls into question the traditional assumption that adrenergic symptoms provide the early warning signs of hypoglycemia, while neuroglycopenic symptoms occur later with more severely low BG levels.

We are also continuing to investigate the accuracy of BG perception and estimation in diabetic patients. One goal is to understand why individual patients differ so greatly in ability to estimate BG and to identify factors that contribute to these differences. Our studies with adult patients found no relationships between accuracy and subject characteristics such as age, gender, and duration of diabetes. It should be pointed out, however, that these studies involved assessment of relatively healthy and well-educated subjects, a population that is not representative of the majority of diabetic patients and may represent optimal levels of accuracy. The disconcertingly high rate of serious errors found in the pediatric study suggests that this is true, and that assessments of accuracy in other diabetic populations are needed.

Studies are just beginning that will examine ability to estimate BG in patient subgroups who may have difficulty recognizing BG extremes due to medications, diabetic complications, or other factors. There is preliminary evidence that patients who show deficient epinephrine response to hypoglycemia are less accurate than patients with effective counterregulatory responses (Cox, Gonder-Frederick, et al., 1989). Another group of interest is the visually impaired population, for whom obtaining SMBG and other objective measures of glucose is sometimes a prohibitively complex and expensive task.

Finally, we are also continuing efforts to develop effective intervention to improve ability to perceive BG. At present, BGAT has been shown to have an immediate positive effect on both BG estimation and metabolic control. The next step in this research is to determine the stability of these improvements over time. An initial test of this question will involve bringing back control and BGAT subjects from the current study 1 year later to assess BG estimation and metabolic control. If no long term differences are found, then we will test the effects of short "booster" training sessions to achieve stable improvement.

It is also important to determine what types of learning experiences contribute to improvements in BG detection. Our current study is testing the utility of an inpatient training procedure in which subjects are connected to the Biostator while BG level is manipulated to high, normal, and low levels. Throughout this protocol, subjects estimate their BG level, and are then given immediate feedback concerning actual BG measurement. Subjects are asked to "pay attention to how this BG level feels to you." Preliminary analysis indicates that this in vivo learning experience enhances the effects of BGAT.

Our long term goal is to develop and apply BGAT training with those subgroups of diabetic patients who have particular difficulty recognizing BG extremes. In some cases, this may involve expanding use of our current BGAT to other populations, such as individuals with a history of sudden-onset or frequent hypoglycemia. In other cases, this will involve development of specifically adapted training programs, such as for children, parents, or visually impaired adults. Although identification of these target populations is important, intervention to improve BG estimation should not be limited to only these patients with special needs. Our studies demonstrate that even patients who are not in these high-risk groups have serious problems in symptom recognition and BG estimation. We recommend that diabetic patients be taught that perceived symptoms can be misleading and that subjective estimations of BG are often in error. Health care practitioners can also encourage patients to systematically test their own accuracy, by estimating BG just prior to self-testing and by measuring actual BG when perceived symptoms occur.

References

Ameil, S.A., Tamborlane, W.V., Simonson, D.C., & Sherwin, R.S. (1987). Defective glucose counterregulation after strict glycemic control of insulin-dependent diabetes melliltus. *The New England Journal of Medicine, 316*, 1376–1383.

Boulton, A., Drury, L., Clarke, B., & Ward, J. (1982). Continuous subcutaenous insulin infusion in the management of painful diabetic neuropathy. *Diabetes Care, 5*, 386–390.

Bulpitt, C.J., Shaw, K.M., Clifton, P., & Bloom, A. (1981). The reduction in symptoms of diabetic patients after treatment in diabetic clinics. *Diabetes Care, 42*, 476–479.

Clarke, W.L., Carter, W.R., Moll, M., Cox, D.J., Gonder-Frederick, L.A., & Cryer, P.E. (1988). Metabolic and cutaneous events associated with hypoglycemia detected by Sleep Sentry. *Diabetes Care, 11*, 630–635.

Clarke, W.L., Cox, D.J., Gonder-Frederick, L.A., Carter, W., & Pohl, S.L. (1987). Evaluating the clinical accuracy of self-blood glucose monitoring systems. *Diabetes Care, 10*, 622–628.

Cox, D., Antoun, B., Gonder-Frederick, L.A., Schroeder, D., Cryer, P., & Clarke, W. (in press). A descriptive study of perceived hypoglycemic symptoms: Adrenergic vs. neuroglycopenic. *Diabetes Care.*

Cox, D.J., Carter, W.R., Gonder-Frederick, L.A., Clarke, W., & Pohl, S. (1988). Blood glucose awareness training in IDDM patients. *Biofeedback and Self-Regulation, 13*, 201–217.

Cox, D.J., Clarke, W.L., Gonder-Frederick, L.A., Pohl, S., Hoover, C., Snyder, A., Zimbleman, L., Carter, W.R., Bobbitt, S., & Pennebaker, J.W. (1985). Accuracy of perceiving blood glucose in IDDM. *Diabetes Care, 8*, 529–536.

Cox, D.J., Gonder-Frederick, L.A., Lee, J.H., Julian, D.M., Carter, W.R., & Clarke, W.L. (1989). Blood glucose awareness training among patients with IDDM: Effects and correlates. *Diabetes Care, 12*, 313–318.

Cox, D.J., Gonder-Frederick, L.A., Pohl, S., & Pennebaker, J.W. (1983). Reliability of symptom-blood glucose relationships among insulin-dependent adult diabetes. *Psychosomatic Medicine, 45*, 357–360.

Cox, D., Herrman, J., Snyder, A., Gonder-Frederick, L., Reschke, J., & Clarke, W. (1988). Stability of reacted Chemstrip bG. *Diabetes Care, 11*, 288–291.

Cox, D.J., Moll, M.E., Gonder-Frederick, L.A., Savory, J., & Jones-Garrison, S. (1988). Accuracy of time-delayed filter-paper blood glucose determination. *Diabetes Care, 11*, 517–518.

Freund, A., Bennett-Johnson, S., Rosenbloom, A., Alexander, B., & Hansen, C. (1986). Subjective symptoms, blood glucose estimation, and blood glucose concentrations in adolescents with diabetes. *Diabetes Care, 9*, 236–243.

Gonder-Frederick, L.A. & Cox, D.J. (1986). Behavioral responses to perceived hypoglycemic symptoms: A report and some suggestions. *The Diabetes Educator, 12*, 105–109.

Gonder-Frederick, L.A., Cox, D.J., Bobbitt, S.A., & Pennebaker, J.W. (1989). Changes in mood state associated with blood glucose fluctuations in insulin-dependent diabetes mellitus. *Health Psychology, 8*, 45–59.

Gonder-Frederick, L.A., Cox, D.J., Pennebaker, J.W., & Bobbitt, S.A. (1986). Blood glucose symptom beliefs in Type I diabetic adults: Accuracy and implications. *Health Psychology, 3*, 327–341.

Gonder-Frederick, L.A., Cox, D.J., Pohl, S.L., & Carter, W. (1984) Patient blood glucose monitoring: Use, accuracy, adherence, and impact. *Behavioral Medicine Update, 6*, 12–16.

Gonder-Frederick, L.A., Julian, D.M., Cox, D.J., Clarke, W.L., & Carter, W.R. (1988). Self-measurement of blood glucose: Accuracy of self-reported data and adherence to recommended regimen. *Diabetes Care, 11*, 579–585.

Gonder-Frederick, L.A., Snyder, A.L., & Clarke, W.L. (in press). Accuracy of detection of hypo- and hyperglycemia by children with Type I diabetes and their parents. *Diabetes Care*.

Hoeldtke, R.D., Boden, G., Shuman, C.R., & Owen, O.R. (1982). Reduced epinephrine secretion and hypoglycemia unawareness in diabetic autonomic neuropathy. *Annals of Internal Medicine, 96*, 459–462.

Koschinsky, T., Dannehl, K., & Gries, F.A. (1988). New approach to technical and clinical evaluation of devices for self-monitoring of blood glucose. *Diabetes Care, 11*, 619–629.

Leventhal, H., Meyer, D., & Nerenz, D. (1980). The common sense representation of illness danger. In S. Rachman (Ed.). *Medical Psychology Vol 2*. New York: Pergamon Press.

Moses, J.L., & Bradley, C. (1985). Accuracy of subjective blood glucose estimation by patients with insulin-dependent diabetes. *Biofeedback and Self-Regulation, 10*, 301–314.

Nerenz, D.R., & Leventhal, H. (1983). Self-regulation theory in chronic illness. In T.G. Burish & L.A. Bradley (Eds.), *Coping with chronic disease: Research and applications*. New York: Academic Press, pp. 13–37.

O'Connell, K.A., Hamera, E.K., Knapp, T.M., Cassmeyer, V.L., Eaks, G.A., & Fox, M.A. (1984). Symptom use and self-regulation in Type II diabetes. *Advances in Nursing Science, 6*, 19–28.

O'Connell, K.A., Hamera, E.K., Schorfheide, A., & Guthrie, D. (1989). Symptom beliefs and actual blood glucose in Type II diabetes. Unpublished manuscript.

Pennebaker, J.W. (1982). *The Psychology of physical symptoms*. New York: Springer-Verlag.

Pennebaker, J.W., Cox, D.J., Gonder-Frederick, L., Wunsch, M.G., Evans, W.S., & Pohl, S. (1981). Physical symptoms related to blood glucose in insulin-dependent diabetics. *Psychosomatic Medicine, 43*, 489–500.

Pohl, S., Gonder-Frederick, L., Cox, D., & Evans, W. (1985) Self-measurement of blood glucose concentration: Clinical significance of patient-generated measurements. *Diabetes Care, 8*, 617–619.

Ryan, C.M. (1988). Neurobehavioral complications of Type I diabetes: Examination of possible risk factors. *Diabetes Care, 11*, 86–93.

Schiffrin, A., & Belmonte, M. (1982). Multiple daily self-glucose monitoring: Its essential role in longterm glucose control in insulin-dependent diabetic patients treated with pumps and multiple subcutaneous injections. *Diabetes Care, 5*, 479–484.

Swets, J.A. (1973). The relative operating characteristic in psychology. *Science, 82*, 990–1000.

Taylor, S.E., & Fiske, S.T. (1978) Salience, attention, and attribution: Top of the head phenomena. In L. Berkowitz (ed), *Advances in experimental social psychology* (Vol. II), pp. 249–288. New York: Academic Press.

White, N., Waltman, S., Krupin, T., & Santiago, J. (1981). Reversal of neuropathic and gastrointestinal complications related to diabetes mellitus in adolescents with improved metabolic control. *Journal of Pediatrics, 99*, 41–45.

Section II

Non-Insulin-Dependent Diabetes

9

Non-Insulin Dependent (Type II) Diabetes: Medical Overview

Bruce R. Zimmerman

Introduction

Non-insulin-dependent diabetes mellitus (NIDDM) frequently is diagnosed in the asymptomatic patient, and therapy is often a weight reduction diet alone or oral hypoglycemic medication without other instructions. In the past, patients were often told they had borderline diabetes and their physicians exhibited little interest in careful follow-up or vigorous treatment. Unfortunately, even asymptomatic patients with moderate hyperglycemia are subject to severe complications of diabetes. Appropriate therapy for NIDDM no longer permits a passive approach to the treatment program. Active involvement with efforts to modify the patient's dietary habits, behavior patterns, medication program, glucose monitoring, and medical follow-up is necessary. These efforts may create behavioral and neuropsychological problems which are as complex as the more commonly studied problems in patients with insulin-dependent diabetes mellitus (IDDM). This chapter will briefly review the medical aspects of NIDDM which must be understood if the behavioral issues are to be addressed.

Diagnosis and Classification

The majority of patients with NIDDM have diabetes diagnosed during routine testing or as part of their evaluation for other medical problems. These patients may have fasting plasma glucose concentrations well above 200 mg/dl without obvious symptoms. Some patients present with typical symptoms of polyuria, polydipsia, and weight loss. A few patients reach medical attention because of the symptoms of a chronic complication of diabetes even though diabetes had not previously been diagnosed. Rarely, a patient presents with nonketotic hyperosmolar coma or even diabetic ketoacidosis precipitated by another illness.

NIDDM is diagnosed following the criteria of the National Diabetes Data Group (National Diabetes Data Group, 1979). Simply stated, these criteria require two fasting plasma glucose levels ≥140 mg/dl or typical symptoms of diabetes and a random plasma glucose ≥200 mg/dl. Although criteria for the diagnosis using an oral glucose tolerance test (GTT) are available, the use of the GTT is generally discouraged except in a research setting, epidemiologic studies, or during pregnancy.

Classification of the type of diabetes is based on clinical judgment. Patients with NIDDM are ketosis resistant even without treatment. There are no specific markers for NIDDM. Plasma insulin concentration, or C-peptide concentration in the insulin-treated patient, will generally demonstrate adequate basal levels and a good response to injected glucagon or a meal. No specific human leukocyte antigen (HLA) type has been found, and islet-cell antibodies are absent. At diagnosis, over 80% of patients with NIDDM are obese and most are diagnosed over age 40 years. NIDDM is much more common in some population groups such as American Indians. A subtype of NIDDM called maturity-onset diabetes of the young (MODY) may be diagnosed in young patients. Other subtypes exist and more will probably be identified in the future (Fagan, Cloutier, & Crowther, 1978). Some adult patients may have a gradual onset of IDDM and may be difficult to distinguish from patients with NIDDM. Generally, a clinical decision regarding appropriate treatment can be made in spite of these problems.

Pathophysiology and Heredity

Neither the exact pathophysiology nor the heredity of NIDDM is established. Identical twin studies have demonstrated over 90% concordance for NIDDM indicating a major heredity component (Barnett, Eff, Leslie, & Pyke, 1981). MODY follows an autosomal dominant inheritance pattern.

Absolute plasma insulin levels may be reduced, normal, or increased in patients with NIDDM. Meal-related insulin secretion is generally reduced relative to the glucose concentration, and the first phase of insulin secretion is blunted. Hyperglycemia in the presence of adequate insulin concentrations is explained by insulin resistance with decreased insulin receptor binding and postreceptor insulin action. Insulin resistance alone does not cause diabetes unless β-cell function is impaired. On the other hand, the β-cell impairment is usually insufficient to cause NIDDM without insulin resistance. Obesity aggravates insulin resistance. Hyperglycemia also impairs insulin secretion and insulin action further aggravating the situation (DeFranzo, Ferrannini, & Koivisto, 1983; Gerich, 1984; Horton, 1983; Kolterman et al., 1981). Although these abnormalities are well established, the primary defect or defects in NIDDM remain a source of controversy.

Management Approach to the Patient

Prevention of the acute symptoms of NIDDM can be accomplished relatively easily. Methods to prevent the chronic complications have not been proven, although available evidence strongly suggests hyperglycemia is the major determinant of the complications. The first step in caring for the patient is to review the medical history and examination, establish the diagnosis of diabetes, exclude secondary causes of diabetes, and determine the baseline status in regard to diabetes control and complications. Second, treatment goals must be selected. Treatment goals include degree of blood glucose control, general well-being day to day, avoidance of serious hypoglycemia, and prevention of the chronic complications of diabetes. Treatment goals serve as a measure of the effectiveness of the treatment program, and failure to achieve the goals mandates a change in the treatment plan. Treatment goals are modified because of old age, other life-threatening illness, impaired mental status, increased risk of hypoglycemia, interactions with other medications, a history of alcohol or drug abuse, and lack of patient cooperation. Goal and treatment selection involves judgment, and there is no universal agreement regarding the best options (Zimmerman and Service, 1988).

Therapeutic options include diet alone, sulfonylureas, and insulin. Data are not available indicating which of these options is most effective in varying circumstances. Generally lesser glucose elevations, older age, and obesity favor dietary therapy, and younger age, higher glucose, and normal weight favor insulin therapy.

In the asymptomatic, obese patient, the initial therapy should be an attempt at weight reduction. If achieved, the blood glucose may be normalized. The success rate of weight reduction programs is very poor, and improvement in these programs is one of the major behavioral challenges in the care of patients with diabetes (Fitzgerald, 1981).

The current recommendations are that the diet be balanced and moderately restricted in calories. Total fat intake should not exceed 30% of calories and less than 10% should be saturated fats. Dietary cholesterol should be less than 300 mg daily. Protein requirement constitutes 12% to 20% of total calories, and the remainder are carbohydrates (Consensus Development Panel, 1987). Carbohydrates have the greatest glucose-raising potential. It appears that mixing carbohydrates with other foods blunts their effect on the blood glucose and that even sucrose may not have an adverse influence when used with a meal (Laine et al., 1987).

The role of exercise in achieving weight reduction and improved glucose control has received renewed interest (Bogardus et al., 1984; Lampman et al., 1987; Schneider et al., 1984). Elderly patients often cannot tolerate a vigorous exercise program, and other medical problems such as coronary artery disease may increase the risk of unrestricted exercise. Recommendations for a specific exercise program are part of the treatment prescription for patients with NIDDM. Development of appropriate recommendations may require a cardiovascular fitness evaluation. Once again, the challenge is to modify long-standing behavior patterns.

Patients with massive obesity respond very poorly to conventional diet and exercise programs. Modified fasts, liquid diets, and very low calorie diets can result in very rapid weight reduction, but the weight loss is rarely maintained. Gastric bypass surgery might be the most effective option in these patients (Flickinger et al., 1984).

When treatment goals are not met by dietary therapy or when the patient is symptomatic from hyperglycemia, oral sulfonylureas or insulin injections must be added to the treatment program. Neither medication has a unique advantage (UK Prospective Study, 1983). In the United States, six different sulfonylureas are available. These are tolbutamide, tolazamide, chlorpropamide, acetohexamide, glyburide, and glipizide. They differ primarily in potency on a milligram basis, duration of action, and metabolism. Sulfonylureas seem to act by inhibiting an ATP-linked potassium transport enzyme leading to β-cell depolarization, calcium influx, and insulin secretion. With chronic treatment, the insulin increase primarily follows glucose stimulation. Sulfonylureas also reduce insulin resistance. However, because hyperglycemia impairs insulin action and secretion, this effect may simply be due to the reduced glucose from enhanced insulin secretion and may not be a direct action unique to sulfonylureas.

Comparative studies have not demonstrated a major advantage of any single preparation. Tolbutamide may be less potent on a maximum dose basis, but otherwise it is unusual for an alternative sulfonylurea to be effective when the first has failed. Hypoglycemia is the most common side effect and may occur more frequently with glyburide and chlorpropamide. The risk of severe hypoglycemia increases in elderly patients. Other side effects include hyponatremia, post alcohol flushing, rashes and severe dermatitis, hepatitis, and pancytopenia. Chlorpropamide is associated with the highest incidence of side effects (Ferner, 1988; Skillman & Feldman, 1981). The University Group Diabetes Program study demonstrated an excess of deaths from cardiovascular disease in patients treated with tolbutamide which causes concern about the safety of sulfonylureas (Goldner, Katterud, & Prout, 1971). Because of problems with study design and lack of supporting evidence, these concerns have been gradually discounted with the passage of time. The major clinical problem with sulfonylurea therapy is secondary failure, occurring in 5% to 20% of patients.

Many insulin preparations are available. They differ primarily by source, time course of action, and purity. The brief nature of this review does not permit a full discussion of these differences or detailed explanation of initiation and adjustment of insulin therapy. Usually insulin therapy can be initiated on an outpatient basis using a single injection of NPH or Lente insulin with 0.2 to 0.5 units/kg body weight daily. The dose is adjusted depending on the pattern of the glucose response. When initiation of therapy is combined with an education program, the patient is usually ready to assume day-to-day care for the diabetes after 3 to 4 days. Many patients with NIDDM can achieve adequate blood glucose control on a single daily injection of insulin with a stable dose and few side effects, in contrast to IDDM where this is unusual. Some patients require more complex insulin programs using mixtures of insulin and/or more than one injection daily. A rare patient has marked insulin resistance and requires well over 100 units of insulin daily. This frustrating circumstance is usually related to uncontrolled eating.

The complete management plan must include patient education, self-monitoring by the patient, and regular follow-up. The value of self-monitoring of blood glucose (SMBG) by one of the fingerstick methods is not as clearly established in NIDDM as in IDDM, but is generally helpful. In the patient achieving treatment goals, follow-up every 3 months is usually adequate.

Chronic Diabetic Complications

In patients with NIDDM, the spectrum of diabetic complications varies from that found in patients with IDDM. Because a long asymptomatic period of hyperglycemia may have existed prior to the diagnosis of diabetes, patients with NIDDM may present with a complication at diagnosis or may develop one soon after diagnosis. Death certificate data often omits the diagnosis of NIDDM, and its full contribution to patient mortality is difficult to ascertain (Ochi, Melton, Palumbo, & Chu, 1985). Accelerated atherosclerosis contributes the most to mortality with at least a doubling of coronary disease incidence, 4-fold increase in peripheral atherosclerosis and 15-fold increase in amputations attributable to diabetes. The increased prevalence of hyperlipidemia, especially hypertriglyceridemia (Zimmerman et al., 1981) and hypertension (Working Group on Hypertension in Diabetes, 1987) in patients with NIDDM aggravates the atherosclerosis. In addition to treating the hyperglycemia, both of these problems must be identified and vigorously treated in these patients.

While the atherosclerosis risk is well recognized, it is often forgotten that patients with NIDDM also develop microvascular complications. In our patient population after 20 years, the cumulative incidence of retinopathy is 30% to 35% (Dwyer et al., 1985) and the cumulative incidence of persistent proteinuria is 25% (Ballard et al., 1988). The incidence of neuropathy has been more difficult to define, but impotence occurs in about 50% of the men 10 years after the diagnosis of NIDDM. Clearly patients with NIDDM have significant morbidity from diabetic complications. The problems are complex and can only be mentioned in this brief review.

Summary

The treatment problems and diabetes-related complications associated with NIDDM can have a major impact on the patient's emotional status and behavior. Unless the potential complexities of these problems are understood, the psychological implications of the diagnosis of NIDDM will be underestimated. Advances in the treatment of NIDDM will only occur when better methods to modify behavior patterns are developed.

References

Ballard, D.J., Humphrey, L.L., Melton, L.J., III, Frohnert, P.P., Chu, C-P., O'Fallon, W.M., & Polumbo, P.J. (1988). Epidemiology of persistent proteinuria in Type II diabetes mellitus: population-based study in Rochester, Minnesota. *Diabetes, 37*, 405–12.

Barnett, A.H., Eff, C., Leslie, R.D.G., & Pyke, D.A. (1981). Diabetes in identical twins: A study of 200 pairs. *Diabetologia, 20*, 87.

Bogardus, C., Ravussin, E., Robbins, D., Wolfe, R., Horton, E., & Sinis, E. (1984). Effects of physical training and diet therapy on carbohydrate metabolism in patients with glucose intolerance and noninsulin-dependent diabetes mellitus. *Diabetes, 33*, 311.

Consensus Development Panel (1987). Consensus development conference on diet and exercise in noninsulin-dependent diabetes mellitus. *Diabetes Care, 10*, 639–644.

DeFranzo, R., Ferrannini, E., & Koivisto, V. (1983). New concepts in the pathogenesis and treatment of noninsulin-dependent diabetes mellitus. *American Journal of Medicine* (Suppl 1A), *74*, 754.

Dwyer, M.S., Melton, L.J., III, Ballard, D.J., Palumbo, P.J., Trautman, J.C., & Chuc C-P. (1985). Incidence of diabetic retinopathy and blindness: A population-based study in Rochester, Minnesota. *Diabetes Care, 8*, 316–322.

Fagan, S.S., Cloutier, M.C., & Crowther, R.L. (1978). Clinical and etiological heterogeneity of idiopathic diabetes mellitus. *Diabetes, 27*, 1112.

Ferner, R.E. (1988). Oral hypoglycemic agents. *Medical Clinics in North America, 72*, 1323–1335.

Fitzgerald, F.T. (1981). The problem of obesity. *Annual Reviews of Medicine, 32*, 221–231.

Flickinger, F.G., Pories, W.I., Meelheim, H.D., et al. (1984). The Greenville gastric bypass. *Annals of Surgery, 199*, 555–562.

Gerich, J. (1984). Assessment of insulin resistance and its role in noninsulin-dependent diabetes mellitus. *Journal of Laboratory and Clinical Medicine, 103*, 497.

Goldner, M.G., Knatterrud, G.L., & Prout, T.E. (1971). Effects of hypoglycemic agents on vascular complications in patients with adult-onset diabetes III clinical implications of UGDP results. *Journal of the American Medical Association, 218*, 1400–1410.

Horton, E.S. (1983) Role of environmental factors in the development of non-insulin-dependent diabetes mellitus. *American Journal of Medicine* (Suppl 5B), *75*, 32–40.

Kolterman, O., Gray, R., Griffin, J., Burstein, P., Insul, J., Scarlett, J., & Olefsky, J. (1981). Receptor and postreceptor defects contribute to the insulin resistance in noninsulin-dependent diabetes mellitus. *Journal of Clinical Investigation, 68*, 957.

Laine, D.C., Thomas, W., Levitt, M.D., et al. (1987). Comparison of predictive capabilities of diabetic exchange lists and glycemic index of foods. *Diabetes Care, 10*, 387–394.

Lampman, R.M., Schteingart, D.E., Santinger, J.T., et al. (1987). The influence of physical training on glucose tolerance, insulin sensitivity, and lipid lipoprotein concentrations in middle-aged hypertriglyceridemic, carbohydrate-intolerant men. *Diabetologia, 30*, 380–385.

National Diabetes Data Group (1979). Classification and diagnosis of diabetes mellitus and other categories of glucose intolerance. *Diabetes, 28*, 1039–1057.

Ochi, J.W., Melton, I.J., III, Palumbo, P.J., & Chu, C-P. (1985). A population-based study of diabetes mortality. *Diabetes Care, 8*, 224–229.

Schneider, S.H., Amoroso, L.F., Khachsdurian, A.K., et al. (1984). Studies on the mechanism of improved glucose control during regular exercise in Type II (noninsulin-dependent) diabetis. *Diabetologia, 26*, 355–360.

Skillman, T.G., & Feldman, J.M. (1981) The pharmacology of sulfonylureas. *American Journal of Medicine, 70*, 361–372.

UK Prospective Study (1983). UK Prospective study of therapies of maturity-onset diabetes I. Effects of diet, sulphonylurea, insulin or biguanide therapy on fasting plasma glucose and body weight over one year (multi-central study) *Diabetologia, 24*, 404–411.

Working Group on Hypertension in Diabetes. (1987). Statement on hypertension in diabetes mellitus. *Archives of Internal Medicine, 147*, 830–842.

Zimmerman, B.R., Palumbo, P.J., O'Fallon W.M., et al. (1981). A prospective study of peripheral occlusive arterial disease in diabetes. III. Initial lipid and lipoprotein findings. *Mayo Clinic Proceedings, 56*(4), 233–242.

Zimmerman, B.R., & Service, F.J. Management of noninsulin-dependent diabetes mellitus. *Medical Clinics in North America, 72*, 1355–1364.

10

Stress, Behavior, and the Autonomic Nervous System in Type II Diabetes Mellitus

Richard S. Surwit, Suzanne L. Ross, and Mark N. Feinglos

Stress has long been shown to have major effects on metabolic activity. Energy mobilization is a primary result of the "fight or flight" response. Stress stimulates the release of a variety of hormones which can result in elevated blood glucose levels. While this is of adaptive importance in a healthy organism, in diabetes, due to a relative or absolute lack of insulin, stress-induced increases in glucose cannot be properly metabolized. Furthermore regulation of these stress hormones is abnormal in diabetes. Thus, stress is a potential contributor to chronic hyperglycemia in this disease although its exact role is unclear. The role of stress in Type II diabetes is of particular importance because, in contrast to Type I diabetes, the pathophysiology of Type II diabetes remains obscure. In this chapter we will review the literature on the effects of stress on hyperglycemia in Type II diabetes and evaluate the possible role of the autonomic nervous system and behavior in the etiology and course of this disease.

The autonomic nervous system is of primary importance in the regulation of carbohydrate metabolism. The effects of the autonomic nervous system on insulin action is both facilitatory and inhibitory. Branches of the right vagus nerve innervate the pancreatic islets, and stimulation of the right vagus causes increased insulin secretion. Stimulation of pancreatic islet cell beta adrenergic receptors also facilitates insulin secretion. Conversely, insulin secretion is inhibited by stimulation of the sympathetic nerves of the pancreas through the activation of alpha adrenergic receptors. Beta adrenergic stimulation also stimulates glucagon release from the pancreatic alpha cells. Glucagon, in turn, stimulates glucose production in the liver. Thus, sympathetic and parasympathetic innervation of the pancreas modulates the normal regulation of carbohydrate metabolism (Clutter, Bier, Shah, & Cryer, 1980; Williams & Porte, 1974; Young & Landsberg, 1979).

The autonomic nervous system has further metabolic effects. Beta adrenergic stimulation promotes the conversion of glycogen to glucose in the liver as well as fat to free fatty acids in adipose tissue. (Free fatty acids are further metabolized to ketoacids in the liver.) Circulating epinephrine present in levels which stimulate those achieved during minor stress can also adversely affect glucose tolerance (Hamburg, Hendler, & Sherwin, 1980). Thus, the autonomic nervous system, particularly the sympathetic branch, has both direct neural as well as indirect hormonal control pathways in the regulation of glucose metabolism (Williams & Porte, 1974).

Stressful stimuli can activate several other neuroedocrine responses which can result in elevated blood glucose levels. Activation of the hypothalamic-pituitary-adrenocortical axis causes release of increased amounts of glucocorticoids, which cause resistance to insulin action, leading to enhanced glucose production by the liver and diminished cellular glucose uptake. Stress-induced release of growth hormone can also cause insulin resistance and beta endorphin which can suppress insulin secretion and elevate glucose levels (Guillemin, 1978).

While it is now known that Type I diabetes results from autoimmune destruction of the pancreatic beta cells, the pathophysiology of Type II diabetes remains obscure. There is now speculation among investigators that the autonomic nervous system is involved in the pathophysiology of Type II diabetes (Feldberg, Pike, & Stubbs, 1985; Giugliano, 1984; Guillemin, 1978; Ipp, Dhorajiwala, Pugh, Moosa, & Rubinstein, 1982; Surwit & Feinglos, 1988). This was foreseen by Claude Bernard who found that hyperglycemia could be produced in normal rabbits by lesioning the area of the hypothalamus. More recently, several researchers have shown that hyperglycemia can be produced by chemical stimulation of the brain with morphine and by a variety of endogenous neuropeptides and can be abolished by bilateral adrenalectomy (Guillemin, 1978; Van Loon & Appel, 1981). Hyperglycemia has also been found to occur from a slow intravenous infusion or epinephrine (Lori, Lori, & Buchwald, 1930) and from the type of stress that results in prolonged sympathetic discharge (Woods, Smith, & Porte, 1981). In this chapter we will investigate the role of stress in the etiology and course of Type II diabetes and review the experimental evidence which suggests that altered sympathetic nervous system activity makes this disease particularly responsive to stress.

The Role of Stress in the Onset of Type II Diabetes Human Studies

There are no controlled studies on how stress might affect the initial onset of Type II diabetes in humans. However, the earliest recognition of how stress seemingly interacts with this disease was from anecdotal reports of diabetes being precipitated by acute life stress (Willis, 1679; Maudsley, 1899). Since the first awareness of the relationship between stress and diabetes, numerous physiologic mechanisms have been postulated to explain how stress disrupts glucose metabolism in diabetes. One line of research has focused on how glucose intolerance can be induced by stress hormones or by stress itself in nondiabetic individuals. Hamburg et al. (1980) gave normal volunteers a low-dose epinephrine infusion which produced elevations in plasma epinephrine similar to those associated with the stress of a minor viral illness. They demonstrated that, under these conditions, there was significant deterioration in glucose tolerance. Using a different type of experimental paradigm, Wing, Epstein, Blair, and Nowalk (1985) investigated the effect of a standardized psychologic stressor on the utilization of a carbohydrate load in normal individuals. Subjects were fed a carbohydrate load and were then exposed to a stressor which involved participation in competitive tasks. They found that an acute psychologic stressor delayed the peak glucose response and, therefore, apparently altered the ability of the subjects to absorb carbohydrates.

Animal Studies

Animal research has provided evidence to suggest that stress affects the "onset" of diabetes. Almost a half century ago, Cannon (1941) described stress-induced hyperglycemia in normal cats. In this early investigation, 12 cats were confined in a holder, for varying lengths of time, which were dependent on the animals' reactions to this novel situation. The cats were given a large quantity of water by stomach tube and urine was drained promptly. In all of the cases, sugar was absent from the urine before the animal became excited; conversely, the stress intervention invariably resulted in glycosuria. Cannon observed an apparent relationship between the animals' emotional state and the onset of the hypoglycemia. Specifically, those animals which appeared to be frightened or enraged developed glycosuria more quickly than animals which responsed to the confinement in a calm manner.

Along a different line, some studies have looked at the stress on an analogue of Type II diabetes which has been chemically or surgically induced. Capponi, Kawada, Varela, and Vargas (1980) studied the "diabetongenic potentiality" of stress by looking at the effect of repeated restraint on adult Sprague–Dawley rats that had been partially surgically pancreatectomized. While few of these animals spontaneously developed diabetes, repeated restraint stress resulted in permanent diabetes in a significant percentage of the pancreatectomized animals.

One of the first observations that stress could contribute to the expression of hyperglycemia in an animal model of spontaneously occurring Type II diabetes was made during metabolic studies of the sand rat (psammomys obesus). The sand rat is a North African rodent that eats an exclusively low-calorie diet of succulent plants in its natural habitat. Those animals that are maintained on a low-calorie, low-carbohydrate diet do not develop diabetes. However, when they are fed laboratory chow and allowed to become obese, a significant percentage of the animals develop an analog of Type II diabetes (Dulin, Gerritsen, & Chang, 1983). Mikat, Hackel, Cruz, and Lebovitz (1972) have shown that stress, as well as diet and obesity, may play a role in the expression of hyperglycemia in these animals. They maintained sand rats on a low-calorie, low-carbohydrate diet of vegetables and saline so that they remained euglycemic. Glucose or saline was then administered to rats either through an esophageal tube or intraperitoneally by injection. Similar procedures were carried out on a group of Sprague–Dawley rats. Blood sample were drawn from all of the animals at intervals of 30 and 120 min and analyzed for glucose and insulin. Sand rats receiving glucose via an intraperitoneal injection and not intubated showed normal glucose tolerance values. However, sand rats experiencing esophageal intubation showed the abnormal glucose tolerance which would be considered typical of diabetes. In contrast, in the Sprague–Dawley rats intubation did not alter normal glucose tolerance values. Thus, it appears that " stress" such as that of intubation precipitates glucose intolerance even in lean, euglycemic sand rats genetically predisposed toward developing diabetes.

Most recently, Surwit and colleagues have shown that altered adrenergic sensitivity might be a biologic marker for the development of Type II diabetes in mice. They demonstrated that C57BL/6J mice that show exaggerated glucose response to epinephrine in the lean state develop true Type II diabetes when allowed to become obese on a hypercaloric diet (Surwit, Kuhn, Cochrane, McCubbin, & Feinglos, 1988).

The Relationship Between Stress and Glycemic Control in Type II Diabetes

Not surprisingly, more attention has been devoted to the effects of stress on established diabetes. Over the last fifteen years, a modest literature has acculated which has focused on the effects of stress in both human and animal models of diabetes. We will begin by reviewing the studies on animal models of type II diabetes.

Animal Studies

Surwit, Feinglos, and colleagues have studied the effects of stress on hyperglycemia in the genetically obese mouse (C57BL/6J, ob/ob), a commonly used model of NIDDM. This animal is a good model of Type II diabetes in humans as it is characterized by a syndrome of obesity, hyperinsulinemia, insulin resistance, hyperglycemia, and glucose intolerance (Dulin et al., 1983). However, there has been some controversy over the degree to which the obese mouse is hyperglycemic. Different laboratories have reported varying "basal" plasma glucose levels ranging from 130 mg/dl to over 300 mg/dl (Beloff-Chain, Freund, & Rookledge, 1975; Dubuc, Cahn, Ristimaki, & Willis, 1982; Grundleger, Godbole, & Thenen, 1980). Surwit, Feinglos, Livingston, Kuhn, and McCubbin (1984) have shown that the degree of hyperglycemia is dependent, in part, on whether the animal is exposed to stressful environmental stimuli. In one experiment, blood samples were drawn from the obese and lean mice following either a rest period or exposure to stress. Stress consisted of restraint in a wire-mesh cage for 60 min punctuated by a 5-min period of shaking. Both lean and obese animals had an increase in plasma glucose levels produced by the stress. This effect was significantly greater in the obese animals than in their lean littermates. Similarly, while plasma insulin decreased in all animals following stress, the decrease was significantly greater in obese animals. A second experiment was conducted to look at the effects of epinephrine on plasma glucose and insulin in both lean and obese animals. The experimental group received an injection of epinephrine bitartrate, and control animals were injected with saline. Blood samples were drawn 1 hr following injection. The results indicated that the effects of epinephrine were analogous to those of stress. That is, epinephrine produced an increase in plasma glucose in all animals with obese mice showing a greater response than their lean littermates. Likewise, epinehprine decreased plasma insulin only in obese mice. These data demonstrate that the expression of hyperglycemia in obese mice is, to some degree, dependent on the animals' exposure to stress. Furthermore, it appears that the differential responsivity of the obese animals to stress may be related to their heightened sensitivity to adrenergic stimulation.

If we assume that environmental stimulation can have a direct effect on the extent of hyperglycemia in animals, there is a possibility of indirect environmental (psychologic) effects which might occur through learning and conditioning. Indeed, there is a substantial literature on the topic of classical conditioning of blood glucose responses in normal animals (see Woods and Kulkosky, 1976, for review). In the majority of these studies, large doses of insulin were used to produce an unconditioned hypoglycemic response (blood glucose from 30 to 50 mg/dl). Other investigators have demonstrated conditioned increases in blood glucose using alterations in this paradigm (Siegel, 1972). Although the sheer number of studies reporting conditioned changes in blood glucose argue persuasively for the existence of this phenomenon, in only one report was insulin assayed, and the effects of these conditioning paradigms on counterregulatory hormones have not been systematically investigated. Furthermore, since normal animals were used as subjects, these studies do not shed light on what role classical conditioning of blood glucose may play in hyperglycemia in diabetes.

Surwit, McCubbin, Livingston, and Feinglos (1985) have demonstrated that by pairing a stressful stimulus known to produce hyperglycemia (shaking) with a previously neutral stimulus (a metronome), ob/ob mice could be trained to show classically conditioned hyperglycemia. Exposure to the metronome alone or the noncontingently presented metronome and shaking, or paired exposure to the metronome and shaking, were repeated seven times over 3 days. On the fourth day, both control and experimental animals were tested for conditioning of stress-induced hyperglycemia by exposure to the metronome alone for 20 min while remaining in their home cages. The training procedure produced acquisition of conditioned hyperglycemia in obese animals only, despite the fact that both lean and obese animals showed a significant rise in plasma glucose as an unconditioned response to shaking. There was no significant change in plasma insulin in either obese or lean animals following any of the experimental manipulations. The obese mouse's tendency to show conditioned hyperglycemia while the lean mouse does not may be related to its greater sensitivity to adrenergic stimulation. In this study, as in earlier studies, the obese mouse showed a significantly greater unconditioned response than the lean mouse. Since a strong unconditioned stimulus must be present for classical conditioning to occur, this animal's tendency to show large hyperglycemic responses to stress may make it more susceptible to classically conditioned hyperglycemia. Most importantly, this phenomenon demonstrates that a purely behavioral or psychologic manipulation such as conditioning can play a major role in the expression of hyperglycemia in at least one animal model of Type II diabetes.

There is also evidence that anxiolytic pharmacotherapy can be used to attenuate the effects of stress on hyperglycemia in Type II diabetes. Surwit et al. (1986) gave lean and obese mice injections of either alprazolam, a triazolobenzodiazepine, or vehicle alone prior to exposure to restraint and shaking stress or to a no stress control period. Blood samples were then drawn and subsequently analyzed for glucose, insulin, and corticosterone. The results indicated that during stress alprazolam significantly lowered plasma glucose in obese but not lean mice, and it also appeared to reduce plasma corticosterone more in obese mice than in lean mice. The implication from these findings is that benzodiazepines might have a role in the modification of stress hyperglycemia in Type II diabetes.

Human Studies

There has been a notable amount of research done with human subjects to look at the relationship between stress and blood glucose. The investigation of the effects of psychologic stress on glucose metabolism in diabetic patients was first undertaken by Hinkle and his co-workers (Hinkle, Evans, & Wolf, 1951a; Hinkle, Evans, & Wolf, 1951b; Hinkle & Wolf, 1952). In this early study, an interview method was used to obtain information about the life histories of 64 "labile" and mild "stable" diabetics, respectively. Each subject participated in a series of interviews which were spaced at approximately weekly intervals over a period of 6 months to 2 years. The patients were observed during both stressful and nonstressful periods during the interview. These investigators emphasized that the initial onset of diabetes often corresponded with a period of serious life stress. Moreover, exacerbations of the illness as defined by increased glycosuria, polyuria, and wight loss in stable diabetics or ketosis and coma in labile patients were also associated with life stressors. Conversely, they noted that remissions of the diabetes, as assessed by fewer symptoms and decreased insulin requirements, tended to occur in "periods of relative secruity." Because these investigators did not carefully characterize their subjects it is difficult to assess the degree to which these results are appropriate to Type II diabetes.

Grant, Kyle, Teichman, and Mendels (1974) looked at the role of stress in terms of the relationship between actual life events and fluctuations in the course of diabetes mellitus. Subjects included 15 patients with "juvenile-onset" diabetes and 22 adult-onset diabetes patients. Life events were measured using a modified version of the Schedule of Recent Events (Holmes & Rahe, 1967). Their results suggested a relationship between life events, particularly those of a negative nature, and changes in diabetic symptomatology. Based on their results, they suggested that there may be "life-event responsive" diabetic patients. However, no attempt was made to differentiate stress responding in Type I and Type II patients.

Also interested in the role of stress with respect to its impact on diabetes, McLesky, Lewis, and Woodruff (1978) investigated the effect of a physical stressor, namely surgery and anesthesia, on glucagon levels in both normal and diabetic patients. The subjects included normal patients, those with IDDM, and individuals with Type II diabetes who were undergoing elective surgery. Serum glucagon and glucose levels were repeatedly sampled during the preoperative, intraoperative, and postoperative periods. Throughout the time sampling period, the diabetic patients showed a clear hyperglycemic response to the surgical stress.

Taken together, these studies indicate a possible adverse relationship between stress and diabetes. However, most studies have failed to delineate whether or not these effects are more prominent in Type I or Type II diabetes. Given this observation there is growing interest in the alteration of the stress response to maintain optimal glycemic control. One behavioral intervention which has been used with this goal in mind is relaxation therapy.

Relaxation Therapy and Type II Diabetes

The investigation of the effects of stressful stimulation upon diabetes control can also be approached by investigating the effects of relaxation techniques which have been designed to reduce or modify an individual's response to stressful environmental stimuli. The use of such techniques in the treatment of diabetes has a long history. Prior to the discovery of insulin, it was common to treat diabetes or obesity, which probably corresponds to what we consider to be Type II diabetes today, with rest and opiates (Osler, 1892). More recently, relaxation techniques have been applied to the treatment of diabetes. Relaxation has been employed in the treatment of a variety of autonomically mediated illnesses (Shapiro and Surwit, 1979). Relaxation appears to decrease adrenocortical activity (Degood & Redgate, 1982; Jevning, Wilson, & Davidson, 1978) as well as circulating levels of catecholamines (Mathew, Ho, Kralik, Taylor, & Claghorn, 1980; Mathew, Ho, Kralik, Taylor, Semchuk, et al., 1980). Thus, relaxation therapy might serve to moderate some of the negative effects of the stress response on metabolic control in some Type II diabetes patients. Moreover, relaxation is not associated with the undue adverse effects caused by andrenergic blockade. There is a growing literature reporting the results of experimental applications of relaxation training in Type II diabetes.

Rosenbaum (1983) introduced four IDDM patients and two Type II diabetes patients, who were being treated with insulin, to the use of a comprehensive stress management program. Biofeedback training proceeded sequentially from frontal EMG, to digital skin temperature, to skin conductance. The family therapy component of this treatment package included a recognition of life events as a potential stressor. Five of the six subjects showed improvement in at least one of the following areas: decreased average plasma glucose, decreased insulin dosage, and increased glucose stability. Unfortunately, since at least four different therapeutic interventions were used simultaneously, it is difficult to attribute any therapeutic effect to relaxation per se. This limitation minimizes but does not invalidate the idea that relaxation played a role in maintaining euglycemia in diabetes.

Lammers, Naliboff, and Straatmeyer (1984) investigated in a more systematic manner the specific effect of progressive muscle relaxation on blood glucose levels in Type II diabetes. Four Type II patients who were receiving insulin and reported experiencing significant stress in their lives served as subjects. The multiple baseline single subject design demonstrated that progressive muscle relaxation significantly lowered blood glucose levels in two of the four subjects during discrete treatment periods. The researchers concluded that progressive muscle relaxation can have a beneficial effect of lowering blood glucose in diabetics, and that this positive response may be especially likely to occur in those patients with initially elevated glucose levels and less stable metabolic control.

While these studies provide suggestive evidence for the utility of relaxation training in the control of plasma glucose in diabetes, they have been relatively uncontrolled and the patient populations reported on have not been adequately defined. There has been one recent report of the controlled application of relaxation training to patients with clearly documented Type II diabetes. Surwit and Feinglos (1983) studied the acute effects of relaxation training on glucose tolerance in a carefully defined population of patients with Type II diabetes. Nine male and three female patients with Type II diabetes in poor control, who were not using insulin, served as subjects. All patients were admitted to a clinical research unit where they remained for 9 days. During the subjects' hospitalization, diet, exercise, and other extraneous stimuli and behaviors were held constant. Half of the patients were assigned to receive instruction in a modified version of progressive relaxation. Each subject was instructed to practice PMR two times per day for 5 days. In addition, all patients in the relaxation group were given five 50-min EMG biofeedback sessions. The other six patients remained in the hospital under conditions identical to that of the treatment group except they did not receive relaxation training. At the end of the week, glucose and insulin tolerance tests were repeated while patients receiving relaxation training practiced the technique with the aid of the cassette tape. While fasting glucose improved for all subjects with hospitalization, glucose tolerance improved significantly in patients who had received relaxation training as compared to controls. The improvement in glucose tolerance was not accompanied by a change in insulin sensitivity, insulin secretion, or plasma glucagon. Plasma cortisol and catecholamines were measured immediately prior to the first and second glucose tolerance test. Subjects receiving relaxation also showed a decrease in plasma cortisol between the first and second glucose tolerance tests, whereas control subjects showed an increase over the same period (Surwit and Feinglos, 1983). Plasma catecholamines decreased in both groups from the first to the second test. However, differences between the groups were not significant.

Altered Adrenergic Sensitivity and Type II Diabetes

There is substantial evidence to support the notion that increased alpha adrenergic sensitivity is a characteristic of Type II diabetes. For example, Kuhn, Cochrane, Feinglos, and Surwit (1987) investigated the contribution of altered peripheral sympathetic function to the exaggerated glycemic response of ob/ob mice to stress. Obese mice and their lean littermates were injected with one of three doses of epinephrine bitartrate or phentolamine mesylate. Epinephrine administration resulted in a dose-related increase in plasma glucose in lean animals in the dose range 1–5 μg/10 g body weight, while plasma glucose responses were maximal at the lowest dose of epinephrine tested in the obese mice, suggesting that the dose–response relationship is altered in obese animals. Moreover, phentolamine, an alpha adrenergic antagonist, produced a greater increase in plasma insulin in ob/ob mice than the lean littermates, suggesting that this increased sensitivity to catecholamines may be largely alpha adrenergic. Altered peripheral responses to sympathetic stimuli are therefore important in the exaggerated glycemic responses of ob/ob mice to stress and may be an etiologic factor in the development of diabetes in these animals. Fujimoto, Sakaguchi, and Ui (1981) observed a similar exaggerated sensitivity to epinephrine in the KK mouse, another animal model of Type II diabetes. Furthermore, they also observed that alpha adrenergic blockage with phentolamine could provoke an exaggerated insulin response in KK mice compared to control mice suggesting that KK, like ob/ob mice, have altered adrenergic sensitivity.

There is also evidence of altered adrenergic sensitivity and responsivity in patients with Type II diabetes. Linde and Deckert (1973) and Robertson, Halter, and Porte (1976) observed that alpha adrenergic blockade with phentolamine increased glucose-stimulated insulin secretion in patients with Type II diabetes, the latter group showing that this increase is five times greater in patients than in normal controls. This suggests that alpha adrenergic stimulation may be having a greater effect on insulin release in diabetic patients than in normals. Most recently, Kashiwagi et al. (1986) demonstrated that selective blockade of alpha-2 receptors increased both insulin secretion and glucose disposal rate following a mixed meal in patients with Type II diabetes. Finally, it has been reported that glyburide, one of the sulfonylurea oral agents used to treat Type II diabetes, binds to alpha-2 receptors in the pancreas suggesting that one effect of this drug on insulin secretion may be due to antagonism of adrenergic activity (Cherksey and Altszuler, 1984). These findings suggest that environmental stress, which activates the sympathetic nervous system, may be particularly deleterious to patients with Type II diabetes and that methods to reduce the effects of stress may have some clinical utility in this disease (Surwit & Feinglos, 1988).

Summary and Conclusions

There is considerable data on how stress affects glycemic control in Type II diabetes. Numerous animal studies exist which suggest that stress can adversely affect glycemic control in this form of the disease. Furthermore, there is evidence from both animals and humans which suggests that individuals with Type II diabetes have altered adrenergic sensitivity in the pancreas (and perhaps other sites as well) which could make them particularly sensitive to stressful environmental stimulation. However, while there is substantial data showing the importance of stress in understanding hyperglycemia in animal models of Type II diabetes, there is no direct evidence that stress plays a role in the expression or control of the human disease. Indirect support for this hypothesis is provided by several studies which show that relaxation can attenuate hyperglycemia in patients.

In summary, there has been speculation for over 300 years that stressful behavioral stimulation may be important in both the etiology and course of diabetes. There is now mounting evidence of autonomic nervous system abnormalities in Type II diabetes in which there is an exaggeration of sympathetic nervous system (SNS) effects upon glucose metabolism. Thus, any behavioral stimulus which excites the autonomic nervous system would impair insulin secretion and glucose utilization, the pathophysiologic hallmarks of the disease (Surwit & Feinglos, 1988). This hypothesis does not require the presence of unusual psychologic stress for metabolic dysregulation to occur in that the metabolic effects of even normal SNS activity appear to be exaggerated. Thus, Type II diabetes may be, in part, a problem of neurally regulated homeostatis in which stress and the autonomic nervous system interact in contributing to the development and/or course of the disease. This model is consistent with the early theoretical speculations of Claude Bernard and the clinical observations of Willis, Osler, and Maudsley. Further investigation will determine its relevance to our understanding of the etiology and treatment of diabetes.

References

Beloff-Chain, A., Freund, N., & Rookledge, K.A. (1975). Blood glucose and serum insulin levels in lean and genetically obese mice. *Hormone and Metabolic Research, 1*, 374–378.

Cannon, W.B. (1941). *Bodily changes in pain, hunger, fear and rage.* New York: MacMillan.

Capponi, R., Kawada, M.E., Varela, C., & Vargas, L. (1980). Diabetes mellitus by repeated stress in rats bearing chemical diabetes. *Hormone and Metabolic Research, 12*, 411–412.

Cherksey, B., & Altszuler, N. (1984). Tolbutamide and glyburide differ in effectiveness to displace alpha- and beta-adrenergic radioligands in pancreatic islet cells and membranes. *Diabetes, 33*, 499–503.

Clutter, W.E., Bier, D.M., Shah, S.D., and Cryer, P.E. (1980). Epinephrine plasma metabolic clearance rates, and physiologic thresholds for metabolic and hemodynamic actions in man. *Journal of Clinical Investigation, 66*, 74–101.

Degood, D.E., & Redgate, E.S. (1982). Interrelationship of plasma cortisol and other activation indexes during EMG bio-feedback training. *Journal of Behavioral Medicine, 5*, 213–224.

Dubuc, P.O., Cahn, P.J., Ristimaki, S., & Willis, P.L. (1982). Starvation and age effects on glycoregulation and hormone levels of C57BL/6J ob/ob mice. *Hormone and Metabolic Research, 14*, 532–535.

Dulin, W.E., Gerritsen, G.C., & Chang, A. (1983). Experimental and spontaneous diabetes in animals. In M. Ellenberg and H. Rifkin (Eds.). *Diabetes mellitus: Theory and practice* (3rd ed.) (pp. 361–408). New York: Medical Examination Publishing Company.

Feldberg, W., Pike, D.A., & Stubbs, W.A. (1985). On the origin of non- insulin-dependent diabetes. *Lancet, 1*, 1263–1264.

Fujimoto, K., Sakaguchi, T., & Ui, M. (1981). Adrenergic mechanisms in the hyperglycaemia and hyperinsulinaemia of diabetic KK mice. *Diabetologia, 20*, 568–572.

Giugliano, D. (1984). Morphine, opioid peptides, and pancreatic islet function. *Diabetes Care, 7*, 92–98.

Grant, I., Kyle G.C., Teichman, A., & Mendels, J. (1974). Recent life events and diabetes in adults. *Psychosomatic Medicine, 36*, 121–128.

Grundleger, M.L., Godbole, V.Y., & Thenen, S.W. (1980). Age dependent development of insulin resistance of soleus muscle in genetically obese (ob/ob) mice. *American Journal of Physiology, 239*, 363–371.

Guillemin, R. (1978). Hypothalamus, hormones and physiological regulation. In E. Debbs-Robin (Ed.). *Claude Bernard and the Internal Environment: A Memorial Symposium* (pp. 137–156). New York: Dekker.

Hamburg, D., Hendler, R., & Sherwin, R.S. (1980). Influence of small increments of epinephrine on glucose tolerance in normal humans. *Annals of Internal Medicine, 93*, 566–568.

Hinkle, L.E., Jr., Evans, F.M., & Wolf, S. (1951a). Studies in diabetes mellitus III: Life history of three persons with labile diabetes, and the relation of significant experiences in their lives to the onset and course of their disease. *Psychosomatic Medicine, 13*, 160–183.

Hinkle, L.E., Jr., Evans, F.M., & Wolf, S. (1951b). Studies in diabetes mellitus IV: Life history of three persons with relatively mild, stable diabetes, and relation of significant experiences in their lives to the onset and course of the disease.

Hinkle, L.E., Jr., & Wolf, S. (1952). Importance of life stress in course and management of diabetes mellitus. *Journal of the American Medical Association, 148*, 513–520.

Holmes, T.H., & Rahe, R.H. (1967). The social readjustment rating scale. *Journal of Psychosomatic Research, 11*, 213–218.

Ipp, E., Dhorajiwala, J., Pugh, W., Moossa, A.R., & Rubinstein, A.H. (1982). Effects of an enkephalin analog on pancreatic endocrine function and glucose homeostasis in normal and diabetic dogs. *Endocrinology, 111*, 461–463.

Jevning, R., Wilson, A.F., & Davidson, J.M. (1978). Adrenocortical activity during meditation. *Hormones and Behavior, 10*, 54–60.

Kashiwagi, A., Harano, Y., Suzuki, M., Kojima, H., Harada, M., Nisho, Y., & Shigeta, Y. (1986). New alpha-2 adrenergic blocker (DG-5128) improves insulin secretion and in vivo glucose disposal in NIDDM patients. *Diabetes, 35*, 1085–1089.

Kuhn, C.M., Cochrane, C., Feinglos, M.N., & Surwit, R.S. (1987). Exaggerated peripheral responsivity to catecholamines contributes to stress-induced hyperglycemia in the ob/ob mouse. *Physiology, Biochemistry and Behavior, 26*, 491–495.

Lammers, C.A., Naliboff, B.D., & Straatmeyer, A.J. (1984). The effects of progressive relaxation on stress and diabetic control. *Behavior Research and Therapy, 22*, 641–650.

Linde, J., & Deckert, T. (1973). Increase of insulin concentration in maturity-onset diabetics by phentolamine (Regitine) infusion. *Hormone and Metabolic Research, 5*, 391–395.

Lori, C.F., Lori, G.T., & Buchwald, K.W. (1930). The mechanism of epinephrine action vs. changes in blood sugar, lactic acid and blood pressure during continuous intravenous injection of epinephrine. *American Journal of Physiology, 93*, 273–283.

Mathew, R.J., Ho, B.T., Kralik, P., Taylor, P., & Claghorn, J.L. (1980). Catecholamines and migraine: Evidence based on biofeedback-induced changes. *Headache, 20*, 247–252.

Mathew, R.J., Ho, B.T., Kralik, P., Taylor, D., Semchuk, K., Weinman, M., & Claghorn, J.L. (1980). Catechol-O-Methythransferase and catecholamines in anxiety and relaxation. *Psychiatric Research, 3*, 85–91.

Maudsley, H. (1899). *The pathology of mind.* New York: Appleton.

McLesky, C.H., Lewis, S.B., & Woodruff, R.E. (1978). Glucagon levels during anesthesia and surgery in normal and diabetic patients. *Diabetes, 27*, 492.

Mikat, E.M., Hackel, D.B., Cruz, P.T., & Lebovitz, H.E. (1972). Lowered glucose tolerance in the sand rat (psammonys obesus) resulting from esophageal intubation. *Proceedings of the Society for Experimental Biology and Medicine, 139*, 1390–1391.

Olser, W. (1892). *The principles and practice of medicine.* New York: Appleton.

Porte, D. & Woods, S. (1983). Neural regulation of islet hormones and its role in energy balance and stress hyperglycemia. In M. Ellenberg and H. Rifkin (Eds.). *Diabetes mellitus: Theory and practice* (3rd ed.) (pp. 267–294). New York: Medical Examination Publishing Company.

Robertson, P.R., Halter, J.B., & Porte, D. (1976). A role for alpha-adrenergic receptors in abnormal insulin secretion in diabetes mellitus. *The Journal of Clinical Investigation, 57*, 791–795.

Rosenbaum, L. (1983). Biofeedback assisted stress management for insulin-treated diabetes mellitus. *Biofeedback and Self-Regulation, 8*, 519–532.

Shapiro, D., & Surwit, R.S. (1970). Biofeedback. In O.F. Pomerleau and J.P.

Brady (Eds.). *Behavioral medicine: Theory and practice* (pp. 45–73). Baltimore: Williams & Wilkins, Co.

Siegel, S. (1972). Conditioning of insulin-induced hypoglycemia. *Journal of Comparative and Physiological Psychology, 78*, 233–241.

Surwit, R.S., & Feinglos, M.N. (1983). The effects of relaxation on glucose tolerance in non-insulin dependent diabetes mellitus. *Diabetes Care, 7*, 203–204.

Surwit, R.S., & Feinglos, M.N. (1988). Stress and autonomic nervous system in type II diabetes: A hypothesis. *Diabetes Care, 11*, 83–85.

Surwit, R.S., Feinglos, M.N., Livingston, E.G., Kuhn, C.M., & McCubbin, J. A. (1984). Behavioral manipulation of the diabetic phenotype in ob/ob mice. *Diabetes, 33*, 616–618.

Surwit, R.S., Kuhn, C.M., Cochrane, C., McCubbin, J.A., & Feinglos, M.N. (1988). Diet-induced type II diabetes in C57BL/6J mice. *Diabetes, 371*, 1163–1167.

Surwit, R.S., McCubbin, J.A., Kuhn, C.M., McGee, D., Gerstenfeld, D.A., & Feinglos, M.N. (1986). Alprazolam reduces stress hyperglycemia in ob/ob mice. *Psychosomatic Medicine, 48*, 278–282.

Surwit, R.S., McCubbin, J.A., Livingston, E.G., & Feinglos, M.N. (1985). Classically conditioned hyperglycemia in the obese mouse. *Psychosomatic Medicine, 47*, 565–568.

Van Loon, G.R., & Appel, N. (1981). Endorphin-induced hyperglycemia is mediated by increased central sympathetic outflow to adrenal medulla. *Brain Research, 204*, 236–241.

Williams, R.H., & Porte, D., Jr. (1974). The pancreas. In R.H. Williams (Ed.). *Textbook of endocrinology* (15th ed.). Philadelphia: Saunders.

Willis, T. (1679). Pharmaceutice rationalis: Or the exercitation of the operation of medicines in humane bodies. *The works of Thomas Willis*. London: Dring, Harper, & Leigh.

Wing, R.R., Epstein, L.H., Blair, E., Nowalk, M.P. (1985). Psychologic stress and blood glucose levels in nondiabetic subjects. *Psychosomatic Medicine, 47*, 558–564.

Woods, S.C., & Kulkosky, P.J. (1976). Classically conditioned changes of blood glucose level. *Psychosomatic Medicine, 38*, 201–219.

Woods, S.C., Smith, P.H., & Porte, D. (1981). The role of the nervous system in metabolic regulation and its effects on diabetes and obesity. In M. Brownless (Ed.). *Handbook of diabetes mellitus. Vol. 3*. (pp. 208–271). New York: Garland.

Young, J.B., & Landsberg, L. (1979). Sympathoadrenal system: The regulation of metabolism. In S.H. Ingbar (Ed.). *Contemporary endocrinology* (Vol. 1.) New York: Plenum Medical Book.

11

Behavioral Strategies for Improving Weight Loss in Obese Type II Diabetic Patients

Rena R. Wing, Leonard H. Epstein, and Marsha D. Marcus

Weight control is considered the treatment of choice for obese patients with Type II diabetes. Weight loss will improve glycemic control in these patients and will reduce coronary heart disease (CHD) risk factors. The problem remains, however, that it is difficult to produce long-term weight loss in these patients. The goal of the chapter is to describe the research that has been conducted to date on weight control interventions for Type II diabetic patients. The chapter will point out differences between diabetic and nondiabetic patients and discuss in detail the treatment strategies that have been tested with Type II diabetic patients.

Obesity as a Risk Factor for the Development of Type II Diabetes

Obesity is a well-established risk factor for the development of Type II diabetes and 60–90% of individuals with Type II diabetes are overweight (West, 1978). In a prospective study of a cohort of 3,737 men in Oslo, Norway, none of the men who were <90% of ideal body weight developed diabetes, compared to 1% of those who were normal weight, 2% of those 10–15% overweight, 4% of those 25–35% overweight, and 13% of those >45% overweight (Westlund & Nicholaysen, 1972).

Recent data suggest that not only is the amount of body fat important in producing diabetes, but also where it is located. Upper body fat obesity, where the weight is in the abdominal area, poses a greater risk for the development of diabetes than lower body fat obesity, where the weight is on the hips (Hartz, Rupley, Kalkhoff, & Rimm, 1983; Ohlson et al., 1985). For example, in a survey of 15,000 female members of TOPS (Take Off Pounds Sensibly), 16.5% of those women who were severely obese and had upper body fat obesity reported diabetes, compared to 6.1% of those women who were equally obese but had lower body fat obesity. Among those women who were not obese, 5.6% of those with upper body fat reported diabetes and 1.9% of those with lower body fat (Hartz et al., 1983). Thus, Type II diabetes was most prevalent in those who were severely obese and had upper body fat distribution.

Obesity also appears to interact with family history in determining the risk of developing diabetes. Data from the Pima Indians, a population group with very high rates of Type II diabetes, show that the incidence of Type II diabetes in those with a body mass index >35 is 3.8% per year in individuals whose parents do not have diabetes. The incidence increases to 6.9% per year in those with one diabetic parent and 9.2% per year in those with two diabetic parents (Bennett, Knowler, Pettitt, Garraher, & Vasquez, 1982).

Thus, individuals who are overweight are at increased risk of developing diabetes, and this risk is particularly elevated in individuals with a family history of diabetes and those with upper body fat obesity. However, to date, there have been no controlled prospective studies to determine whether weight reduction in these individuals will decrease their risk of developing diabetes.

Benefits of Weight Control

While it is not known whether weight reduction can prevent the development of Type II diabetes, it is well established that weight loss will improve glycemic control in patients with the disease. Numerous metabolic ward studies have demonstrated that just 10 days of a very low calorie diet will dramatically improve glycemic control in patients with Type II diabetes (Greenfield, Kolterman, Olefsky, & Reaven, 1978; Henry, Scheaffer, & Olefsky, 1985).

However, it remains unclear whether it is weight loss per se, or calorie restriction, that is responsible for the improvement. Henry et al. (1985) studied 30 obese Type II diabetic patients during a 40-day very low calorie diet (300 kcal/day). These patients lost 4.6 kg within the first 10 days on the diet, 7.1 kg after 20 days, and 10.5 kg after 40 days. In contrast to this steady pattern of weight loss, almost all of the improvement in blood glucose occurred within the first 10 days. Fasting glucose decreased from 297 mg/dl at pretreatment to 158 mg/dl by day 10 and averaged 139 mg/dl on day 40. Thus, 87% of the reduction in fasting glucose occurred within 10 days.

Twelve of the subjects were refed for 40 days at a calorie level designed to produce weight maintenance. Weight increased slightly (17.8 kg loss to 16.3 kg loss, $p < .02$) and there was some worsening in control (FBS = 167 mg/dl after 40 days of refeeding). However, blood glucose levels remained markedly improved over pretreatment levels. Thus, it appears that both calorie restriction and weight loss per se may contribute to the improvement in glycemic control.

There appear to be several physiological mechanisms responsible for the improvement in glycemic control. Henry et al. (1985) demonstrated that the improvements in control were strongly correlated with decreases in hepatic glucose output. There are also improvements in insulin sensitivity and insulin secretion with weight loss. In subjects with fasting blood glucose levels <200, and a hyperinsulinemic response to an oral glucose load, a decrease in insulin levels is often observed. In contrast, in patients with more severe hyperglycemia and a hypoinsulinemic response, an increase in insulin secretion may be observed (Savage et al., 1979; Stanik & Marcus, 1980).

Diabetic patients also experience significant improvements in CHD risk factors with weight loss. Improvements in triglycerides (Hughes, Gwynne, Switzer, Herbst, & White, 1984) and cholesterol (Henry, Wiest-Kent, Scheaffer, Kolterman, & Olefsky, 1986) have been noted. Others have reported no change in total cholesterol, but an improvement in the LDL/HDL ratio (Hughes, Gwynne, Switzer, Herbst, & White, 1984). Levels of several coagulation proteins are increased in diabetic patients and may contribute to their increased risk of CHD (Colwell et al., 1976). Decreases in Factor VIII coagulant activity and serum fibrinogen with weight loss have recently been reported (Hughes et al., 1984).

These improvements in CHD risk factors are of marked importance in diabetic patients. Numerous epidemiological studies have shown that diabetic patients are at increased risk of coronary heart disease (Kannel, 1982). However, the risk for an individual with diabetes is greatly reduced in the absence of other CHD risk factors. For example, the 8-year probability of a female aged 50, with diabetes, developing CHD is 25/1000 if the woman has a favorable profile on other CHD risk factors. The risk increases to 298/1000 if the woman is a smoker, with elevated blood pressure, cholesterol, and EKG-abnormalities (Kannel, 1982). Thus, weight loss is a particularly important intervention strategy for Type II diabetic patients since it will not only improve glycemic control, but also will reduce other CHD risk factors.

The majority of research on the benefits of weight reduction has focused on the acute effects of weight loss. Moreover, there has been no effort to determine how much weight is needed to produce these benefits. To answer these questions, Wing and colleagues (Wing, Koeske, et al., 1987) studied the long-term benefits of weight loss in 114 patients treated in their behavioral weight loss programs. These authors found that weight loss during the 12–16-week behavioral program correlated $r = .55$ with HbA_1 changes over the same time period. The correlation between weight loss from pretreatment to 1 year and changes in HbA_1 over the year was similar ($r = .51$). However, the regression line predicting weight loss and changes in HbA_1 at the two time points differed tremendously (Figure 11.1). As seen in Figure 11.1, a weight loss of 5 kg was associated with a 0.6% reduction in HbA_1 at posttreatment, but only a 0.1% reduction in HbA_1 at 1 year. These data suggest that the long-term benefits of weight loss are not as great as the acute effects.

However, even at 1-year follow-up, modest weight losses of 15–30 lbs or 30+ lbs produced significant long-term changes in HbA_1. As seen in Table 11.1, patients who lost 15–30 lbs reduced their HbA_1 from 9.8% to 8.7%. Patients who lost 30+ lbs had even more marked improvements in HbA_1 and achieved HbA_1 levels within the normal range (normal = 6.1 ± 0.5%). This normalization occurred despite the fact that patients remained 20% above ideal body weight. Changes in hypoglycemic medication were also related to weight reduction, and as can be seen, those who lost 30+ lbs. achieved their improvements in HbA_1 with all patients off medication. Finally, modest weight losses of 15 lbs or more produced long-term changes in insulin, triglycerides, and HDL-cholesterol (Table 11.2).

These data should be encouraging to patients and health care pro-

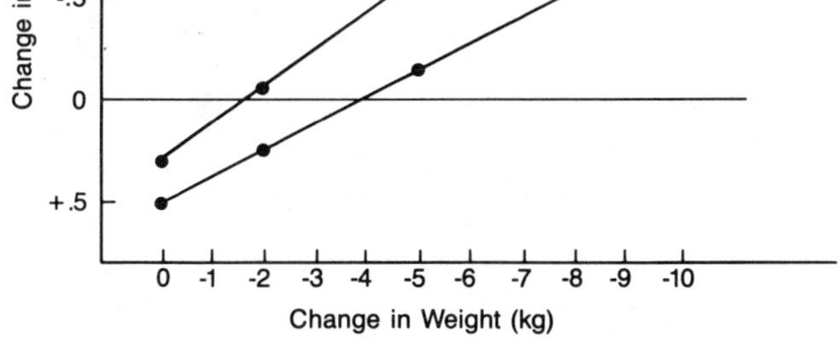

Figure 11.1. Relationship between weight loss and changes in HbA_1 from pretreatment to posttreatment and from pretreatment to 1-year follow-up.

Table 11.1. Change in Weight and Glycemic Control 1-Year After Treatment in a Behavioral Weight Control Program

	Lost				
	30+ lb (>13.6 kg)	15–30 lb (6.9–13.6 kg)	5–15 lb (2.4–6.8 kg)	0–5 lb (0–2.3 kg)	Gained
N	6	21	42	22	23
Weight (kg)					
Pre	97.8	97.3	97.1	97.2	97.5
1 year	70.8*	87.4*	91.5*	96.0*	100.3*
HbA_1 (%)					
Pre	9.7	9.8	9.8	9.8	9.8
1 year	7.1*	8.7*	9.8	10.4*	10.6**
% with reductions in medication	100	63	46	40	16

Adapted from Wing et al. (1987) *Archives of Internal Medicine, 147,* 1749–1753.
*$p<.001$
**$p<.01$

fessionals alike. They suggest that diabetic patients need not achieve ideal body weight to experience long-term improvements in glycemic control and CHD risk factors. Rather, weight losses of 15–30 lbs or 30+ lbs appear sufficient to produce long-term improvements.

Weight Loss and Mood

Participation in a behavioral treatment program not only improves physiological outcome, but may also help improve mood in obese Type II diabetic patients (Salata, Marcus, Nowalk, & Blair, 1986). The mean

Table 11.2. Effect of Weight Losses at 1 Year of 15 Pounds or More on Glycemic Control and Serum Lipid Levels

	Lost>30 lb		Lost 15–30 lb	
	Pre	1 year	Pre	1 year
FBS (mg/dl)	186	109***	191	162*
Insulin (μu/ml)	21.1	2.9***	18.2	10.5**
Triglycerides (mg/dl)	194.4	87.3***	194.4	154.5**
HDL-C (mg/dl)	38.2	48.8***	38.8	41.3*

Adapted from Wing et al. (1987) *Archives of Internal Medicine, 147,* 1749–1753.
*$p<.05$
**$p<.01$
***$p<.001$

score on the Beck Depression Inventory averaged 11.1 ± 6.7 (mean ± SD) in the first 99 diabetic patients who entered our treatment program; 25% of these patients reported moderate or severe symptomatology (BDI ≥ 16). Self-reported depression decreased significantly during treatment in the behavioral weight control program; the average score on the BDI was 6.5 ± 6.4 at posttreatment and, despite some recidivism, remained significantly ($p < .001$) below baseline levels at 1 year (8.8 ± 7.6). Moreover, only 10% of patients reported moderate or severe depressive symptomatology at posttreatment and 17% at 1 year.

The best predictors of changes in mood from pretreatment to posttreatment were initial BDI score and change in percent overweight; taken together, these variables explained 48% of the variance. The effects on long-term changes in mood were weaker; the best predictors were change in glycemic control and initial BDI score, but together these variables explained only 13% of the variance. These data suggest that improvements in mood may occur in part due to weight loss and improved control, but perhaps also because participation in a behavioral treatment program is a positive experience for Type II diabetic patients.

Differences Between Diabetic and Nondiabetic Patients Participating in Weight Control Studies

Given the benefits of weight reduction for obese Type II diabetic patients, clinicians and researchers may wish to develop treatment programs specifically for these patients. It is important to recognize that participants in programs for diabetic patients differ in several ways from those who participate in standard behavioral weight control programs. Most notable is the fact that participants in programs for diabetic patients are older and often less healthy than the general obese population. The average patient in our program for diabetics is 53 years of age, whereas those patients treated in general obesity programs have averaged 39–44 years of age (Brownell, Heckerman, & Westlake, 1979; Foreyt et al., 1982; Jeffery, Wing, & Stunkard, 1978). Moreover, 50% of the diabetic patients in our program are on medication for hypertension. Approximately 60% of our patients are treated with oral medication for their diabetes; 20% with insulin and 20% with diet only. About one third of our patients are males, whereas 18–22% of patients in general obesity program are males (Brownell et al., 1979; Foreyt et al., 1982; Jeffery et al., 1978).

These differences between obese diabetic and nondiabetic participants should be kept in mind when designing intervention programs. The age and health of the diabetic patients may make intense exercise programs questionable. In addition, since improvements in blood pressure and blood sugar occur with weight loss, it is necessary to monitor these parameters regularly and to make adjustment in medication as needed. The input of a physician is important in monitoring diabetic patients and assisting in medication adjustments.

Moreover, while there have been few studies comparing the weight loss of diabetic and nondiabetic patients treated in the same weight loss program, the limited data available suggest that diabetic patients may have more difficulty losing weight than nondiabetics. Henry et al. (1986) studied 10 obese Type II diabetic patients and 5 obese nondiabetic controls who were fed a 300-kcal/day diet for 36 days while inpatients on a metabolic ward. The nondiabetic patients lost significantly more weight than the diabetic patients (35.6 vs. 24.4 lbs, $p<.01$). However, since the nondiabetic patients were heavier than the diabetics at pretreatment, this difference may have contributed to their larger weight losses.

Wing, Marcus, Epstein, and Salata (1987) compared the weight loss of 12 overweight Type II diabetic patients and their overweight nondiabetic spouses. The diabetic and nondiabetic group included an equal number of males and females and the groups were comparable in age, weight, and percent overweight. Since the study used spouse pairs, the diabetic and nondiabetic patients were also similar in socioeconomic status.

Both patient and spouse were treated together in a behavioral weight control program. The nondiabetic spouse lost significantly more weight than the diabetic patients over the 20-week program (29.5 vs. 16.5 lb, $p<.01$). As seen in Figure 11.2, the differences emerged by week 5 and became greater over the course of the program.

The differences in weight loss did not seem to be due to differences in medication, since diabetics on diet only ($N = 6$), oral medication ($N = 3$), and insulin ($N = 3$), all had similar weight losses (7.6, 7.0, and 7.8 kg, respectively). Rather the differences seemed to be due to the magnitude of caloric restriction. While patients and spouses were instructed to restrict their intake by 1000 kcal/day, the diabetic patients restricted their intake by only 709 kcal/day, whereas the spouses cut back by 1172 kcal/day ($p<.02$).

It remains unclear why the diabetic patients were less successful at caloric restriction. Perhaps, their past training with exchange system diets and the emphasis placed on eating three meals and one or two snacks/day made it more difficult for them to restrict their intake. Alternatively diabetic patients may be hungrier and have more difficulty restricting intake. A third possibility is that the diabetic patients were less motivated than their spouses; the latter may have been eager to help the diabetic patients by modeling the appropriate behaviors. Further study with groups of unrelated diabetic and nondiabetic patients is needed to replicate these findings and to try to understand why dia-

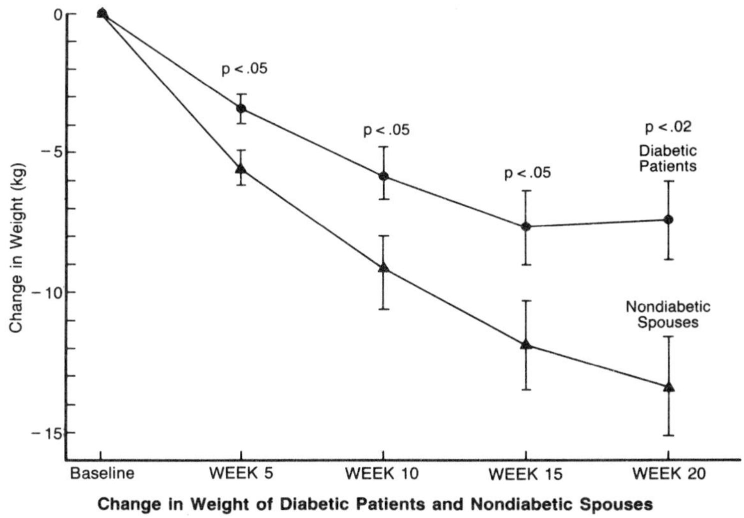

Figure 11.2. Weight loss of diabetic patients and their nondiabetic spouses. Reprinted from Wing, Marcus, Epstein, & Salata (1987). *Diabetes Care, 10*(5), 563–566.

betic patients have more trouble losing weight. However, these differences between diabetic and nondiabetic should be kept in mind when designing programs for these patients or interpreting data from previous studies.

Overview of Early Studies on Dietary Interventions for Type II Diabetic Patients

While weight loss is an important therapeutic approach to the management of obese Type II diabetic patients, there are actually few controlled trials comparing different weight loss therapies or comparing weight loss to other approaches in the treatment of Type II diabetes. Even fewer of these studies have evaluated long-term effects. Wing (1985) reviewed six studies that included at least 1 year of follow-up; five of the six were uncontrolled clinical reports which were difficult to interpret because of the varying length of follow-up and the lack of information on the number of dropouts. Kempner, Peschel, and Schlayer (1958), for example, reported the results for a cohort of 100 diabetic patients fed a rice diet for at least 3 months. Follow-up occurred 3–11 years later (mean = 22 months), at which time the mean weight loss was 7.3 kg. Streja, Boyko, and Rabkin (1981) presented short-term (mean = 66 days) and long-term (mean = 32 months) data on 66 participants out of an original sample of 82 patients (80%). All patients were seen for 1 hr and taught the exchange system for meal planning. Additional contact, if any, was not described. The average short-term weight loss was 4.1 kg and the long-term weight loss was 2.37 kg. Stanik and Marcus (1980) followed seven patients, who were treated with a 600-kcal diet in a hospital setting for 1–3 months and lost 11 kg initially. Four of the seven regained all the weight and the other two maintained their losses, but no average weight loss data are presented. These studies are described briefly to illustrate the diversity of results that have been reported in the diabetes literature, the diversity of diets that have been used, and the methodological problems encountered in these studies.

Perhaps the most interesting data available are from the University Group Diabetes Program (1971), a major multicenter study comparing placebo, oral medication, and insulin therapy in the treatment of Type II diabetic patients. All patients were also placed on a diet designed to achieve normal body weight. Eight hundred twenty-three patients participated in this study and 654 had completed 5 years of follow-up at the cut-off date. Weight data were presented for 510 patients. At entry, these patients were 33% above ideal body weight. Patients in the placebo and diet condition had an average weight loss of 1.9 kg at 3 months, 2.4 kg at 6 months, and maintained a loss of 1.3 kg over the full 4¾ years of the study. Patients in the other conditions lost 0.7–1.8 kg at 3 months, but regained this weight and were approximately 1 kg above baseline values at 4¾ years. Unfortunately, the dietary intervention in the UGDP is not described in detail; it would appear that little emphasis was placed on the diet and the intervention was quite weak. The poor long-term weight losses obtained in this study highlight the need for more careful examination of techniques for promoting weight loss in obese diabetic patients.

Behavioral Weight Control Versus Nonbehavioral Treatments

Three studies have compared behavioral and nonbehavioral approaches to weight control in the treatment of Type II diabetic patients. Rainwater and colleagues (1982) compared a behavioral weight control program to a conventional program in the treatment of obese male diabetic patients. Both programs were offered during a 5-day inpatient stay. The behavioral program produced greater weight losses initially (− 3.8 vs. − 0.8% of body weight) and at 6-month follow-up (− 3.3 vs. 3.7% body weight) than the conventional program.

In contrast, Rabkin, Boyko, Wilson, and Streja (1983) found better results with nutrition education than behavior modification. The nutrition education program included a 1-hour individual counseling session, followed 6 weeks later by a 15-min visit. The behavioral program was conducted by the same nutritionist and involved weekly group sessions for 6 weeks. Patients in the nutrition education program lost 1.7 kg after 6 weeks, compared to -0.36 kg for the behavioral condition ($p<.10$). At 12 weeks, the nutrition education group had lost 3.0 kg compared to -0.9 kg in the behavioral condition, $p<.01$. Given that the behavioral condition had more therapist contact than the nutrition education condition, the results are quite surprising.

The behavioral weight loss programs used in both the Rabkin et al. (1983) and the Rainwater et al. (1982) study were atypical for behavioral programs. Usually, behavioral programs are conducted in an outpatient setting, with meetings held weekly for 10–20 weeks (Brownell & Wadden, 1986; Jeffery et al., 1978). Moreover, the therapist in behavioral programs is usually someone with training and experience in running this type of program. Since both duration of treatment (Brownell & Wadden, 1986) and therapist experience (Jeffery et al., 1978) have been related to outcome, these factors may explain the poor results obtained in the behavioral interventions.

A more traditional behavioral weight control program was tested by Wing and colleagues (Wing, Epstein, Nowalk, Koeske, & Hagg, 1985), in a study comparing behavior modification to nutrition education and standard care control. The behavioral program involved weekly meetings for 16 weeks. All patients in the behavioral condition were given a calorie goal designed to produce a 2-lb/week weight loss (usually 1200–1800 kcal/day) and taught to self-monitor their caloric intake. Information was presented about the calorie value of protein, fat, and carbohydrates, and patients were encouraged to decrease their intake of fat and increase consumption of complex carbohydrates. Exercise, particularly walking, was stressed and patients were taught to gradually increase their exercise until they were using 1000 kcal/week in new exercise (this would equal walking 2 miles/day for 5 days/week). Behavioral techniques including stimulus control, preplanning, relapse prevention, and problem-solving, were also taught. Patients deposited $85 at the start of the study and were refunded portions of their deposit contingent on weight loss.

The nutrition education condition was also seen weekly for 16 weeks, to control for frequency of contact. These patients received information regarding diabetes, diet, and exercise that was comparable to that given to the behavioral condition; however, they were not taught to use any of the behavioral strategies for changing eating and exercise. Patients in the nutrition education condition were placed on an exchange system diet at a calorie level equivalent to that used in the behavioral condition. They were also encouraged to exercise but were not given specific strategies to use to increase their exercise nor asked to self-monitor intake or exercise. The $85 deposited was refunded to these patients contingent only on attendance.

The standard care condition was seen only monthly to more closely approximate the contact schedule usually used in the treatment of Type II diabetic patients (who are usually seen only once every 3–4 months). These patients received identical information to that given to the nutrition education condition.

Fifty-three patients (20 males, 33 females) were recruited for this study and 50 (94%) completed the full 1-year study. These patients were 55 years of age on average and 60% above ideal weight (mean = 96.4 kg); 25% were treated with diet only and 75% with oral medication. Weight losses over the 16-week program were significantly greater in the behavioral condition than in either nutrition education or standard care control (6.3, 3.9, and 2.9 kg, respectively). Significant differences were still apparent at 6-month follow-up, but overall weight losses from pretreatment to 1 year did not differ significantly (– 1.78, 3.03, and 3.42 kg) for the behavioral, nutrition education, and standard care control conditions (Figure 11.3).

Physiological parameters improved significantly during the 4-month intervention. There were significant decreases in fasting blood glucose, HbA_1, and insulin. In addition, cholesterol decreased significantly and HDL-cholesterol increased; systolic and diastolic blood pressure also decreased. However, none of these improvements in physiological parameters were significantly affected by treatment condition. Changes in blood sugar, HbA_1, and insulin were significantly correlated with weight loss, but changes in lipids and blood pressure were not.

Unfortunately, most of these improvements were not maintained at 1-year follow-up. Only insulin and HDL-C showed significant long-

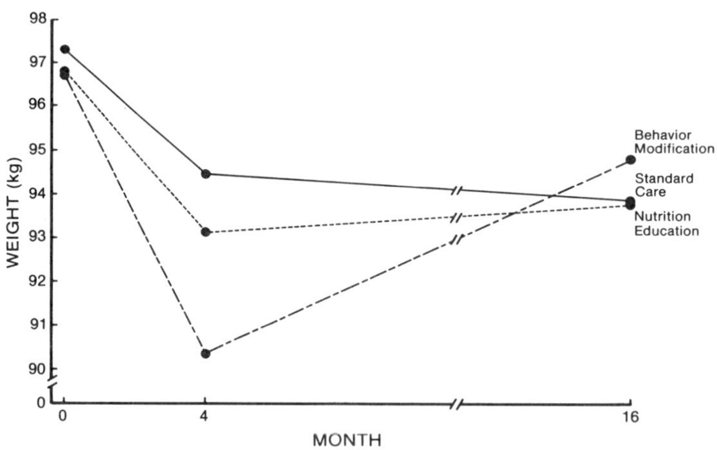

Figure 11.3. Weight loss of diabetic patients treated with behavior modification, nutrition education, or standard care. Reprinted from Wing, Epstein, Nowalk, Koeske, & Hagg (1985). *Journal of Consulting and Clinical Psychology*, *53*, 111–122.

term improvements, again with no differences between conditions. However, weight loss at 1 year was significantly correlated with improvements in fasting blood sugar, HbA_1, insulin, triglycerides, cholesterol, and diastolic blood pressure.

During the first 4 months of the program, patients reported marked improvements in exercise and reduction in consumption of foods high in fat and sugar. These changes were associated with weight loss. Although improvements were also significant from pretreatment to 1 year, patients reported backsliding during the period after the program. These data suggest that if our treatment program could be improved to produce better maintenance of behavior change, it might be possible to also produce better maintenance of weight loss and, consequently, better long-term improvements in the physiological parameters. Subsequent research efforts have been designed to try to accomplish this goal.

Exercise

One approach to improving long-term weight loss might be to focus more heavily on the exercise component within the behavioral weight loss program. Four previous studies with nondiabetic patients have shown that the combination of diet plus exercise produces better long-term weight loss than diet only (Dahlkoetter, Callahan, & Linton, 1979; Epstein, Wing, Koeske, & Valoski, 1984; Harris & Hallbauer, 1973; Stalonas, Johnson, & Christ, 1978). However, previous studies with diabetic patients have been less clear on this issue. Bogardus et al. (1984) compared diet only and diet plus exercise and found no difference in weight loss (−9.9 vs. −11.1 kg) over a 12-week intervention. Improvements in glycemic control were also similar in the two treatment conditions. This study used a 600-kcal/day diet, and it is possible that maximum rates of weight loss were obtained with this diet, overshadowing any effects of exercise.

Hartwell, Kaplan, and Wallace (1986) randomly assigned 32 men and 44 women to 10-week behavior modification programs focusing on diet only, exercise only, or diet plus exercise, or to an education only control group. The diet only condition lost more weight than the other conditions both at the end of the 3-month intervention (−2.5 kg for diet only; −0.24 kg for diet plus exercise, −0.70 kg for exercise only, and +0.28 kg for control) and at 3-month follow-up (−3.5 kg for diet only; −0.24 kg for diet plus exercise, −1.4 kg for exercise only, and +1.0 kg for control). The diet only group also experienced the greatest improvements in HbA_1. It is difficult to explain the relatively modest weight losses that were achieved in all treatment conditions in this study and to reconcile the findings on diet and exercise with the results of the literature on nondiabetics. Perhaps the difference is due to the fact that Hartwell et al. (1986) had the diet plus exercise condition work for 5 weeks on diet followed by 5 weeks of exercise, whereas the previous studies stressed diet and exercise throughout. It is possible that 5 weeks is too brief a period to allow patients to really modify eating or exercise habits.

Our group has recently completed two studies which were designed to determine whether adding exercise to a behavioral weight control program would improve the outcome for Type II diabetic patients. In the first study (Nowalk, Wing, Epstein, Paternostro, & Kriska, 1984), 25 subjects were randomly assigned to either a diet plus moderate exercise condition, which involved an exercise program based on walking or to diet plus placebo exercise condition, which involved light stretching and calisthenics. Both conditions exercised twice a week as a group and once a week on their own. The diet plus moderate exercise condition walked a 3-mile route at each of their exercise sessions. Both conditions were given intake, exercise, and weight loss goals, taught to self-monitor caloric intake, and instructed in behavior change strategies.

Both groups had excellent attendance at the exercise sessions, and differences in caloric expenditure, based on heart rate–work load curves, were documented. However, there was no evidence that participation in the moderate exercise program improved weight loss or glycemic control compared to that found in the placebo control. Weight losses during the initial 10-week program averaged 8.5 kg for the moderate exercise group and 7.3 kg for the placebo exercise condition. At 1-year follow-up, weight loss averaged 7.8 kg for the moderate exercise condition and 4.0 kg for the placebo condition.

In an effort to understand these data, we examined patients' self-reported activity, as indicated on the Paffenbarger Activity Questionnaire (Paffenbarger, Wing, & Hyde, 1978). We found that the patients in the walking condition reported greater increases in walking from pretreatment to posttreatment than the placebo condition, but both groups had similar, significant increases in overall activity (walking plus other activity) from pretreatment to posttreatment. At 1-year follow-up, increases in activity were also similar. Thus, it appears that patients who participated in the placebo exercise program made other more general changes in their activity level.

As a result, a second study was conducted to try to maximize the difference between conditions (Marcus et al., 1987). Two more extreme conditions were compared: a diet only condition, that was asked to maintain their current level of activity, and a diet plus exercise condition, that exercised three times per week as a group, walking a 3-mile route at each session, and a fourth time each week on their own. Both groups attended group sessions 3 times/week for 10 weeks, 1 time per week for weeks 10–20, and then periodically over the year of follow-up. The exercise group walked at each of these sessions, while the diet only group used them to practice diet-related skills.

Self-reported data indicated that this study produced more dramatic differences between the two conditions in activity level. Subjects in the diet plus exercise group increased their overall caloric expenditure from 619 kcal/week at baseline to 1522 kcal/week at posttreatment and continued to expend 1561 kcal at 1 year. In contrast, the diet only condition maintained a low level of activity throughout (668 kcal at pretreatment, 816 kcal at posttreatment, and 853 kcal at 1 year).

The combination of diet plus exercise produced greater weight losses at every time point studied. At week 10, patients in the diet plus exercise group lost 9.2 kg on average, compared to 5.6 in the diet only condition ($p < .01$); at 1 year follow-up, the diet plus exercise group had lost 7.9 kg compared to 3.7 kg in the diet only ($p < .01$).

There were significant improvements in HbA_1 at posttreatment and 1 year, but these changes were similar in the two treatment conditions. However, at 1-year follow-up, a far greater percentage of patients in the diet plus exercise condition had decreases in medication than in the diet only condition (83% vs. 38%, $p < .05$). These data suggest that adding exercise to a behavioral weight loss program can increase weight loss in Type II diabetic patients. Moreover, while improvements in glycemic control were similar, patients treated with diet and exercise were able to achieve these significant improvements in glycemic control while off medication.

Self-Monitoring Blood Glucose

The weight reduction techniques described above are applicable to both diabetic and nondiabetic patients alike. One strategy that is unique to the former and might help to improve dietary adherence is self-monitoring of blood glucose (SMBG).

Self-monitoring techniques are now available that allow diabetic patients to prick their finger and use a drop of blood to determine their current blood glucose level. The blood glucose information is accurate and is available to the patient within 1 min. This information can serve as feedback to the patients on the success of their efforts to control blood glucose and as a basis for making decisions about whether further behavior changes are needed (Wing, Epstein, Nowalk, & Lamparski, 1986).

To determine whether adding SMBG techniques to a behavioral weight loss program would improve weight loss and/or glycemic control, Wing and colleagues (Wing, Epstein, Nowalk, Scott, et al., 1986) recruited 50 Type II diabetic patients and randomly assigned them either to our standard behavioral weight loss program or to a weight control program that included self-monitoring of blood glucose. The weight loss condition focused on weight loss as the goal of therapy. Their contracts were refunded contingent on weight loss and changes in eating and exercise habits. Blood glucose levels were checked at weekly treatment meetings and used as the basis for adjusting diabetes medication or insulin; however, patients were not given goals for blood sugar and no praise or reinforcement was given for blood sugar control.

Patients in the weight loss plus SMBG condition were given monitoring equipment and taught to monitor their blood glucose four times/week (two preprandial and two postprandial measures). Since blood glucose levels are quite stable in Type II diabetic patients, this schedule is considered sufficient to allow patients to determine their current level of glycemic control. Patients in the weight loss plus SMBG condition were given goals for blood sugar control and were refunded portions of their deposit for complying with SMBG and achieving improvements in glycemic control. These patients were taught to observe relationships between diet, exercise, weight, and glycemic control, and to make changes in their diet and exercise if glucose levels were elevated.

There was no evidence from this study that adding SMBG to the program improved outcome. Weight losses of the two conditions did not differ significantly at posttreatment (−6.8 kg for weight control condition and −5.8 kg for weight loss plus SMGB condition) or 1 year (−8.2 kg for weight loss condition and −4.1 kg for weight loss plus SMBG condition). Changes in HbA_1 and reductions in medication were also similar in the two treatment conditions. The failure to achieve effects of monitoring did not seem to be due to problems with accuracy or compliance to these techniques. A better explanation seemed to be that patients were monitoring their glucose levels, but were not using the information to make changes in their intake or exercise. Therefore, a second study was designed to provide more extensive training in how to use the information from self-monitoring (Wing, Epstein, Nowalk, & Scott, 1988).

Patients in this second study were all provided with meters for monitoring their blood glucose and asked to complete 12 SMBG readings/ week. In addition, all patients participated in our standard behavioral weight control program and were given calorie and exercise goals and taught strategies for changing these behaviors.

Half of the patients were randomly assigned to a self-monitoring only condition; these patients recorded their blood glucoses but were not given goals for blood sugar nor instructions on how to use the SMBG information to adjust intake or exercise behaviors. In contrast, patients assigned to the self-regulation condition were given extensive training in how to use the information from glucose monitoring. During the initial weeks of their program, these patients were given homework assignments designed to illustrate the effect of diet and exercise on blood sugar. Later, they were given goals for blood sugar and asked to determine which of their readings were within the "fair" or "good" range. If blood glucose readings were outside this range, patients were instructed to earn a specified number of points by making behavior changes. For example, if one, two, or three readings were outside the goal, patients were instructed to achieve three, four, or five points, respectively. Points could be obtained by increasing exercise (1 point for each 10 min of additional exercise), decreasing intake (1 point for each 50 calories of additional reduction), increasing fiber, or decreasing sugar. It should be noted that patients were not instructed to alter their diabetes medication. Rather, to maintain similarity between the two conditions, all medication changes were made by a physician using a standard algorithm.

Again, this study provided no evidence that training in SMBG and specific instructions in how to use the SMBG information improved outcome. Both groups experienced improvements in weight (-7 kg for self-monitoring only and -5.1 kg for self-regulation condition) and HbA_1 (-2.1% and -1.6%, respectively) at posttreatment. At 1-year follow-up, weight loss averaged 3.7 and 3.9 kg in the two conditions. Neither condition achieved long-term changes in HbA_1.

There are several explanations for the failure to find an effect of SMBG training in these studies. It may be that for Type II diabetic patients, the majority of improvements in control occurs very quickly after starting a diet and that further changes in blood glucose are not closely related to changes in diet and exercise. Thus, despite improvements in intake and exercise, some patients may experience no change or even deterioration in glycemic control. Alternatively, the feedback provided from SMBG may not be sufficient to promote long-term changes in behavior. Patients may see their glucose increasing, know what they are supposed to do, but not make the necessary behavior changes. Further research is needed to distinguish between these alternatives.

Spouse Support

In a recent study of regimen adherences in Type II diabetic patients, Glasgow and Toobert (1988) reported that family support was the strongest and most consistent predictor of adherence. Therefore, efforts to teach other members of the family to be supportive of the diabetic patients' efforts may help to promote long-term dietary adherences.

Several investigators have tried to use the spouse as a source of ongoing social support for nondiabetic participants in behavioral weight loss programs. Brownell and colleagues (Brownell, Heckerman, Westlake, Hayes, & Monti, 1978) found that patients who were treated with their spouse lost 13.6 kg at 6-month follow-up, while those treated without their spouse lost 8.6 kg and those whose spouses refused to participate lost 6.8 kg. Subsequent efforts to replicate these findings have produced mixed results (Brownell & Stunkard, 1981; Pearce, LeBow, & Orchard, 1981).

However, in previous studies of spouse support, the overweight patients was given treatment in a behavioral weight control program, and the spouse, who may or may not have been overweight, was seen as a "helper." Although the spouse was asked to keep records of whether the patient was completing the self-monitoring assignments and was instructed in ways to reinforce the patients' efforts, the spouse was not asked to make changes in his/her own behavior.

Based on the successful interventions of Epstein and colleagues (e.g., Epstein, Wing, Koeske, Andrasik, & Ossip, 1981) that show that targeting both an overweight parent and child for weight loss is more effective than targeting either the child or parent alone, we reasoned that better long-term effects might be obtained if both the patient and spouse were targeted for weight loss.

To test this possibility, we (Marcus et al., 1988) recruited 49 obese Type II diabetic patients, all of whom had overweight spouses (with or without diabetes) who were willing to participate in our behavioral treatment program. These patients were randomly assigned to be treated alone or with their spouse. In the latter condition, both patients and spouses were given intake and exercise goals, and contracts were refunded for weight loss and homework completion in both the patient and the spouse. In addition, the couples program included training in listening skills, and strategies for offering and eliciting social support.

Forty-three of the 49 couples completed the full year of study. Weight losses of patients treated alone or with the spouse did not differ at posttreatment (9.1 vs. 8.7 kg) or at 1-year follow-up (5.3 vs. 3.8 kg). There was thus no evidence to support the hypothesis that treating the patient together with the spouse would improve outcome. As expected, spouses who participated in the program lost more weight than those who were excluded (14.2 vs. 2.3 kg at posttreatment and 7.6 vs. 1.7 kg at 1 year), and as discussed earlier, the participating spouses also lost more weight than the patients.

When we examined the correlation between the long-term weight loss of patients and spouses, we found that the correlations at 1-year were nonsignificant in both groups. Thus, the long-term outcome for the patient appeared independent of the spouses' outcome in both treatment conditions. These data raise questions about whether, in the long term, spouse support is really an important factor in weight control.

Very Low Calorie Diet Regimen

Recently, we have also been studying the use of very low calorie diets (VLCD) in the treatment of Type II diabetic patients. These diets, which limit consumption to 400 kcal/day of high-quality protein, have been shown to be safe when used for limited periods of time, with careful medical monitoring and in carefully selected patients (Wadden, Stunkard, & Brownell, 1983). These diets are also very effective in producing initial weight loss. A randomized, controlled trial by Wadden and Stunkard (1986) showed, however, that patients treated with very low calorie diets alone lost weight initially (mean = 14.1 kg), but rapidly regained their weight losses (weight loss at 1-year follow-up of 4.6 kg). In contrast, patients treated with a very low calorie diet in combination with behavior modification lost a great deal of weight initially (−19.3 kg) and maintained a loss of 12.9 kg at 1-year follow-up. The combination condition produced better results than behavior modification alone at the end of treatment, but not at 1-year follow-up. Behavior modification alone produced losses of 14.3 kg at the end of treatment and 9.5 kg at follow-up. Thus, while the combination of behavior modification plus VLCD was more successful than VLCD alone, it remains unclear whether it is more successful than behavior therapy alone in the long term.

To answer this, and investigate the effectiveness of a VLCD diet with Type II diabetic patients, we (Wing, Salata, Marcus, Nowalk, & Miaskiewicz, 1988) recruited 36 Type II diabetic patients and randomly assigned them either to our standard behavioral weight loss program or to a behavioral program which included 8 weeks on the VLCD. Both groups met weekly for 20 weeks. At the end of the 20-week program, the patients in the combined condition had lost 18.5 kg, compared to 9.8 kg ($p < .002$) in the behavior modification only condition. Both conditions had significant improvement in HbA_1, but these improvements were obtained with 93% of patients in the combination condition off medication (and treated with diet only) compared to only 33% of the behavioral group ($p < .001$). Long- terms data are not yet available, but the key question is whether this combination program is also effective in the long term.

Predictors of Outcome

In addition to systematically examining the effect of specific components of behavioral weight loss programs, our group has also tried to identify patients characteristics that might be associated with outcome.

Analyses were conducted across studies ($N = 178$) to determine whether sex, age (<40 yrs, >40 yrs), years diabetic (<2 yrs, 2–5 yrs, ≥5 yrs), percent overweight (<40%, 40–59%, 60–80%, >80%), medication (diet, oral, insulin), or fasting blood glucose (<200 mg/dl, >200 mg/dl) were related to outcome in our program. These analyses showed that the only variable related to short- or long-term weight loss was sex; males lost more weight in our program than females (9.5 kg for males and 6.3 kg for females at posttreatment and 7.0 kg vs. 3.8 kg at 1 year). Males, however, did not have greater changes in body mass index or percent overweight. The finding that males lose more weight than females has been reported previously for both diabetic (Heitzmann, Kaplan, Wilson, & Sandler, 1987) and nondiabetic (Jeffery et al., 1978) subjects and seems to be due in part to differences in initial body weight.

It is of interest to note that we have found no evidence that patients treated with insulin have more difficulty losing weight. Previous studies, including the UGDP (1971), have suggested that insulin therapy may impede weight loss, and a recent study found that patients on insulin lost less weight during 6-weeks on a very low calorie diet regimen (Harris, Davidson, & Bush, 1988). In contrast, we find the weight losses of patients treated with diet only, oral medication, or insulin are 8.7 kg, 6.7 kg, and 7.4 kg, respectively, at posttreatment and 5.5 kg, 4.1 kg, and 5.5 kg, respectively, at 1 year. None of these weight losses differ significantly from each other.

The difference between previous studies and our study may be due to differences in treatment duration. Moreover, in our program, we measure glucose at weekly intervals and adjust medication as needed to maintain good control. This frequent adjustment may help reduce occurrences of hypoglycemia and/or hyperinsulinemia.

We have also tried to determine whether any of these pretreatment patient characteristics affect the magnitude of change in glucose for a given weight loss. Previous studies suggested that recent onset patients (diagnosis made <2 years previously) benefited more from weight reduction than those patients who have had diabetes for 5 years or more (Nagulasparen, Savage, Bennion, Unger, & Bennett, 1981). However, we find no evidence to support this.

Rather, the pretreatment characteristic which had the greatest effect on improvement in control in our studies was initial blood glucose level; patients who were in the worst control to begin with experienced the greatest improvements in control.

We have also examined the effect of family history of diabetes on outcome. As discussed above, family history of diabetes appears to interact with obesity in determining the incidence of Type II diabetes, but data are not available on whether patients with a family history of Type II diabetes experience less improvement in control with a given weight loss. To examine this, we compared the response of 44 patients who had no parental history of diabetes, 25 with one diabetic parent, and 8 with 2 diabetic parents. We found that short- and long-term weight losses of these three groups were similar, as were the improvements in control (Wing, Epstein, Nowalk, Scott, & Gooding, 1987).

Finally, we have examined behavioral factors that might be related to outcome. All patients in our program complete the Eating Behavior Inventory (EBI) at pretreatment, posttreatment, and 1-year follow-up. The EBI (O'Neil et al., 1979) is a self-report instrument that asks about frequency of use of specific behavioral weight control strategies (e.g., recording intake, daily weighing, shopping from a list). We (Guare, Gooding, Blair, & Burton, 1988) found no relationship between pretreatment scores on the EBI and success in the program. However, patients who made the greatest improvements in eating behaviors from pretreatment to posttreatment ($r = -.33$, $p < .001$) and from pretreatment to 1 year ($r = -.25$, $p < .001$) experienced the greatest weight losses. Moreover, we identified four strategies that seemed to be most clearly related to weight loss at both time points. The four key strategies were: I eat foods that I believe will aide me in losing weight; I record the type and quantity of food I eat; I refuse food offered to me by others; I eat and just can't seem to stop (scored in reverse). Perhaps these four techniques should be given greater stress in behavioral treatment strategies, and other techniques, that were not related to weight loss, should be deemphasized.

Conclusion

It is important that greater attention be given to the development of effective weight control programs for Type II diabetic patients. This is a patient group that clearly can benefit from weight reduction, in terms of improvements in glycemic control, changes in other CHD risk factors, and improvements in mood. From the research conducted to date, it appears that treatment programs combining behavior modification, diet, and exercise produce the best long-term results. Further study is needed to determine whether the use of the VLCD is also warranted. Other strategies that have been examined, including involving the spouse in the treatment program and providing training in self-monitoring of blood glucose, appear to have little or no effect on outcome.

At present, it is unclear whether the strategies used in treating diabetic patients should differ in any way from those used with nondiabetics. The data discussed above suggest that diabetics may have more difficulty losing weight than nondiabetics, but the mechanism explaining this difference is not established. Moreover, diabetic patients seem to respond to interventions, such as very low calorie diets, in a manner similar to nondiabetics. As noted above, these patients do require more medical supervision for frequent adjustment in diabetes and hypertensive medications.

There are many important issues remaining in this area of investigation. The first, of course, is the development of more effective weight loss interventions. While some of the studies discussed above have produced weight losses of approximately 10 kg at 1 year, these results are still far from ideal. Second, it remains unclear whether modest weight losses maintained over 3–5 years will produce continued improvements in glycemic control. The effects of weight loss appear to be most dramatic initially and the long-term impact is unclear. Thus, it may be important to study ways in which weight loss and/or periodic episodes of caloric restriction can be used to promote long-term glycemic control. Finally, it is important to know whether weight reduction in patients at risk for diabetes could prevent or postpone the onset of this disease.

References

Bennett, P.H., Knowler, W.C., Pettitt, D.J., Garraher, M.J., & Vasquez, B. (1982). Longitudinal studies of the development of diabetes in the Pima Indians. In E. Eschwege (ed.) *Advances in diabetes epidemiology* (p. 65–74). Amsterdam: Elsevier Biomedical Press.

Bogardus, C., Ravussin, E., Robbins, D.C., Wolfe, R.R., Horton, E.S., & Sims, E.A.H. (1984). Effects of physical training and diet therapy on carbohydrate metabolism in patients with glucose intolerance and non-insulin-dependent diabetes mellitus. *Diabetes, 33,* 311–318.

Brownell, K.D., Heckerman, C.L., & Westlake, R.J. (1979). The behavioral control of obesity: A descriptive analysis of a large-scale program. *Journal of Clinical Psychology, 35,* 864–869.

Brownell, K.D., Heckerman, C.L., Westlake, R.J., Hayes, S.C., & Monti, P. M. (1978). The effect of couples training and partner cooperativeness in the behavior treatment of obesity. *Behavior Research and Therapy, 16,* 323–334.

Brownell, K.D., & Stunkard, A.J. (1981). Couples training, pharmacotherapy, and behavior therapy in the treatment of obesity. *Archives of General Psychiatry, 38,* 1224–1229.

Brownell, K.D., & Wadden, T.A. (1986). Behavior therapy for obesity: Modern approaches and better results. In K.B. Brownell & J.P. Foreyt (Eds.), *Handbook of Eating Disorders: Physiology, Psychology, & Treatment of Obesity, Anorexia and Bulimia.* (pp. 180–198). New York: Basic Books.

Colwell, J.A., Halushka, P.V., Sarji, K., Levine, J., Sagel, J., & Raghaven, M. G. (1976). Altered platelet function in diabetes mellitus. *Diabetes, 25*(Suppl 2), 826–831.

Dahlkoetter, J., Callahan, E.J., & Linton, J. (1979). Obesity and the unbalanced energy equation: Exercise vs. eating habit change. *Journal of Consulting and Clinical Psychology, 47,* 898–905.

Epstein, L., Wing, R., Koeske, R, Andrasik, F., & Ossip, D. (1981). Child and parent weight loss in family-based behavior modification programs. *Journal of Consulting and Clinical Psychology, 49,* 674–685.

Epstein, L.H., Wing, R.R., Koeske, R., & Valoski, A. (1984). Effects of diet plus exercise on weight change in parents and children. *Journal of Consulting and Clinical Psychology, 52,* 429–437.

Foreyt, J.P., Mitchell, R.E., Garner, D.T., Gee, M., Scott, L.W., & Gotto, A. M. (1982). Behavioral treatment of obesity: Results and limitations. *Behavior Therapy, 13,* 153–161.

Glasgow, R.E., & Toobert, D.J. (1988). Social environment and regimen adherence among Type II diabetic patients. *Diabetes Care, 11,* 377–386.

Greenfield, M., Kolterman, O., Olefsky, J.M., & Reaven, M. (1978). The effect of ten days of fasting on various aspects of carbohydrate metabolism in obese diabetic subjects with significant fasting hyperglycemia. *Metabolism, 27*(12), 1839–1852.

Guare, J., Gooding, W., Blair, E., & Burton, L. (1988). Which behaviors should we change? *Diabetes, 37,* 17A.

Harris, M.D., Davidson, M.B., & Bush, M.A. (1988). Exogenous insulin therapy slows weight loss in Type II diabetic patients. *International Journal of Obesity, 12*(2), 149–156.

Harris, M.B., & Hallbauer, E.S. (1973). Self-directed weight control through eating and exercise. *Behavior Research and Therapy, 11,* 523–529.

Hartwell, S.L., Kaplan, R.M., & Wallace, J.P. (1986). Comparison of behavioral interventions for control of Type II diabetes mellitus. *Behavior Therapy, 17,* 447–461.

Hartz, A.J., Rupley, D.C., Kalkhoff, R.D., & Rimm, A.A. (1983). Relationship of obesity to diabetes: influence of obesity level and body fat distribution. *Preventive Medicine, 12,* 351–357.

Heitzmann, C.A., Kaplan, R.M., Wilson, D.K., & Sandler, J. (1987). Sex differences in weight loss among adults with Type II diabetes mellitus. *Journal of Behavioral Medicine, 10*(1), 197–211.

Henry, R.R., Scheaffer, L., & Olefsky, J.M. (1985). Glycemic effects of intensive caloric restriction and isocaloric refeeding in noninsulin-dependent diabetes mellitus. *Journal of Clinical Endocrinology and Metabolism, 61*(5), 917–925.

Henry, R.R., Wiest-Kent, T.A., Scheaffer, L., Kolterman, O.G., & Olefsky, J. M. (1986). Metabolic consequences of very-low-calorie diet therapy in obese non-insulin-dependent diabetic and nondiabetic subjects. *Diabetes, 35,* 155–164.

Hughes, T.A., Gwynne, J.T., Switzer, B.R., Herbst, C., & White, G. (1984). Effects of caloric restriction and weight loss on glycemic control, insulin release and resistance, and atherosclerotic risk in obese patients with Type II diabetes mellitus. *American Journal of Medicine, 77,* 7–17.

Jeffery, R.W., Wing, R.R., & Stunkard, A.J. (1978). Behavioral treatment of obesity: The state of the art 1976. *Behavior Therapy, 9,* 189–199.

Kannel, W.B. (1982). Diabetes as a risk factor for atherosclerotic cardiovascular disease. In B.N. Brodoff & S.J. Bleicher (Eds.). *Diabetes and the Heart* (pp. 735–740). Baltimore: Williams & Wilkins.

Kempner, W., Peschel, R.L., & Schlayer, C. (1958). Effect of rice diet on diabetes mellitus associated with vascular disease. *Postgraduate Medicine, 24,* 359.

Marcus, M.D., Wing, R.R., Nowalk, M.P., Salata, R., Bayles, M., Pambianco, G., & Guare, J. (1987). Adding exercise to a diet program improves weight loss, but not glycemic control, in Type II diabetic subjects. *Diabetes, 36,* 88A.

Marcus, M.D., Wing, R.R., Nowalk., M.P., Blair, E., Guare, J., & McDermott, M. (1988). Spouse support in the treatment of Type II diabetes. *Diabetes, 37,* 17A.

Nagulesparan, M., Savage, P.J., Bennion, L.J., Unger, R.H., & Bennet, P.H. (1981). Diminished effect of caloric restriction on control of hyperglycemia with increase in known duration of Type II diabetes mellitus. *Journal of Endocrinology and Metabolism, 53*,(3), 560–568.

Nowalk, M.P., Wing, R.R., Epstein, L.H, Paternostro, M., & Kriska, A. (1984). Exercise intensity in weight loss programs for Type II diabetic. *Diabetes, 33*, 19A.

Ohlson, L.O., Larsson, B., Svarsudd, K., Welin, L., Eriksson, H., Wilhelmsen, P., Bjorntorp, P., & Tibblin, G. (1985). The influence of body fat distribution on the incidence of diabetes mellitus. *Diabetes, 34*, 1055–1058.

O'Neil, P.M., Currey, H.S., Hirsch, A.A., Malcolm, R.J., Sexauer, J.D., Riddle, F.E., & Taylor, C.I. (1979). Development and validation of the eating behavior inventory. *Journal of Behavioral Assessment, 1*, 123–132.

Paffenbarger, R.S., Wing, A.L., & Hyde, R.T. (1978). Physical activity as an index of heart attack risk in college alumni. *American Journal of Epidemiology, 108*, 161–175.

Pearce, J., LeBow, M., & Orchard, J. (1981). Role of spouse involvement in the behavioral treatment of overweight women. *Journal of Consulting and Clinical Psychology, 49*, 236–244.

Rabkin, S.W., Boyko, E., Wilson, A., & Streja, D.A. (1983). A randomized clinical trial comparing behavior modification and individual counseling in the nutritional therapy of non-insulin-dependent diabetes mellitus: Comparison of the effect on blood sugar, body weight and serum lipids. *Diabetes Care, 6*, 50–56.

Rainwater, N., Ayllon, T., Fredericksen, L.W., et al. (1982). Teaching self-management skills to increase diet compliance in diabetics. In R. Stuart (Ed.). *Adherence, compliance and generalization in behavioral medicine.* New York: Brunner/Mazel.

Salata, R., Marcus, M., Nowalk, M., & Blair, E. (1986). Mood and glycemic control in Type II diabetic patients in behavioral weight control programs. *Diabetes, 35*, 21A.

Savage, P.J., Bennion, L.J., Flock, E.V., Nagulesparan, M., Mott, D., Roth, J., Unger, R.H., & Bennett, P.H. (1979). Diet-induced improvement of abnormalities in insulin and glucagon secretion and in insulin receptor binding in diabetes mellitus. *Journal of Clinical Endocrinology and Metabolism, 48*, 999–1007.

Stalonas, P.M., Johnson, W.G., & Christ, M. (1978). Behavior modification for obesity: The evaluation of exercise, contingency management, and program adherence. *Journal of Consulting and Clinical Psychology, 46*, 463–469.

Stanik, S., & Marcus, R. (1980). Insulin secretion improves following dietary control of plasma glucose in severely hyperglycemic obese patients. *Metabolism, 29*, 346–350.

Streja, D., Boyko, E., & Rabkin, S.W. (1981). Nutrition therapy in non-insulin-dependent diabetes mellitus. *Diabetes Care, 4*, 81–84.

University Group Diabetes Program (1971). Effects of hypoglycemic agents on vascular complications in patients with adult-onset diabetes. *Journal of the American Medical Association, 218*, 1400.

Wadden, T.A., & Stunkard, A.J. (1986). Controlled trial of very low calorie diet, behavior therapy, and their combination in the treatment of obesity. *Journal of Consulting and Clinical Psychology, 54*, 482–488.

Wadden, T.A., Stunkard, A.J., & Brownell, K.D. (1983). Very low calorie diets: Their efficacy, safety, and future. *Annals of Internal Medicine, 99,* 675–684.

West, K.M. (1978). *Epidemiology of diabetes and its vascular lesions.* New York: Elsevier.

Westlund, K., & Nicholaysen, R. (1972). Ten-year mortality and morbidity related to serum cholesterol. *Scandinavian Journal of Clinical and Laboratory Investigation, 30,* 3–24.

Wing, R.R. (1985). Improving dietary adherence in patients with diabetes. In L. Jovanovic & C.M. Peterson (Eds.), *Nutrition and Diabetes* (pp. 161–186). New York: Liss.

Wing, R.R., Epstein, L.H., Nowalk, M.P., Koeske, R., & Hagg, S. (1985). Behavior change, weight loss and physiological improvements in Type II diabetic patients. *Journal of Consulting and Clinical Psychology, 53,* 111–122.

Wing, R.R., Epstein, L.H., Nowalk, M.P., & Lamparski, D.M. (1986). Behavioral self-regulation in the treatment of patients with diabetes mellitus. *Psychological Bulletin, 99,* 78–79.

Wing, R.R., Epstein, L.H., Nowalk, M.P., & Scott, N. (1988). Self-regulation in the treatment of Type II diabetes. *Behavior Therapy, 19,* 11–23.

Wing, R.R., Epstein, L.H., Nowalk, M.P., Scott, N., & Gooding, W. (1987). Family history of diabetes and its effect on treatment outcome in Type II diabetes. *Behavior Therapy, 18,* 283–289.

Wing, R.R., Epstein, L.H., Nowalk, M.P., Scott, N., Koeske, R., & Hagg, S. (1986). Does self-monitoring of blood glucose levels improve dietary compliance for obese patients with Type II diabetes? *The American Journal of Medicine, 81* 830–836.

Wing, R.R., Koeske, R., Epstein, L.H., Nowalk, M.P., Gooding, W., & Becker, D. (1987). Long-term effects of modest weight loss in Type II diabetic patients. *Archives of Internal Medicine, 147,* 1749–1753.

Wing, R.R., Marcus, M.D., Epstein, L.H., & Salata, R. (1987). Type II diabetic subjects lose less weight than their overweight nondiabetic spouses. *Diabetes Care, 10*(5), 563–566.

Wing, R.R., Salata, R., Marcus, M., Nowalk, T., & Miaskiewicz, S. (1988). A very low calorie diet (VLCD) plus behavior modification in the treatment of Type II diabetes. *Diabetes, 37,* 110A.

12

Cognitive Function in Non-Insulin-Dependent Diabetes

Lawrence C. Perlmuter, Steven H. Goldfinger, Anne R. Shore, and David M. Nathan

Patients with non-insulin-dependent diabetes mellitus (NIDDM) are likely to show selective cognitive decrements relative to age-matched controls—a relationship that has been shown in some but not all studies (cf., Mattlar, Falck, Ronnemaa & Hyyppa, 1985; Perlmuter et al., 1984). While such decrements in cognitive performance might be the result of any of several disease-related alterations in biologic function, a primary etiology may be impaired glucose control (Reaven & Thompson, 1988). The influence of glucose levels and regulation on learning and memory has been demonstrated in humans (Perlmuter, Tun, Sizer, McGlinchey & Nathan, 1987) and animals, diabetic and nondiabetic (Gold & Stone, 1988).

The purpose of this chapter is to delineate the nature of the relationship between NIDDM and cognitive function. With advancing age there is a steady, albeit slight, increase in fasting glucose levels as well as a tendency toward glucose intolerance (Andres, 1971); both of these changes, in more exaggerated degrees, occur (National Diabetes Data Group, 1979) in NIDDM. Thus, a better understanding of the relationship between NIDDM and cognitive function may help to identify the contribution of glucose metabolism to cognitive decline in normal aging as well as in diabetes.

Diabetic patients are required to continuously monitor and actively regulate their behaviors in order to limit hyperglycemic and hypoglycemic episodes and to avoid those behaviors that aggravate disease-related complications. Thus, the study of cognition in NIDDM may help guide the development of instructional programs for cognitively disadvantaged NIDDM patients, thereby enhancing patient performance through increased program effectiveness.

Compliance with instructional objectives relevant to self-care in general and glucose control in particular depends in part on memory and motivation. Indeed, the extent to which patients *attempt* to conform to instructional guidelines may be as or even more important than the degree of *success* in reaching normoglycemia per se. Irrespective of glycemic level, efforts at glycemic control appear to reduce the incidence and severity of certain complications of diabetes mellitus (Rand et al., 1985).

Methodological Considerations

Information derived from performance on cognitive tests as well as responses to self-report questionnaires may each be limited in the accuracy with which they reflect routine memory problems. Both types of instruments are subject to confounds from various sources. However, these instruments, used jointly, may provide a more accurate picture of cognitive functioning than either alone. Self-report questionnaires and laboratory or psychometric instruments may not be equivalently sensitive to cognitive deficits in their various forms; thus, the information derived from these test procedures may be discrepant. That is, performance deficits observed on cognitive laboratory tests may be harbingers of routine memory problems that have not yet reached (self) reportable levels, or performance on cognitive tests may be associated with only subtle deficits whose impact on highly practiced behaviors can be compensated for or simply ignored.

In addition, poor performance on cognitive tests may simply reflect low motivation or a lack of familiarity with the test procedure. Furthermore, test procedures may generate reactive effects such that poor performance on one test may diminish an individual's motivation, thereby degrading performance on subsequent tests (Perlmuter & Monty, 1986).

Self-report measures are also subject to a variety of confounds. For example, self-reports of memory problems may be affected by habituation, so that individuals no longer notice memory difficulties. Elevated levels of depression associated with a chronic disease such as NIDDM (Tun, Perlmuter, Russo & Nathan, 1987) may exaggerate or, in some individuals, even eradicate the perception of routine memory difficulties. Since self-reports depend on memory, the reported information may be contaminated by the very memory deficits they are designed to index. Moreover, in the interest of maintaining self-esteem, an individual's self-reports may be distorted intentionally.

Despite the aforementioned limitations, cognitive testing, (including the use of self-reports) currently provides the most comprehensive procedures for the assessment of cognitive function. The results derived from studies using performance and/or self-report procedures to investigate cognitive function in NIDDM will be reviewed below.

Cognitive Function in NIDDM

One of the earliest investigations into the association between diabetes mellitus (DM) and cognitive function was reported by Miles and Root (1922). As with many of the early studies, insulin-dependent and non-insulin-dependent diabetic patients were evaluated, but not separately. Performance on a variety of cognitive tests was impaired in diabetic patients by 5–20%. Patients reported memory loss and poor ability to concentrate. Meuter, Thomas, Gruneklee, Gries, and Lohmann (1980) evaluated cognitive function in NIDDM and IDDM patients, and reported results separately for each of these groups. A comprehensive test battery was used, the results of which were factor analyzed, accounting for 68% of the total variance. Factors included speed of reaction, memory concentration, visual perception, and quality of performance. With respect to reaction time and memory-concentration factors, performance was significantly poorer for the NIDDM group relative to a control group matched for age, gender, and education. For the factors of visual perception and the quality of performance, no significant effects of NIDDM were found.

Two studies were designed to describe the scope of cognitive difficulties in DM. In one of these, Lichty and Connell (1988) selected tasks that were presumed to reflect varying levels of cognitive complexity. Generally, IDDM patients performed as well as age-matched conrols, but NIDDM patients differed significantly on a number of tasks from age-matched controls. Specifically, accuracy of performance on a simple same/different number comparison task was significantly poorer in NIDDM patients relative to controls, as was accuracy on the digit symbol substitution task. On an analogies test designed to measure reasoning and problem-solving, performance was significantly less accurate in NIDDM. The two groups did not differ in speed of responding on any of the above tasks. On a paired associate task designed to evaluate secondary memory, NIDDM patients performed significantly poorer than controls.

On the other hand, NIDDM and controls performed similarly on a test of (verbal) primary memory. There were no significant differences on a frequency judgment task that is thought to depend on automatic processing—a putative process the parameters of which remain theoretically nebulous (Naveh-Benjamin, 1988).

Lichty and Connell (1988) proposed that NIDDM-related deficits are, in general, less likely on simple tasks but can be expected on more difficult cognitive tasks, especially if the latter involve a speed component. However, given the significant difference in accuracy between NIDDM and controls on the very simple number comparison task, this hypothesis may be premature.

Reaven and Thompson (1988) reported results from a comprehensive test battery that was factor analyzed. Four factors were identified accounting for about 75% of the total variance. One factor reflected simple motor speed (e.g., finger tapping), while a second factor was considered to reflect simple verbal ability (e.g., vocabulary and digit span). Performance as indexed by these factors was similar in NIDDM patients and age-matched controls. On the other hand, factors reflecting reasoning and learning (e.g., delayed recall) as well as complex visuospatial factors (e.g., digit symbol and trail making) were reflected in significantly poorer performance in NIDDM patients. Reaven and Thompson (1988) concluded that even relatively healthy NIDDM patients are more likely to reveal greater cognitive deficits than age-matched controls, but these are generally restricted to so-designated complex tasks.

To determine that the NIDDM-related cognitive deficits were not merely secondary to hypertension or cardiovascular disease which may be associated with measurable cognitive difficulties (cf., Elias, Robbins, Schultz, & Streeten, 1986; Farmer et al., 1987; Solomon et al., 1983), independent analyses were performed in NIDDM patients without clinical hypertension, elevated blood pressures (greater than 150/90 mm of Hg) or cardiovascular abnormalities. A subanalysis of NIDDM patients free of these abnormalities was then compared with an age-matched control group who met similar exclusion criteria. The four cognitive factors that had been identified previously were reanalyzed in these newly constituted groups. The subanalysis replicated the overall results reported earlier.

The results of Lichty and Connell, and Reaven and Thompson remain in some disagreement about the extent to which simpler cognitive processes are affected in NIDDM. To clarify the relationship between NIDDM and cognitive impairment, the most fruitful strategy may be the continued examination of various response measures in order to better define the scope of NIDDM-related cognitive problems. With that objective we will turn to a study (Perlmuter et al., 1984) that examined serial-list learning in NIDDM and age-matched controls. The task required the learning of a list of words in a fixed sequence. NIDDM patients required significantly more trials to reach the level of performance attained by the controls, i.e., learned more slowly. Within the number of trials presented, significantly fewer NIDDM patients than controls learned the entire list perfectly.

On the other hand, certain functions appear to be spared in NIDDM. When required to briefly remember a string of digits just long enough to report these back in the order in which they had been presented (forward digit span), performance was similar in both groups. However, when presented with the additional requirement to reverse the sequence of digits prior to report (backward digit span), NIDDM patients performed significantly poorer than controls. Apparently, attentional and immediate memory functioning were adequate to support equivalent levels of performance in both groups on the forward digit span. However, the added requirement of holding the digits in memory long enough to recite them in the reverse direction revealed a NIDDM-related deficit—a longer term memory deficit that may also have contributed to poorer serial learning.

Improving Performance Through Choice

Since there is evidence that arousal and motivational levels may be attenuated with advanced age (Furchtgott & Busemeyer, 1979; Weisz, 1983), we examined the possibility that NIDDM may have further weakened the process of motivation that in turn influences cognitive performance. The next study (Perlmuter & Nathan, 1988) examined the role of motivation in enhancing performance on a recognition task. The participants were 211 diabetic men and women between the ages of 55 and 74 years. They were selected from the longitudinal study conducted at the Massachusetts General Hospital in Boston. Age-matched controls ($N = 37$) were drawn from outpatient clinics at the same hospital. Parenthetically, many of the recruits in this study also participated in other studies of NIDDM, aging, and cognitive performance at the Massachusetts General Hospital, reported by Perlmuter and his associates in this chapter.

The task (Perlmuter & Monty, 1982) involved the presentation of 20 lines of words, in which the to-be-learned target word (one per line) was accompanied by one or three unrelated "background" words. Participants were instructed to study target words; no explicit mention was made of background words; hence the learning of these contextual stimuli may be considered "incidental."

On half the lines in this task, target words had been selected by the experimenter; that is, target words had been underlined and participants reunderlined and studied them (force lines). On the remaining lines, participants underlined the (target) word they wished to learn (choice lines). Choice and force lines were intermixed on the page. After studying the targets, an "old–new" recognition test was presented. All of the target and background words were presented individually in random order. An equal number of new words were also included in the test. The proportion of target words and the proportion of background words correctly recognized were the dependent measures. A mixed analysis of variance was used to analyze the recognition data which involved the following variables: NIDDM vs. control, choice vs. force, target vs. background, line length 2 vs. 4 words per line. All variables were within subjects except NIDDM.

The relevant features of the results are as follows: choice targets (mean % correct = 80 ± 21) were recognized better than force targets (60 ± 26%), choice background words (50 ± 25%), or force background words (36 ± 22%). Also, choice background words were recognized better than force background words. All effects were significant at $p<.05$, or better. While NIDDM was not a significant main effect, it was involved in two important interactions: NIDDM × Target/Background; NIDDM × Choice × Line Length.

On two-word force lines, NIDDM patients correctly recognized only 57% of the targets whereas controls recognized 74%, $p<.05$. When individuals selected their own target words on two-word lines, choice improved performance significantly—relative to force lines—for NIDDM patients who attained 75% correct recognition, whereas controls showed 74% correct recognition.

On four-word force lines, performance was relatively poor for both NIDDM (61% correct) and controls (60% correct). The greatest benefit of choice occurred when selections were made from four alternatives. Controls attained 94% correct target recognition while NIDDM patients reached only 85% correct, $p<.05$. Moreover, the *improvement* from four-word force to choice lines was significantly greater for controls than for NIDDM patients. When all of these data were reanalyzed with false alarms as a covariate, the results remained essentially unchanged.

In summary, these results show that choice enhances the recognition of chosen target words and nonchosen (rejected) background words, but not to equivalent levels. Similar effects have been reported with young subjects (Perlmuter & Monty, 1982). While the opportunity to choose improves target learning for NIDDM patients, the magnitude of the effects are somewhat less than they are for controls. Apparently, NIDDM attenuates the motivational effects of choice.

While the results are compatible with the notion that choice has motivational effects (Perlmuter & Monty, 1977), they nevertheless present a theoretical problem. That is, since motivation is presumed to operate as a generalized enhancer of performance (Brown, 1961), it would be expected to show similar beneficial effects with respect to performance on choice and force lines, which it did not. To examine the differential effects of choice, the following analysis is proposed.

Motivation and the Improvement in Performance

To examine the way in which choice affects performance with respect to learning of target and background stimuli in NIDDM and controls, we performed additional analyses (Perlmuter, Goldfinger, Sizer, &

Monty, 1989). The basic notion tested in these analyses is that when individuals learn target materials it is necessary, first, to distinguish or *differentiate* between target and background stimuli. Differentiation facilitates the allocation of attentional resources to target and background stimuli, in the appropriate proportions. Thus, in the process of learning target words, background words are learned concurrently, but to a different level. For example, the learning of a word (target) is often accompanied by learning its place-on-the-page (background stimulus). Acquisition of background information increases with target learning (Schulman, 1975).

The process of differentiation is presumed to be demanding of effort. Consequently, when motivation is low, the effectiveness of differentiation is diminished and interference from background stimuli may result in poorer performance, as in normal aging (Kausler & Kleim, 1978). Choice as an enhancer of motivation is expected to increase the effectiveness of differentiation, while NIDDM, which appears to be associated with a diminution in motivation, should decrease the magnitude of differentiation.

To assess the magnitude of differentiation, a difference score (mean target recognition minus mean background recognition) was calculated for choice and force lines separately.

Results showed that (target minus background) difference scores were significantly greater in the choice condition (mean difference = 30 ± 23%) than in the force condition (25 ± 22%), $t(247) = 2.98$, $p < .01$. Thus, as predicted, choice facilitates the magnitude of differentiation. In NIDDM (mean = 26 ± 19%), differentiation scores were smaller than in controls (mean = 33 ± 11%), $t(246) = 2.23$, $p < .05$. This finding is consistent with the generally decreased effectiveness of choice as a motivator in NIDDM patients.

Since differentiation is presumed to reflect a routine cognitive strategy, target/background difference scores should predict performance on other tasks. The median difference score was used to identify "low" (below median) and "high" (equal or above median) differentiators. Separate medians were calculated for force lines and choice lines because they differed significantly. Also, controls were eliminated from these analyses because, following the median splits, the small number of participants in each subgroup might have produced unreliable results. Performance on five cognitive tasks was compared for low versus high differentiators.

One test of the differentiation process involved an analysis of simple (lift) mean reaction times derived from a task in which individuals released a key in response to a tone and struck a second key located 13 cm to the right of the first. Thirty trials were presented. Mean lift (key release) times were analyzed separately from movement times—the time required to reach the second key. Results (Table 12.1) showed

Table 12.1. Mean Performance of Low and High Differentiators on Force and Choice Lines (diabetics only; force/choice = within-subject factor)

	Force		Choice	
	Low	High	Low	High
Simple reaction time (ms)	476 ± 100	437 ± 88	468 ± 101	446 ± 90
	$t(167) = 2.69$ $p < .01$		$t(167) = 1.51$ $p > .05$	
Digit symbol substitution	37.5 ± 11.8	42.6 ± 10.8	39.3 ± 11.2	41.0 ± 11.9
	$t(200) = 3.20$ $p < .01$		$t(200) = 1.08$ $p > .05$	
Digit span backward	4.22 ± 1.45	4.87 ± 1.39	4.60 ± 1.54	4.50 ± 1.36
	$t(204) = 3.28$ $p < .01$		$t(204) = 0.49$ $p > .05$	
Digit span forward	6.71 ± 1.36	6.62 ± 1.46	6.72 ± 1.51	6.61 ± 1.32
	$t(204) = 0.44$ 02p>.05		$t(204) = 0.57$ $p > .05$	
Movement time (ms)	477 ± 177	432 ± 158	481 ± 191	431 ± 144
	$t(167) = 1.75$ $p > .05$		$t(167) = 1.97$ $p > .05$	

that NIDDM patients with low difference scores (force lines) released the key more slowly than those with high difference scores. The slowing of behavior is one of the markers for cognitive decline in normal aging (Light, 1975) and appears to be associated with poorer differentiation.

Another test of the predictive utility of the differentiation process derived from an analysis of performance on the digit symbol test. Performance on this test decreases with age and in NIDDM (Tun et al., 1987). The test reflects a number of putative processes including distractability (Erber, 1986). Results showed that NIDDM patients with high difference scores (force lines) correctly transcribed significantly more symbols than those with low difference scores (Table 12.1). Apparently, individuals who are more successful at distinguishing or differentiating between target stimuli and background stimuli (high difference scores) are also more proficient at overcoming interference from background stimuli and therefore show better digit–symbol performance.

The next task (background digit span) required individuals to hold a string of digits in memory long enough to reverse the order of their output relative to the sequence in which they had been presented. Results showed that individuals with high difference scores correctly stored longer strings of digits in memory than those with low difference scores (Table 12.1). These results extend the predictive utility of differentiation to an untimed task.

On the other hand, two measures that are relatively unaffected by practice or learning (forward digit span, a measure of working memory capacity, and movement times) were not predicted by difference scores (Table 12.1).

If differentiation is a (learned) cognitive strategy, then it would be expected that individuals with more years of education or with higher vocabulary scores might have learned to differentiate more effectively. On the other hand, those with high difference scores might pursue more formal education or engage more frequently in tasks that would increase vocabulary. While the direction of causality is unclear, those with high difference scores had more years of formal education (low, $M = 11.6 \pm 3.6$; high, $M = 12.7 \pm 2.8$; $t(207) = 2.40$, $p < .05$), as well as higher vocabulary scores (low, $M = 39.2 \pm 14.9$; high, $M = 48.5 \pm 14.7$; $t(198) = 4.43$, $p < .01$).

It is apparent that difference scores from force lines are predictive of performance on various tasks, while scores derived from choice lines are not. It is assumed that difference scores from force lines reflect the typical strength of the differentiation process, whereas such scores from choice lines have been inflated by choice and their predictive utility has thereby been diminished. It will be recalled that difference scores were greater on choice than on force lines.

In summary, it appears that in addition to other variables, reduced motivation mediates poorer performance in NIDDM. To the extent that differentiation is an effort demanding process, its diminished strength in NIDDM is consistent with reduced motivation, lessened ability to concentrate and generally poorer performance. Indeed, it is not surprising that individuals with a chronic disease such as NIDDM are less responsive motivationally to an opportunity to choose, when control over their lives is undermined chronically.

NIDDM and Information Retrieval From Long-Term Memory

The results presented to this point have been derived from tasks in which NIDDM patients and controls were instructed to encode and then retrieve recently learned information from memory. If encoding is compromised as it may be in NIDDM, the quality of the information to be retrieved is necessarily diminished. To minimize possible restrictions in the quality of performance attributable to encoding, the next study examined the recall of information learned much earlier, perhaps even prior to the (onset) diagnosis of NIDDM.

Perlmuter et al. (1987) compared the performance of NIDDM patients and age-matched controls on a measure of verbal fluency, a task sensitive to specific neuropsychological pathologies (Borkowski, Benton, & Spreen, 1967). The verbal fluency task involved generating as many words as possible beginning with the letters "S" or "F" within a limited time interval. While no significant retrieval deficit was found with respect to the number of unique words each group generated, NIDDM patients *repeated* significantly more words than controls. It is plausible that NIDDM patients forgot the previous recitations or that they were less attentive to their own recitations. Indeed, one age-related sign of cognitive decline is the poorer recognition that a particular utterance was self-generated (see McFarland, Warren, & Crockard, 1985). Whether increased repetitions are primarily attributable to forgetting or are secondary to reduced behavioral monitoring (Perlmuter & Langer, 1982) remains to be investigated. In any case, the phenomenon appears to be more prevalent in NIDDM.

NIDDM and Self-Reported Memory Problems

We selected tasks to provide analogues for evaluating some of the cognitive processes that may be required for the execution of daily activities. To assess, more directly, possible NIDDM influences on daily cognitive functioning, we turned to a self-report procedure (Tun et al., 1987). The participants were recruited from the longitudinal study at the Massachusetts General Hospital. Self-reported memory problems, depression, and cognitive performance were examined.

Compared to an age-matched outpatient control group, NIDDM patients reported more frequent memory problems on the Short Inventory of Memory Experiences (SIME), and more severe problems on the Memory Problem Inventory (Perlmuter, Tenney, & Smith, 1980). Next, the subscales of the SIME were examined separately and these showed that momentary absentmindedness, problems recognizing people, and recalling errands were more frequently encountered by NIDDM patients than by controls, p's $< .05$. In addition, NIDDM patients tended to report more frequent problems in recalling conversations, $p = .06$.

To examine other variables that might be associated with self-reported memory problems, depression scores and performance on selected cognitive tests were examined next. Results showed that NIDDM patients were significantly more depressed than controls, as measured by the overall score on the Zung Depression Scale. Examination of a number of cognitive tasks (some of which were described previously by Perlmuter et al., 1984) revealed significantly poorer performance by NIDDM patients on the backward digit span and digit symbol substitution tests, and on a serial list learning task; however, no significant differences were found on the forward digit span or on a simple reaction time task. Scores on the two self-report memory problem questionnaires were each correlated significantly with performance on the serial-list learning task and on the reaction time measure, such that increased frequency or severity of problems was associated with poorer performance. SIME scores were also correlated with performance on the backward digit span. Higher depression scores were significantly correlated with more frequent and severe memory problems. Higher depression scores also correlated significantly with poorer performance on the digit symbol, serial learning, and reaction time tasks.

When depression scores were statistically controlled (partial correlation), correlations between the SIME and performance measures were no longer significant. Self-reports and cognitive performance appear to be relatively independent. Apparently, the relationship between test performance and self-reported memory problems is mediated through depression.

We performed multiple regression analyses to determine the extent to which self-reported memory problems and poorer cognitive performance in NIDDM were secondary to elevated depression. After the effects of depression were removed, NIDDM accounted for poorer performance only on the digit symbol task and on serial-list learning; after controlling for depression, NIDDM was no longer a significant predictor of self-reported memory problems. Thus, the depression associated with NIDDM appears to account for some, but not all, of the cognitive problems that accompany the disease. The mediating role of depression in a chronic disease such as NIDDM (Geringer, Perlmuter, Stern, & Nathan, 1988) or parkinsonism (Dakof & Mendelsohn, 1986) raises questions about the interpretation of results from other studies (e.g., Reaven & Thompson, 1988) which purport to show that NIDDM is associated with a rather broad set of cognitive problems. Such studies must consider the role of confounders before conclusions are drawn about the targeted relationships. On the other hand, if the objective of the research is to characterize the cognitive functioning of NIDDM patients versus controls, then it may be acceptable to directly compare the respective groups, while explicitly recognizing that such patients differ from controls in more than one respect.

Failures to Find NIDDM-Related Cognitive Deficits

The only other study (Mattlar et al., 1985) to assess self-reported difficulties associated with daily living as well as neuropsychological and cognitive functioning failed to find an association between NIDDM and test performance. This outcome was especially surprising in view of the significantly higher depression scores in the NIDDM patients. A number of tasks such as lifting, bedmaking, and so on, were reported by NIDDM patients to be more difficult to perform. Whether this report of increased difficulty reflects higher depression or greater physical impairments in NIDDM cannot be deduced.

The failure (Mattlar et al., 1985) to find a NIDDM-related cognitive decrement may be the consequence of stringent exclusion criteria whereby more than 60% of NIDDM patients were ineligible to participate because of hypertension, or the use of insulin therapy. This latter exclusion may have little impact on the results since Perlmuter et al. (1984) showed that cognitive function was similar irrespective of therapy, including insulin. While excluding hypertensive patients may help focus on the specific role of diabetes, such a sample would be atypical, admitting only about 40% of its potential subjects.

Robertson-Tchabo, Arenberg, Tobin, & Plotz, (1986) also failed to find a NIDDM-associated cognitive deficit in a group of men, the majority of whom were college educated. In addition to assessing vocabulary scores, an untimed test of memory for designs was used. Analyses of the error scores failed to distinguish NIDDM patients from controls either cross sectionally or longitudinally. The only other study to examine the association between NIDDM and cognitive functioning cross sectionally and longitudinally found cross-sectional effects but no evidence, in a 3-year period, for a more rapid decline in cognitive function in NIDDM patients relative to age-matched controls (Perlmuter & Nathan, 1988).

The reasons for the lack of association between NIDDM and cognitive function in Robertson-Tchabo et al. are not apparent. However, the participants were more educated on average than those in other studies and the limited cognitive protocol may have failed to be sensitive to subtle cognitive decrements, even over a 12-year period. Further, as the authors suggest, it is possible that treatment for NIDDM began earlier in their subjects than it might have for other individuals who are not members of a longitudinal study on aging in which continual medical monitoring occurs. However, this speculation remains as such since no measures of metabolic control or disease duration were presented.

Cognitive Function and Metabolic Control in NIDDM

We reported that (Perlmuter et al., 1984) higher levels of hemoglobin Alc were weakly associated, albeit significantly, with slower learning on a serial learning task. Fasting glucose levels showed a similar (inverse) relationship with performance, but the correlation was not significant. Reaven and Thompson, (1988) found that fasting plasma glucose concentration as well as hemoglobin Alc were negatively associated with the reasoning/learning factor only. On the other hand, Lichty and Connell (1988) found no association between glucose levels at the time of testing and cognitive performance.

In summary, there appears to be an association between levels of chronic glucose control and cognitive function in NIDDM. Whether acute glucose levels affect cognitive function is not clear.

Another metabolic variable that we studied was the effects of elevated triglycerides on cognitive function (Perlmuter et al., 1988). Triglycerides are not only elevated in NIDDM but they also appear to be an independent risk factor for atherosclerosis. The cognitive performance of NIDDM patients with high triglyceride levels (>250 mg/dl) was compared with that of NIDDM patients with low triglyceride levels (≤250 mg/dl). NIDDM patients with triglyceride levels greater than 500 mg/dl were eliminated from the analyses because they were suspected of having a genetic form of hyperlipidemia.

Performance (Table 12.2) of the high triglyceride group was significantly worse than that of the low triglyceride group on the backward digit span, the digit symbol substitution task, and a simple reaction time measure. Performance on the forward digit span was in the predicted direction, but failed to reach significance.

We also investigated whether the low and high triglyceride groups differed on selected biomedical variables that could confound the relationship between lipids and cognitive function. There were no significant differences between low and high triglyceride groups in fasting plasma glucose, hemoglobin Alc, obesity, presence of background retinopathy, or peripheral vascular disease. In addition, there were no differences in these groups with respect to chronological age, disease duration, age at diagnosis of NIDDM, or type of therapy used. The high triglyceride group, however, showed significantly higher choles-

Table 12.2. Cognitive Test Performance: Comparisons of Low and High Triglyceride Groups

	Low Triglyceride	High Triglyceride	
Digit symbol substitution	$\bar{X}=41.3 \pm 12.2$ ($N=177$)	$\bar{X}=34.4 \pm 8.8$ ($N=41$)	$t=3.43$ $^*p<.005$
Digit span forward	$\bar{X}=6.7 \pm 1.4$ ($N=184$)	$\bar{X}=6.4 \pm 1.5$ ($N=43$)	$t=1.05$ $^*p>.05$
Digit span backward	$\bar{X}=4.6 \pm 1.5$ ($N=184$)	$\bar{X}=3.9 \pm 1.3$ ($N=43$)	$t=2.85$ $^*p<.01$
Reaction time	$\bar{X}=457.5 \pm 91.2$ ($N=156$)	$\bar{X}=500.1 \pm 155.0$ ($N=32$)	$t=2.10$ $^*p<.05$

*2-tailed probability.

terol levels and also included significantly more patients with hypertension.

To determine whether the relationship between triglyceride levels and performance was confounded by the aforementioned biomedical variables, we conducted separate covariance analyses for each of these. Significantly poorer performance in the high triglyceride group remained evident even when these covariates were entered. However, with plasma glucose as the covariate, the difference in reaction time between low and high triglyceride groups became only marginally significant ($p = .05$). When obesity served as the covariate, reaction times no longer differed significantly between low and high triglyceride groups. Therefore, elevated triglyceride levels in NIDDM appear to be a risk factor for cognitive dysfunction, with relative independence of glucose control or other physiological sequelae of NIDDM.

Summary and Conclusion

To characterize cognitive status in NIDDM is difficult for two reasons. First, even among those studies that report poorer performance in NIDDM, there are inconsistencies. Some studies failed to find any evidence for diminished performance in NIDDM. Second, unless statistically controlled, elevated depression levels can confound the basic relationship between NIDDM and cognitive performance. For example, after controlling for depression, the significantly greater severity and frequency of routine memory problems in NIDDM was no longer significant. Moreover, the scope of cognitive decline was reduced after depression was controlled. Notwithstanding these limitations, performance on relatively complex tasks including digit symbol, paired associate, serial learning, and problem-solving reflect significant NIDDM-related deficits. On simpler tasks such as reaction time and the forward—but not the backward—digit span, performance is generally similar in NIDDM and controls.

While poor glucose control (hemoglobin Alc) within NIDDM is associated with significantly poorer performance on more complex tasks, such effects are relatively weak. Other NIDDM-related variables including type of therapy, disease duration, or age at onset are not significantly associated with performance. On the other hand, elevated levels of triglycerides within NIDDM are associated with a variety of cognitive problems.

Finally, performance can be significantly improved by increasing the individual's perception of control; however, such motivational interventions appear to be somewhat less effective in NIDDM than in controls. Whether interventions to reduce depression and to increase glucose control can forestall or reverse NIDDM-related cognitive problems remains to be investigated.

Acknowledgments. Research support for this work was provided by the National Institute on Aging (Grant, AGO2300) and VA Medical Research Service. The contributions of Nancy Sizer, M.S., to this research are acknowledged gratefully.

References

Andres, R. (1971). Aging and diabetes. *Medical Clinics in North America, 55,* 835–845.

Borkowski, J.G., Benton, A.L., & Spreen, O. (1967). Word fluency and brain damage. *Neuropsychologia, 5,* 135–140.

Brown, J.S. (1961). *The motivation of behavior.* New York: McGraw-Hill.

Dakof, G.A., & Mendelsohn, G.A. (1986). Parkinson's disease: The psychological aspects of a chronic illness. *Psychological Bulletin, 99,* 375–387.

Elias, M.F., Robbins, M.A., Schultz, N.R., Jr., & Streeten, D.H.P. (1986). A longitudinal study of neuropsychological test performance for hypertensive and normotensive adults: Initial findings. *Journal of Gerontology, 41,* 503–505.

Erber, J.T. (1986). Age-related effects of spatial contiguity and interference on coding performance. *Journal of Gerontology, 41,* 641-644.

Farmer, M.E., White, L.R., Abbott, R.D., Kittner, S.J., Kaplan, E., Wolz, M.M., Brody, J.A., & Wolf, P.A. (1987). Blood pressure and cognitive performance. *American Journal of Epidemiology, 126,* 1103–1114.

Furchtgott, E., & Busemeyer, J.K. (1979). Heart rate and skin conductance during cognitive processes as a function of age. *Journal of Gerontology, 34,* 183–190.

Geringer, E.S., Perlmuter, L.C., Stern, S.A., & Nathan, D.M. (1988). Depression and diabetic neuropathy: A complex relationship. *Journal of Geriatric Psychiatry and Neurology, 1,* 11–15.

Gold, P.E., & Stone, W.S. (1988). Neuroendocrine effects on memory in aged rodents and humans. *Neurobiology of Aging, 9,* 709–717.

Kausler, D.H., & Kleim, D.M. (1978). Age differences in processing relevant versus irrelevant stimuli in multiple-item recognition learning. *Journal of Gerontology, 33,* 87–93.

Lichty, W., & Connell, C. (1988). *Cognitive functioning of diabetics versus nondiabetics.* Presented at the 96th Annual Convention of the American Psychological Association at Atlanta, Georgia.

Light, K.C. (1975). Slowing of response time in young and middle-aged hypertensive patients. *Experimental Aging Research, 1,* 209–227.

Mattlar, C., Falck, B., Ronnemaa, T., & Hyyppa, M.T. (1985). Neuropsychological cognitive performance of patients with Type-2 diabetes. *Scandinavian Journal of Rehabilation Medicine, 17,* 101–105.

McFarland, C.E., Jr., Warren, L.R., & Crockard, J. (1985). Memory for self-generated stimuli in young and old adults. *Journal of Gerontology, 40,* 205–207.

Meuter, F., Thomas, W., Gruneklee, D., Gries, F.A., & Lohmann, R. (1980).

Psychometric evaluation of performance in diabetes mellitus. *Hormone and Metabolic Research Supplement, 9,* 9–17.

Miles, W.R., & Root, H.F. (1922). Psychologic tests applied to diabetic patients. *Archives of Internal Medicine, 30,* 767–777.

National Diabetes Data Group (1979). Classification and diagnosis of diabetes mellitus and other categories of glucose intolerance. *Diabetes: The Journal of the American Diabetes Association, 28,* 1039–1057.

Naveh-Benjamin, M. (1988). Recognition memory of spatial location information: Another failure to support automaticity. *Memory & Cognition, 16,* 437–445.

Perlmuter, L.C., Goldfinger, S.H., Sizer, N.R., & Monty, R.A. (1989). Choosing to improve performance. In P.S. Fry (Ed.), *Psychology of Helplessness and Control.* Amsterdam: North-Holland Publishers.

Perlmuter, L.C., Hakami, M.K., Hodgson-Harrington, C., Ginsberg, J., Katz, J., Singer, D.E., & Nathan, D.M. (1984). Decreased cognitive function in aging non-insulin-dependent diabetic patients. *The American Journal of Medicine, 77,* 1043–1048.

Perlmuter, L.C., & Langer, E.J. (1982). The effects of behavioral monitoring on the perception of control. *Clinical Gerontologist, 1,* 37–43.

Perlmuter, L.C., & Monty, R.A. (1977). The importance of perceived control: Fact or fantasy? *American Scientist, 65,* 759–765.

Perlmuter, L.C., & Monty, R.A. (1982). Contextual effects on learning and memory. *Bulletin of the Psychonomic Society, 20,* 290–292.

Perlmuter, L.C., & Monty, R.A. (1986). Vicissitudes of measurement: Depression tests, a case in point. *Journal of Social and Clinical Psychology, 4,* 475–487.

Perlmuter, L.C., & Nathan, D.M. (1988). Cross sectional and longitudinal analyses of cognitive and biomedical functioning in NIDDM. Unpublished manuscript. Tufts School of Dental Medicine.

Perlmuter, L.C., Nathan, D.M., Goldfinger, S.H., Russo, P.A., Yates, J., & Larkin, M. (1988). Triglyceride levels affect cognitive function in non-insulin dependent diabetics. *The Journal of Diabetic Complications, 2,* 210–213.

Perlmuter, L.C., Tenney, Y.J., & Smith, P.A. (1980). The evaluation and remediation of memory problems in the aged. Technical Report 80-02. Geriatric Research, Educational and Clinical Center, Veterans Administration Outpatient Clinic, Boston, MA.

Perlmuter, L.C., Tun, P., Sizer, N., McGlinchey, R.E., & Nathan, D.M. (1987). Age and diabetes related changes in verbal fluency. *Experimental Aging Research, 13,* 9–14.

Rand, L.I., Krolewski, A.S., Aiello, L.M., Warram, J.H., Baker, R.S., & Maki, T. (1985). Multiple factors in the prediction of risk of proliferative diabetic retinopathy. *The New England Journal of Medicine, 313,* 1433–1438.

Reaven, G.M., & Thompson, L.W. (1988). Reduced cognitive function in older patients with non-insulin-dependent diabetes: Relationship to severity of hyperglycemia. *Diabetes, 37* (Suppl 1), 4A.

Robertson-Tchabo, E.A., Arenberg, D., Tobin, J.D., & Plotz, J.B. (1986). A longitudinal study of cognitive performance in noninsulin dependent (Type II) diabetic men. *Experimental Gerontology, 21,* 459–467.

Schulman, A.I. (1975). Recognition memory and the recall of spatial location. *Memory and Cognition, 3,* 256–260.

Solomon, S., Hotchkiss, E., Saravay, S.M., Bayer, C., Ramsey, P., & Blum, R.S. (1983). Impairment of memory function by antihypertensive medication. *Archives of General Psychiatry, 40,* 1100–1112.

Tun, P.A., Perlmuter, L.C., Russo, P., & Nathan, D.M. (1987). Memory self-assessment and performance in aged diabetics and non-diabetics. *Experimental Aging Research, 13,* 151–157.

Weisz, J.R. (1983). Can I control it? The pursuit of veridical answers across the life span. In P.B. Baltes & O.G. Brim, Jr. (Eds.), *Life span development and behavior,* New York: Academic Press.

13

Affective Disorders and Diabetes Mellitus

Edith S. Geringer

In 1684, Thomas Willis wrote of diabetes mellitus (DM) that "Sadness, or long sorrow, as likewise convulsions, and other depressions and disorders of the animal spirits are used to generate or foment this morbid disposition" (Willis, 1684). An increased prevalence of depression among diabetics has been observed by Maudsley (1899); and Menninger (1935), Dunbar (1943) and Koranyi (1979) found DM occurred twice as frequently in a population of psychiatric patients as in the general population. However, as recently as 1983, there had not been a clear systematic study of the relationship between DM (insulin-dependent or non-insulin-dependent) and depression (Lustman, Amado, & Wetzel, 1983; Wilkinson, 1981). Likewise, there have been suggestions of an increased association between DM and manic-depressive illness (Lilliker, 1980; van der Velde & Gordon, 1969), although the evidence for this is controversial.

Affective disorders are disorders of mood. The two most common affective disorders are major depression (unipolar depression) and bipolar disorder (manic-depressive illness) (Weissman & Boyd, 1983). There are many possible mechanisms underlying an association between DM and affective disorders. In the last several years an explosion of research in psychoneuroendocrinology has provided tantalizing glimpses into the biologic underpinnings of this relationship (Carroll, Curtis, & Mendels, 1976; Cameron, Kronfol, Greden, & Carroll, 1984; Crammer & Gillies, 1981; Hudson et al., 1984; Kronfol, Greden, & Carroll, 1981; Mueller, Heninger, & McDonald, 1969; Schlesser, Winokur, & Sherman, 1980). Depression may also occur as a psychologic response to a chronic illness, or in response to a particular diabetic complication (e.g., blindness, neuropathy). Depression in diabetics may occur coincident with life stresses independent of diabetes, or, as in anyone, on the basis of a genetic predisposition to depression. While depression may sometimes seem to be an understandable response to a difficult illness, its accurate diagnosis and treatment is essential. Diabetic patients may be at increased risk of hyperglycemia and the subsequent development of microvascular complications (Lustman, Griffith, Clouse, & Cryer, 1986) when depression is inadequately treated. Treatment of depression also results in improved quality of life and compliance with medical regimens (Eraker, Kirscht, & Becker, 1984; Wing, Epstein, & Nowalk, 1986).

This chapter will explore the relationship between DM and the major affective disorders (major depression and bipolar disorder). It will focus on the evidence for an increased association between depression and affective disorders, possible mechanisms underlying this association, and the particular issues involved in the treatment of these disorders in diabetics. As very little of this literature applies only to non-insulin-dependent diabetics (NIDDM), the focus will be on studies done with adult populations since this age range encompasses most patients with NIDDM.

Definitions of Affective Disorders

Before beginning a discussion of affective disorders and diabetes it is helpful to clarify the definitions of depression and bipolar disorder. Depression may range from normal feelings of sadness, disappointment, or discouragement, to despondency or grief, to a clinical disorder of mood. Major depression, the most common psychiatric depressive syndrome (Weissman & Boyd, 1983), is an acute syndrome characterized by the presence of a depressed or hopeless mood and four of eight neurovegatative symptoms of depression for at least two weeks. Table 13.1 lists the criteria for major depression found in the *Diagnostic and Statistical Manual*, Third Edition, Revised (DSM-III-R) of the American Psychiatric Association (1987). The neurovegetative symptoms of depression include changes in appetite, sleep pattern, energy level, interest, and concentration. In medically ill patients, major depression can be difficult to diagnose accurately as many of the neurovegetative symptoms may also be caused by physical illness. Major depression should also be distinguished from dysthymia, a state of chronic depression which lasts at least 2 years and is severe enough to impair functioning but never severe enough to warrant a diagnosis of major depression.

The lifetime risk of an episode of major depression is approximately 9%–26% for women and 5%–12% for men (American Psychiatric Association, 1987). The point prevalence of major depression is 4.5%–9.3% for women and 2.3%–3.2% for men. The different rates of depression for men and women are well documented and have been re-

Table 13.1. Criteria for Major Depressive Episode (DSM-III-R)

A. At least five of the following symptoms have been present during the same 2-week period and represent a change from previous functioning; at least one of the symptoms is either (1) depressed mood or (2) loss of interest or pleasure (do not include symptoms that are clearly due to a physical condition, mood-incongruent delusions or hallucinations, incoherence, or marked loosening of associations).

1. depressed mood (or can be irritable in children and adolescents) most of the day, nearly every day, as indicated by subjective account or observation by others
2. markedly diminished interest or pleasure in all, or almost all, activities most of the day, nearly every day, as indicated by subjective account or observation by others of apathy most of the time
3. significant weight loss or weight gain when not dieting (e.g., more than 5% of body weight in a month), or decrease or increase in appetite nearly every day (in children, consider failure to make expected weight gains)
4. insomnia or hypersomnia nearly every day
5. psychomotor agitation or retardation nearly every day (observable by others, not merely subjective feelings of restlessness or being slowed down)
6. fatigue or loss of energy nearly every day
7. feelings of worthlessness or excessive or inappropriate guilt (which may be delusional) nearly every day (not merely self-reproach or guilt about being sick)
8. diminished ability to think or concentrate, or indecisiveness, nearly every day (either by subjective account or as observed by others)
9. recurrent thoughts of death (not just fear of dying), recurrent suicidal ideation without a specific plan, or a suicide attempt or a specific plan for committing suicide

B. 1. It cannot be established that an organic factor initiated and maintained the disturbance

2. The disturbance is not a normal reaction to the death of a loved one (uncomplicated bereavement)

C. At no time during the disturbance have there been delusions or hallucinations for as long as 2 weeks in the absence of prominent mood symptoms (i.e., before the mood symptoms developed or after they have remitted)

D. Not superimposed on schizophrenia, schizophreniform disorder, delusional disorder, or psychotic disorder NOS viewed elsewhere (Weissman & Klerman, 1977). Risk factors for the development of major depression include a family history of depression or alcoholism, a disruptive or negative home environment during childhood, recent negative life events, the absence of an intimate confiding relationship, being female, and giving birth in the prior 6 months (Weissman & Boyd, 1983). Patients with episodes of major depression without periods of mania are classified as unipolar depressed.

In medically ill patients, estimates of depressive symptoms vary from 12%–36% for medical outpatients to 11%–32% for medical inpatients (Rodin & Voshart, 1986). Major depression has been reported to have a lifetime prevalence of 5.8% in primary care medical patients and 36% of Crohn's patients, and a 1-month prevalence of 6.1% in a primary care population (Helzer, Chammas, Norland, Stillings, & Alpers, 1984; Hoeper, Nycz, Cleary, Reiger, & Goldberg, 1979; Schulberg et al., 1985).

Bipolar disorder is characterized by abnormally intense mood swings. In order to be given a diagnosis of bipolar disorder (also called manic-depressive illness) a person must have periods of mania. Mania is a period of time in which the mood is euphoric, expansive, elated, or irritable; the mood causes a marked impairment of social or occupational functioning and three of a possible seven behavioral features are present. Table 13.2 lists the diagnostic features of mania as defined by the DSM-III-R. The behavioral features include pressured speech, impulsivity, and distractibility. Most people who experience periods of mania also experience periods of depression, but this is not universal. Bipolar disorder can be distinguished by the use of the DSM-III-R criteria from normal variations in mood, which everyone experiences, and from cyclothymia, a mood disorder in which a person is usually depressed or elated, but never meets the full criteria for a manic or depressive episode. Bipolar illness is thought to have a different genetic basis from unipolar illness.

The lifetime risk of bipolar disorder is about 0.4%–1.2% (American Psychiatric Association, 1987) and is equal for men and women. The major risk factor is a family history of the illness, and there are suggestions that it occurs more frequently among those in upper socioeconomic classes (Weissman & Boyd, 1983).

There are no reliable estimates of the prevalence of bipolar disorder in general medical populations.

Epidemiology of Affective Disorders and Diabetes Mellitus

Major Depression

Although many studies have looked at psychologic aspects of DM, few have specifically investigated the syndrome of major depression and

Table 13.2. Criteria for Manic Episode (DSM-III-R)

Note: A "Manic Syndrome" is defined as including criteria A, B, and C below. A "Hypomanic Syndrome" is defined as including criteria A and B, but not C, i.e., no marked impairment.

A. A distinct period of abnormally and persistently elevated, expensive, or irritable mood

B. During the period of mood disturbance, at least three of the following symptoms have persisted (four if the mood is only irritable) and have been present to a significant degree

1. inflated self-esteem or grandiosity
2. decreased need for sleep, e.g., feels rested after only 5 hours of sleep
3. more talkative than usual or pressure to keep talking
4. flight of ideas or subjective experience that thoughts are racing
5. distractibility, i.e., attention too easily drawn to unimportant or irrelevant external stimuli
6. increase in goal-directed activity (either socially, at work or school, or sexually) or psychomotor agitation
7. excessive involvement in pleasurable activities which have a high potential for painful consequences, e.g., the person engages in unrestrained buying sprees, sexual indiscretions, or foolish business investments

C. Mood disturbance sufficiently severe as to cause marked impairment in occupational functioning or in usual social activities or relationships with others, or to necessitate hospitalization to prevent harm to self or others

D. At no time during the disturbance have there been delusions or hallucinations for as long as 2 weeks in the absence of prominent mood symptoms (i.e., before the mood symptoms developed or after they have remitted)

E. Not superimposed on schizophrenia, schizophreniform disorder, delusional disorder, or a psychotic disorder NOS

F. It cannot be established that an organic factor initiated and maintained the disturbance. *Note*: Somatic antidepressant treatment (e.g., drugs, ECT) that apparently precipitates a mood disturbance should not be considered an etiologic organic factor

DM. Among recent reviews of the psychologic aspects of DM (Jacobson & Leibovich, 1984; Lustman et al., 1983; Rodin, 1983; Wilkinson, 1981), Lustman's focuses specifically on the issue of depression in diabetes (Lustman et al., 1983). He notes that most of the early studies in this area suffer from methodologic flaws which include retrospective design, unspecified diagnostic criteria for depression, and reliance on inadequate measures of illness such as projective tests which have low reliability and validity. He concludes that "Thus far, there has not been a systematic description of any relationship between diabetes and depression" (p. 69).

Since then, several studies have looked at the relationship between diabetes and depression in a more systematic manner. Because of the limited number of studies in this area, studies on both insulin-dependent and non-insulin-dependent diabetics will be discussed. As will be seen, the rates of depression do not appear to differ significantly between the two groups of diabetics.

Surridge et al., in 1984, studied a group of 50 insulin-dependent diabetics aged 16 to 60 (mean age of 38.1 years.). Patients were assessed for overall psychiatric diagnosis with an open-ended psychiatric interview. In addition, they were rated on the Beck Self-Assessment Scale for Depression and the Hamilton Rating Scale for Depression. He found that 31 of 50 patients reported energy loss and increased fatigue with considerable functional impairment in two thirds of the affected patients. This constellation of symptoms was significantly related to depressed mood as reported on the Hamilton and Beck scales, and the author concluded that fatigue, energy loss, and current depression may be used as a single measure of functional impairment. None of the patients studied, however, were currently depressed, although 12 (24%) reported prior histories of severe vegetative depression.

The study has several methodologic difficulties. The generalizability is limited because the diagnoses were based on a single clinician's psychiatric interviews using nonspecific diagnostic criteria. The subject selection criteria were not clear either. This last may be particularly important, as the mean Hamilton score of the patients in this study was one quarter of the usual population mean, making it questionable whether this was a representative sample of patients.

Tun, Perlmuter, Russo, and Nathan (1987) studied memory deficits in a group of 119 non-insulin-dependent diabetics aged 55–75 and a group of 25 age-matched controls. As part of the protocol, they obtained Zung Self-Rated Depression surveys on their study population and found diabetics were significantly more depressed at all ages than controls. This was true for both somatic and psychological subscales of the Zung. Interestingly, self-reported memory problems were mediated by depressive status (although diabetics performed more poorly on some memory tests independent of affective status). Further refinement of Zung scores in the same study population by Geringer et al (Geringer, Perlmuter, Stern, and Nathan, 1988) revealed that 19% of the diabetic women had Zung scores in the clinically depressed range.

These data are one of the only estimates of depression in a NIDDM population. There are several limitations in generalizability, however.

The data is based on a self-report measure which may lead to underestimation of the prevalence of depression. The Zung scale also gives an estimate of the prevalence of depressive symptoms, which may not be indicative of rates of major depression. The Zung has, however, been shown to be valid in assessing depression when DSM-III based criteria for depression are used (Schaefer et al., 1985).

Another study which investigated the prevalence of depression in diabetics was done by Lustman et al. in 1986a. They randomly selected 114 insulin and non-insulin-dependent diabetic adults from an outpatient clinic and assessed the presence of psychiatric illness with the Diagnostic Interview Schedule (DIS), a structured psychiatric diagnostic interview designed to give a psychiatric diagnosis based on DSM-III criteria. This diagnostic method has been validated in a diabetic population (Lustman, Harper, Griffith, & Clouse, 1986b). Lustman et al. found that 71% of the patients had a lifetime history of at least one psychiatric diagnosis. Major depression had occurred in 33% of the patients, and 16 of the patients (14%) were suffering from an episode of major depression at the time of the study. There were no differences in rates of depression between Type I and Type II diabetics, and no increase in severity of diabetic complications in the depressed patients. The depressed patients showed significantly increased levels of glycosalated hemoglobin (HbA_{1c}), which indicates poorer diabetic control. This was particularly true for those who were depressed in the 6 months prior to the study.

This study is one of the first to give an estimate of depression in diabetics based on well-defined criteria for depression. The authors caution that the study population may be sicker than most diabetic populations and thus might not be comparable to more typical outpatients. However, the rates of depression found in the study are comparable to those found in other medically ill populations. The study also raises questions about the relationship of depression to glycemic control. Unfortunately, the study does not give data on gender differences in depression and diabetes, which makes it more difficult to compare this data with other populations.

Wilkinson et al. (1987) screened 211 consecutive insulin-dependent diabetic outpatients for psychiatric disorder with the General Health Questionnaire (GHQ). A subsample of 69 of the 194 patients that completed the study were then interviewed with a structured interview (Clinical Interview Schedule), including all those specified as psychiatric cases by the GHQ. The study found that 18% of the population was psychiatrically impaired on both measures, and that the confidence limits of these measures was quite wide. They also found that women had twice the GHQ score of men.

Although this study does not address depression specifically, it does give an estimate of psychiatric illness in a diabetic population. The estimate is at the lower end of the spectrum of psychiatric illness in medical patients. The use of a self-report screening measure might bias the sample toward underreporting of symptoms. The authors themselves suggest caution in extrapolating from the work to a larger population.

More recently, Popkin, Callies, Lentz, Colon, and Sutherland (1988) assessed the prevalence of psychiatric disorders in 75 consecutive insulin-dependent diabetic pancreatic transplant candidates. All candidates had diabetes at least 10 years and nephropathy with albuminuria. Psychiatric illness was assessed by the DIS. Overall, 59% of the candidates received a psychiatric diagnosis. A lifetime prevalence of major depression was present in 23% of the women and 26% of the men. The lifetime prevalence of depression among the 25–44-year-olds was 29.8%, a significantly higher prevalence than the 12.5% reported in a comparable population. Popkin et al. could not attribute the rates of depression to gender, age, duration of illness, or the presence of diabetic complications. The rates of depression are similar to those found by Lustman et al. (1986a) who used a similar methodology.

Taken together, these results suggest that there is a higher prevalence of major depression, when investigated by studies using DSM-III-based diagnostic criteria, in Type I and Type II diabetics, than in the general population. The prevalence of depression in diabetics is at the higher end of the spectrum when compared to patients with other medical illness. Table 13.3 shows the differing rates of depression in diabetic, general medical, and general populations.

Bipolar Disorder

Only a handful of studies have looked at the prevalence of DM in patients with bipolar disorder, although there have been anecdotal reports of a link between the two (Lilliker, 1980). In 1969, van der Velde and Gordon studied 59 hospitalized bipolar disorder patients and reported that half of those over 40 years old had abnormal oral glucose tolerance tests (blood sugar sum over 600 mg/100 cc). Although affective state did not correlate with blood glucose, the authors suggested that a correlation existed between affective disorder and glucose metabolism. They postulated that the manic state leads to an increased demand for insulin with a subsequent exhaustion of insulin reserves in the pancreas. Hyperglycemic glucose tolerance tests were found in 20% of a comparison group of schizophrenics.

Although this work is provocative, it suffers from several problems. There were no clear criteria for the diagnosis of bipolar disorder. In addition, the subject and control selection criteria were not specified. The clinical impact of the hyperglycemic glucose tolerance tests was not addressed, particularly with regard to whether treatment for diabetes was initiated and the affective consequences of this. In addition, al-

Table 13.3. Epidemiology of Depression and Bipolar Disorder

	Lifetime Prevalence	Point Prevalence
General Population		
Major depression	5%–12% (men)	2.3%–3.2% (men)
	9%–26% (women)	4.5%–9.3% (women)
Bipolar disorder	0.4%–1.2%	
Medical Population		
Depressive symptoms		
Medical outpatients		12%–36%
Medical inpatients		11%–32%
Diabetics	24%	
Major depression		
Primary care outpatients	5.8%	6.1%
Crohn's patients	36%	
Diabetics		
IDDM[a]	24–25%	
IDDM and NIDDM[a]	33%	14%
NIDDM		19% (women)
Bipolar disorder		
Diabetics	10%	50% (> age 40)

[a]IDDM = insulin-dependent diabetes mellitus; NIDDM = non-insulin-dependent diabetes mellitus.

though body weight was not correlated with glucose tolerance, diet and activity, both of which may influence glucose tolerance, were not controlled.

In 1980, Lilliker retrospectively reviewed the charts of 203 manic-depressive patients admitted over a 10-year period to a state psychiatric hospital and reported that 10% were diabetic. Patients were classified as diabetic if they were on a diabetic diet and diabetes could be further substantiated by a physician's chart review (elevated fasting blood glucose and diabetic medical history). Additionally, the prevalence of diabetes (defined by being on a diabetic diet) was compared across psychiatric diagnoses for 4508 psychiatric inpatients treated over a 6-year period. The prevalence of diabetes ranged from 0.7% in personality disorders to 3.8% in those with a transient situational disturbance. In contrast, diabetes was present in 12.4% of the manic-depressives.

These findings are interesting, but the study has some methodologic weaknesses. The most obvious are the retrospective design and sole reliance on chart review for case identification. Diabetic control was not addressed although this may negatively impact on a patient's affective state (Lustman et al., 1986a). Further, the population was not controlled for length of hospitalization and frequency of medical examinations. One might expect chronic patients (i.e., schizophrenic patients) to receive fewer medical checkups, spuriously underestimating medical problems in the chronic population. Finally, obesity and diabetic family history, known risk factors for diabetes, were not controlled in each population.

In sum, although there is anecdotal evidence of an increased prevalence of DM in bipolar disorder, this is not yet substantiated by research.

Mechanisms Underlying the Association of Diabetes and Depression: Why Do Diabetics Get Depressed?

The data presented above indicate that major depression is much more prevalent in diabetics than in the general population, and that depression occurs in diabetics at one of the highest rates among those with chronic medical illness. Does this mean that there is a unique relationship between depression and DM, or are diabetics depressed because of the psychological hazards of coping with a chronic illness? An investigation of the possible mechanisms underlying depression in diabetes can shed some light on these questions.

Depression has been ascribed to many etiologies, including biological, cognitive, psychologic, and environmental ones. We will consider the evidence for depression in diabetes as due to biologic abnormalities, chronic pain, psychologic stress, and emotional loss.

Depression in DM as an Organic Affective Disorder

This hypothesis implies that depression occurs in diabetics as a consequence of biologic changes associated with diabetes, or as a consequence of biologic abnormalities common to both depression and diabetes.

Neuroendocrine Links

In recent years, there has been an enormous increase in our understanding of the biologic alterations associated with major depression. Many of these changes have been found in neuroendocrine functions, particularly in the regulation of the hypothalamic-pituitary-adrenocortical axis (HPA). HPA dysregulation in depression is manifested by abnormal cortisol production. Although early investigators thought elevations in cortisol might be due to nonspecific stress factors (Mason, 1968; Sachar, 1967; Rubin, 1967), it is now generally accepted that cortisol is elevated in at least some patients with major depression (Ettigi & Brown, 1977). The elevation appears more frequently in depressed patients with specific types of depressive disorders (Schlesser et al., 1980). Some depressed patients have increased 24-hr urinary cortisol production (Ettigi & Brown, 1978; Pryce, 1964), increased urinary free cortisol (Ettigi & Brown, 1977; Rubin, Poland, Lesser, Winston, & Blodgett, 1987) and increased plasma cortisol (Poland, Rubin, Lesser, Lane, & Hart, 1987; Rubin, et al., 1987; Sachar, Asnis, Halbreich, Nathan, & Halpern, 1980) compared to nondepressed controls. Cortisol levels in the cerebrospinal fluid of depressed patients have been less consistent (Ettigi & Brown, 1977), as have urinary and serum cortisol levels in manic patients (Ettigi & Brown, 1977; Rubin, 1967).

Most investigators have also found a flattened diurnal fluctuation of cortisol in depressed patients. Normally, cortisol is maximally secreted in the early morning hours (McEwen, 1975). In some patients with major depression, there is an increase in the number and frequency of bursts of cortisol in the afternoon and evening (Sachar et al., 1973, 1980), although this has not always been replicated (Rubin et al., 1987). Some depressed patients also have abnormal responses to the dexamethasone test (DST). Dexamethasone is a synthetic corticosteroid which usually suppresses the natural production of cortisol for 24 hours following its administration. In about half of all depressed patients, the DST shows an early escape of suppression, that is, patients show a return to baseline levels of cortisol earlier than would be expected (Carroll et al., 1976, 1981; Sachar et al., 1980). The presumptive etiology is the hypersecretion of cortisol in depression (Poland et al., 1987; Rubin et al., 1987). The test has some limitations in distinguishing depressed patients from other psychiatric patients (Arana, Baldessarini, & Ornsteen, 1985) and may have some usefulness in classifying familial subtypes of depressed patients (Schlesser et al., 1980). Future studies are needed to clarify which depressed patients show cortisol abnormalities.

It is also generally accepted that a relative insulin resistance occurs during depression and resolves with treatment of depression (Carroll, 1969; Mueller et al., 1969; Ettigi & Brown, 1977; Sachar, Finklestein, & Hellman, 1971; Sachar et al., 1980), although this finding has not been universal (Herzberg, Coppen, & Marks, 1968; Pryce, 1964). Insulin resistance was most often assessed by measuring the glucose response to exogenous insulin. Early studies in this area did not distinguish between types of depression (i.e., neurotic vs. psychotic) although some investigators found insulin resistance did not occur in neurotic depressives (Mueller et al., 1969). A blunted growth hormone response to insulin-induced hypoglycemia has also been seen in some depressed patients (Greden, Sachar, Altman, & Sassin, 1975).

Insulin resistance in depression is correlated with late afternoon hypersecretion of cortisol (Sachar et al., 1980). The clinical implications of this for nondiabetic depressed patients are not clear. While it has been suggested that depressed patients may present with hyperglycemia (Jenike, 1982), others have not found a correlation between hypercortisolemia and elevated blood glucose in depression (Rihmer & Arato, 1982). Some of these endocrine abnormalities also occur in nondepressed diabetics. Diabetics have been shown to have increased plasma cortisol in some studies (Faiman & Moorhouse, 1967; Lentle & Thomas, 1964) but not in others (Asfeldt, 1972; Serio, Tarquini, Contini, Bucolassi & Toccafondi, 1968). This is difficult to interpret as hyper and hypoglycemia can influence cortisol production.

Others have studied the DST in diabetics. Hudson et al., (1984) found 43% of nondepressed diabetics did not suppress cortisol on a DST. This was a much higher prevalence of nonsuppression compared to normal controls. Nonsuppression correlated with increased glycosalated hemoglobin but did not correlate with age, sex, type of diabetes, body weight, mean glucose, change in glucose, mood, or presence of diabetic complications. This was a well-controlled study that excluded all patients with hypoglycemic reactions (these reactions can cause a compensatory increase in cortisol).

Cameron (1984) found similar results in a study of 54 Type I and Type II diabetics. Fifty-five percent were nonsuppressors on DST, and there was poor test–retest reliability between DSTs on the same patient. He concluded that the DST does not have much clinical usefulness in diabetics. Cameron also reported flattened circadian secretion of cortisol in diabetics with an elevated trough of cortisol and a normal peak (in contrast to depressives who show both elevated peaks and troughs).

Taken together, these results imply that diabetics and depressives share some abnormalities in cortisol production and, by implication, may share some common HPA dysregulation. One might then expect to find these abnormalities intensified in depressed diabetics. Although cortisol production has not been studied specifically in depressed diabetics, there have been reports that blood sugar levels in diabetics vary with depression. Evidence for this comes from case reports of hyperglycemia in depressed insulin and non-insulin-dependent diabetics which resolved with treatment of depression (Crammer & Giles, 1981, Fakhri, 1966; Kronfol et al., 1981; Nelson, Orr & Sullivan, 1982–83; Normand & Jenike, 1984; Thomas, Goldney, & Phillips, 1983). Some of these patients were treated with electroconvulsive shock therapy (ECT) and some with antidepressants. These reports suggest that depression increases insulin resistance in diabetics. The mechanism is likely to be through increased levels of cortisol seen in depression since cortisol antagonizes insulin (Kronfol et al., 1981). Blood sugar then normalizes when depression is treated because the hypercortisolemia of depression also resolves with treatment.

It is also possible that lower blood sugars following treatment for depression are due to independent effects of the treatment rather than neuroendocrine correlates of improved depression. In this regard, Fakhri suggested that ECT itself had a curative effect on new onset NIDDM (Fakhri, Fadhli, & el Rawi, 1980). This study has been criticized on numerous methodologic grounds (Pyke & Watkins, 1980) which include biased patient selection, inadequate characterization of mood, and numerous uncontrolled factors including diet and weight. It has also been suggested that the initial hyperglycelmia on which the diagnosis of diabetes in this study was based was due to depression rather than true diabetes (Jenike, 1982). It seems unlikely that ECT is a cure for diabetes as others have found acutely increased glucose following ECT treatments in depressed diabetics (Finestone & Weiner, 1984; Yudofsky & Rosenthal, 1986).

In general, glucose regulation in diabetics seems more labile when combined with depression. There may also be an increase in insulin resistance mediated through hypercortisolemia in some depressed diabetics. This is based on case reports and awaits studies adequately controlled for diet and activity for further validation.

In summary, it appears that there are common endocrine abnormalities in diabetics and some depressed patients, particularly with regard to cortisol production. These are summarized in Table 13.4.

Blood Sugar and Mood

Although, as noted above, there have been numerous case reports of altered glucose metabolism in depressed diabetics, there are remarkably few studies of blood sugar and mood. Yet both chronic hyperglycemia and hypoglycemia can result in depression regardless of etiology (Leigh & Kramer, 1984), and may have an independent association with mood.

A study done in 1979 by Kymiss, Shatin, and Brown, (1979) stands virtually alone in this area. They looked at the relationship between blood sugar and depression in 4994 community mental health clinic outpatients. Fifty-four patients (10%) had fasting blood sugars greater than 145 mg% a cut-off taken as presumptive evidence of DM. The psychiatric diagnoses of the 54 patients with hyperglycemia (made by psychiatric residents in accordance with DSM-II criteria) were compared with the psychiatric diagnoses of 250 randomly selected control patients from the total clinic population. The same distribution of affective disorders was found in both groups. No one specific psychiatric disorder was associated with hyperglycemia.

These findings refute the idea that hyperglycemia is associated with depressive disorders, and by implication, that DM is associated with clinical depression. However, the study failed to identify well-controlled diabetics and therefore may have missed an association between diabetes and depression. The study also only looked at a single blood

Table 13.4. Neuroendocrine and Neurotransmitter Changes in Depression, Diabetes and Depressed Diabetics

	Major depression	Diabetes	Depressed Diabetics
Neuroendocrine Function			
Cortisol	increase		
urinary free	increase		
24-hr urinary	increase		
plasma	increase	increase	
diurnal fluctuation	flattened	flattened	
secretory bursts	increase in number and frequency		
dexamethasone test	early escape of suppression	early escape of suppression	
Insulin resistance	increase	increase (IDDM[a])	increase (IDDM, NIDDM[a])
Growth hormone insulin-induced hypoglycemia	blunted response		
Glucose	?	increase	increase intensified

Neurotransmitter	Depression	Streptozotocin-Induced Diabetes	Effect on HPA[a]
Norepinephrine	decrease	increase in brainstem decrease in forebrain	decrease tonic cortisol secretion
Serotin	decrease	decrease	may control diurnal cortisol release

[a]IDDM = insulin-dependent diabetes mellitus; NIDDM = non-insulin-dependent diabetes mellitus; HPA = hypothalamic-pituitary-adrenal axis.

sugar determination. While this is appropriate for a screening study, it does not adequately assess the relationship between chronic hyperglycemia or hypoglycemia, labile blood sugar, and mood shifts, a constellation of factors more likely to be seen in diabetics. For example, the rate of change of blood sugar is more likely to produce psychiatric symptoms (including affective ones) than a single abnormal blood sugar (Ettigi & Brown, 1978).

The relationship between blood sugar and depression is not clear at this time, and it is not yet known whether blood sugar levels per se contribute independently to depression.

Neuroendocrine Dysregulation and Neurotransmitters

If there is the potential for a common HPA dysregulation in DM and some depressive syndromes, then it is reasonable to wonder whether there is a biologic abnormality that could lead to both processes. There are fascinating hints that such an abnormality may exist.

The neurotransmitters norepinephrine and serotonin have been implicated in the pathogenesis of affective disorders. According to the catecholamine hypothesis of affective disorder, depression is caused by a relative functional deficiency of catecholamine (norepinephrine) neurotransmitters and mania is associated with an excess (Schildkraut, Schatzberg, Mooney, & Orsulak, 1983). Others have added an indoleamine hypothesis, namely, that some depressions are caused by a relative functional deficiency of serotonin (5-HT), an indoleamine neurotransmitter (Spring, Chiodo, & Bowen, 1987). These hypotheses have yet to be fully substantiated and the nature of norepinephrine (NE) and 5-HT changes in affective disorders are likely to be far more complex than a simple deficiency state (Hyman, 1988). It is generally agreed, however, that there is some functional decrease in NE and 5-HT during depression (Schildkraut et al., 1983).

Catecholamines are also important in HPA regulation. NE tonically inhibits cortisol secretion by the inhibition of corticotropin releasing factor at the level of the hypothalamus. Serotonin has been implicated in the control of diurnal cortisol fluctuation; serotonin biosynthesis blockade abolishes diurnal cortisol release (McEwen, 1975). Again, this probably occurs at the hypothalamic level. Some invesitigators see cortisol hypersecretion in depressed patients as evidence for relative 5-HT and NE deficiencies in depression (Frohman, 1975). Specific evidence for a link between HPA dysregulation and altered NE in depression has been suggested by the finding that in major depression only DST nonsuppressors have elevated concentrations of NE metabolites in cerebrospinal fluid (Roy, Pickar, De Jong, Karoum, & Linnoila, 1988). Table 13.4 summarizes the presumptive neurotransmitter abnormalities in depression, and their relation to the HPA axis.

The possible link between neurotransmitter abnormalities in depression and diabetes come from recent reports that experimentally induced diabetes in rats causes abnormalities in neurotransmitter metabolism. In a series of studies MacKenzie and Trulson showed that brain tryptophan (precursor of 5-HT) and 5-HT metabolism are decreased in streptozotocin-induced diabetic rats (MacKenzie & Trulson, 1978a, 1978b, 1978c; Trulson & MacKenzie, 1980). These changes were reversed by the administration of insulin, not dependent on glucose level, and partially mediated through alterations in the enzyme which controls synthesis of 5-HT. Trulson has recently shown that streptozotocin-induced diabetes decreases forebrain NE turnover rate in rats (Trulson & Himmel, 1985), again this was reversible with insulin. Bitar, Koulu, Rapoport, and Linnoila (1986) have reported an increase in brainstem NE in streptozotocin-induced diabetic rats. These findings open the possibility that diabetes may cause alterations in neurotransmitters that affect mood. Thus, abnormalities in NE or 5-HT metabolism might lead to both the mood and HPA dysregulation in depression and diabetes.

It is obviously not possible, at this time, to definitely say there is evidence for a common abnormality in depression and diabetes, but Trulson and MacKenzie's work suggests a promising link between the neurotransmitter and neuroendocrine changes that occur in both processes. Investigations of neurotransmitter alterations in diabetic patients will help to clarify these relationships. Longitudinal studies that follow neuroendocrine and neurotransmitter functions in both diabetics and depressed patients will also help clarify whether the common abnormalities cited here are causally related.

Diabetic Neuropathy, Depression, and Chronic Pain

The frequent association between depression and chronic pain syndromes (Blumer & Heilbronn, 1982) suggests another etiologic mechanism for the presence of depression in diabetics. In diabetics, pain is often a component of peripheral neuropathy. If depression occurs in diabetics as a result of chronic pain, one might hypothesize that depression occurs more frequently in diabetics with painful peripheral neuropathy. Depression has in fact been commonly clinically observed in patients with diabetic peripheral neuropathy (a heterogeneous syndrome affecting motor, sensory and autonomic pathways (Brown & Greene, 1981)). Ellenberg has observed that "depression and irritability seem to constitute a symptom 'sui generis' of diabetic neuropathy" (Ellenberg, 1976).

Additional evidence for an association between depression and painful neuropathy comes from the clinical syndrome of diabetic neuropathic cachexia. This syndrome, which occurs almost exclusively in males, is characterized by acute onset, severe weight loss, exquisite neuropathic pain, severe depression, and impotence (Archer, Watkins, & Thomas, 1983; Blau, 1983). The etiology is unknown.

There are, however, aside from these clinical observations, no direct studies documenting or refuting an increased prevalence of depression in diabetic neuropathy. This may be a result of the small number of studies that have assessed depression in diabetes at all.

Additional, albeit indirect, evidence for a link between depression and diabetic neuropathy comes from the successful treatment of painful diabetic neuropathy with tricyclic antidepressants (TCA). Case reports (Davis, Lewis, & Gerich, 1977; Gade, Hofeldt, and Treece, 1980; Hoogwerf, 1985; Khurana, 1983; Mitas, Mosley, & Drager, 1983) and double-blind, crossover, placebo-controlled trials (Gomez-Perez, Rull, & Dies, 1985; Kvinesdal, Molin, Froland, and Gram, 1984; Max et al., 1987; Turkington, 1980) have shown that TCAs reduce painful neuropathic symptoms in patients who present for symptomatic relief.

The implications of this for a link between depression per se and diabetic neuropathy are not clear. Antidepressants have been used effectively in the treatment of a variety of chronic pain syndromes, making it less likely there is a unique action in diabetic neuropathy (France, Houpt, & Ellinwood, 1984). Many of the case reports and studies on tricyclics and diabetic neuropathic pain do not give any information as to whether the patients were depressed. Depression was assessed by Turkington, who found that relief of pain paralleled relief of depression, as judged by a depression index and clinical interviews. This was interpreted as evidence that neuropathic pain was a depressive equivalent. In contrast, Max et al. (1987) found clear-cut relief of neuropathic symptoms independent of depression. Many of the patients in Max's study who were depressed reported neuropathic symptomatic relief with TCA treatment but remained depressed (most likely due to inadequate blood levels of TCA). Depression in the study was assessed by three depression rating scales and a psychiatric interview based on DSM-III criteria. Unfortunately, the individual depressive diagnoses were not reported.

Some light may be shed on the relationship between depression and diabetic neuropathy by an examination of the relationship between chronic pain and depression. The nature of the relationship between chronic pain syndromes and depression is controversial. Extensive reviews (Hendler, 1984; Romano, and Turner, 1985; Turk, and Salovey, 1984) have described the inconsistencies and methodologic flaws in the literature, and a detailed review of the literature is beyond the scope of this discussion. In general, it appears that there is a wide spectrum of views on the nature of the relationship between depression and pain. Some see depression as a normal consequence of the psychologic effects of chronic pain (Hendler, 1984), while others have proposed that a substantial proportion of pain patients, particularly those whose complaints outweigh demonstrable organic pathology, are primarily depressed (Blumer & Heilbronn, 1982). Effective antidepressant treatment of chronic pain syndromes is often cited as indirect evidence for a biologic link between pain and depression, as TCAs affect 5-HT metabolism, 5-HT has been implicated in the pathology of depression, and pain transmission involves neural pathways mediated by 5-HT (France, et al., 1984; Woolf & Wall, 1983). Arguments against this come from the observation that the doses of TCAs needed to treat pain syndromes are much lower than those needed to treat depression (Feinmann, 1985). Romano has proposed that pain and depression may be a final common pathway of independent biologic processes (Romano & Turner, 1985).

In diabetes, as we have seen, there may be abnormalities in 5-HT metabolism, which may influence the perception of pain. Additionally, diabetics are reported to have lower pain thresholds than normal control subjects, an effect which is reproduced by glucose infusions into healthy subjects (Morley, Mooradian, Levine, & Morley, 1984). This suggests that pain tolerance may be lower in diabetics, perhaps intensifying the vulnerability to depression in those diabetics with painful symptoms.

The question then arises as to whether depression in diabetic neuropathy occurs secondary to a chronic pain syndrome, whether pain represents a manifestation of a primary depression, or whether depression occurs in neuropathy independent of painful symptoms. Longitudinal studies of diabetics with neuropathy are needed to provide the answer. Max's study implies that the two processes are separable, at least in some patients, but it is not clear to what extent these patients were depressed and what the temporal relationship was between depression and neuropathy.

Additional evidence for an independent relationship between diabetic neuropathy and depression comes from our own work. We (Geringer et al., 1988a) reported self-rated depression scores in the clinically depressed range in a group of elderly NIDDM women with diabetic peripheral neuropathy Depression was correlated with severity of neuropathy (assessed by an objective physiologic measure), but not with neuropathic symptoms (including pain). In other work, we found an association between self-rated depression, objective evidence of neuropathic impairment, and peripheral vascular disease in NIDDM men. This occurred independent of reports of pain or severity of other diabetic complications (Geringer, Perlmuter, Stern, & Nathan, 1988b).

This raises the possibility that depression might occur in conjunction with diabetic neuropathy as a result of a common organic process which occurs in the periphery as well as the central nervous system. Consistent with this hypothesis, Perlmuter et al. (1984) have reported a correlation between cognitive difficulties and neuropathy in elderly non-insulin-dependent diabetics. Microvascular abnormalities have been implicated in the pathogenesis of diabetic neuropathy (Brown & Greene, 1981), and others have noted the importance of central nervous system vascular insults in the genesis of depression (Post, 1962; Robinson, Lipsey, & Price, 1985). An examination of this hypothesis awaits a longitudinal investigation of the prevalence of depression and vascular disease in patients with painful and nonpainful diabetic neuropathy.

Depression and Psychologic Factors in Diabetes

Thus far, we have considered physiologic processes that may be etiologically related to the prevalence of depression in diabetes. No discussion of depression in diabetes would be complete without attention to some of the psychologic factors that impact on the lives of people who suffer with DM.

The psychologic issues raised by DM have been extensively reviewed elsewhere (Dunn & Turtle, 1981; Jacobson & Leibovich, 1984; Lustman et al., 1983; Rodin, 1983; Wilkinson, 1981). Diabetics must carefully regulate their most basic activities, i.e., eating, with a consequent loss of the sense of autonomy and control over their bodies. Diabetes is an illness not immediately apparent to a casual observer, yet many patients feel stigmatized by having a chronic disease. This leads some diabetic patients to keep high blood sugars in order to avoid the public humiliation of a hypoglycemic episode. On the other hand, diabetic patients often feel guilty for past or current dietary indiscretions (particularly with mounting evidence that strict glucose control may delay the onset of complications) when complications do appear. Diabetics live with an uncertain future, and the present is often clouded by anticipation of visual, renal, and other functional losses. All of these issues are added to the pain, disability, heightened attention to physical processes, and role changes that accompany any chronic illness (Jacobson & Leibovich, 1984).

Some additional issues are present in diabetics with NIDDM. Patients with NIDDM are often obese, and the diagnosis of diabetes may precipitate a crisis over the realization that lifelong eating habits cannot be controlled. Many patients with NIDDM are elderly and face an increase in psychologic difficulties on this basis alone. Depression is quite common in elderly patients. Estimates of the prevalence of depressive symptoms in elderly populations range from 13%–24% in community surveys to 34%–46% of elderly medical inpatients, based on screening self-report measures (Katon, 1984; Magni, De Leo, & Schifano, 1985). Elderly people account for 25% of all suicides although they constitute only 13% of the population (Ban, 1984). In one review, despite the observation that many of the epidemiologic studies on elderly people suffer from sampling errors, biased patient selection, and inconsistent and unspecified criteria for the diagnosis of depression, depression was described as one of the most prevalent and important medical conditions in later life (Ruegg, Zisook, & Swerdlow, 1988).

If this were not enough, elderly patients who are medically ill are at increased risk of depression (Ruegg et al., 1988). This may have something to do with the life cycle task in later life. According to Erikson (1963) the crucial issue facing elderly people is the attainment of ego integrity, or a sense of completeness and integration about one's life. The alternative, if this is not achieved, is despair, manifested by the sense that time is too short. It is easy to see how a medical illness, with the implicit threat of disability and death, might intensify the despair felt at this time of life.

In addition, elderly people are coping with the inevitable loss of friends, relatives, spouses, and their own physical attributes. The psychologic experience of loss, in one way or another, has been linked with many psychologic theories of depression. Loss of a meaningful object, loss of self-esteem, loss of rewarding situations, and loss of the sense of powerfulness have all been implicated in the etiology of depression (Bibring, 1953; Freud, 1957; Fordyce, 1976; Seligman, 1972). All of these types of loss may occur in elderly people, particularly those who are ill.

Another problem for older diabetics is social isolation. Social isolation, common in elderly populations, is likely to intensify if one cannot easily walk or see. Social isolation, not surprisingly, has also been linked to depression (O'Neil, Lancee, & Freeman, 1986; Kaplan, Roberts, Camacho, & Coyne, 1987), and to an increase in mortality (Berkman & Syme, 1979) independent of age, sex, and health status. Social support, on the other hand, is reported to mitigate some of the deleterious effects of stress on health (Cohen, Teresi, and Holmes, 1985; McKay et al., 1985; Nuckolls, Cassel, & Kaplan, 1972; Sarason, Sarason, Potter, and Antoni, 1985) in populations of young men, pregnant women, medical outpatients, and inner-city elderly.

This brings us to consideration of stress as a risk factor for depression in diabetics. Stress has been reported to be a risk factor for depression in several studies (Brown, Bifulco, and Harris, 1987; Lewinsohn, and Amenson, 1978; O'Neil, et al., 1986), although none of these studies looked specifically at diabetics. Stress has, however, been studied in the control of DM. The pioneering work in this area was done by Hinkle and Wolf in a series of experiments in the early 1950s (Hinkle & Wolf, 1950, 1952). They measured blood glucose and ketone bodies in diabetics (Type I and II) and normal control subjects during interviews in which stressful material (previously determined for each individual) was discussed. They found an elevation in ketone bodies during stress in both groups and lowered glucose in diabetics. They concluded that stress increased the lability of diabetic control. The study has been criticized for poor patient selection and poorly specified stressors (Wilkinson, 1981), but it does suggest that meaningful psychologic stimuli may impact diabetic control. Along the same lines, relaxation training has improved glucose tolerance in patients with IDDM and NIDDM (Landis et al., 1985; Surwit, and Feinglos, 1983) in uncontrolled case reports.

Increased stress has also been implicated as a factor in the onset of Type I and Type II diabetes (Bradley, 1979; Kisch, 1986; Robinson & Fuller, 1985), although one report did not support this (Grant, Kyle,

Teichman, & Mendels, 1974). Stress was assessed in these studies with a self-report questionnaire for recent stressful life events. This methodology has been criticized for having poor reliability, excessive reliance on self-report measures of stress, and poorly defined illness criteria (Cohen, 1981). Barglow, Hatcher, Edidin, and Sloan-Rossiter (1984) have detailed the methodologic shortcomings of the current research on stress and diabetes and conclude that valid findings are yet to appear. The extent to which stress may influence diabetic control and depression in diabetics remains to be determined.

Depression in diabetics may also arise as a secondary result of diabetic complications. We have already discussed the possible contribution of pain in diabetic neuropathy to depression. Diabetics are at risk of losing vision, an event which often precipitates a grief reaction and can be a severe blow to self-esteem. Diabetics may feel especially guilty about visual loss in the light of recent findings that poor metabolic control (presumably linked to dietary indiscretions) accelerates diabetic retinopathy (Nathan, Singer, Godine, Hodgson-Harrington, & Perlmuter, 1986). This loss (as well as the loss of other functional capacities) may result in the inability to work or maintain one's usual family role, with a consequent loss of further self-esteem. Diabetics are at risk for renal damage and possible reliance on dialysis; depression may come from the loss of independence experienced with this complication. Diabetics are also at increased risk for sexual dysfunction. Estimates of impotence in diabetic men range from 40%–59% (Martin, 1981) in population surveys. (Nathan, Singer, Godine, & Perlmuter, (1986) found impotence in 71% of older NIDDM patients compared to 11% of age-matched control patients. In another study, anorgasmia was reported in 35% of diabetic women versus 6% of control women (Kolodney, 1971). Impotence brings with it a blow to masculinity and self-esteem, with depression a frequent result. Sexual dysfunction can create marital difficulties which lead to depression. Autonomic neuropathies, presumed to be the etiology of diabetic sexual dysfunction, can cause humiliation and loss of self-esteem through decreased bowel and bladder control.

With all of the potential difficulties for diabetics noted above, one may wonder why all diabetics are not depressed. It is important to remember that each individual patient experiences the events surrounding his or her illness in a unique way. The meaning of illness (and each potential complication) will vary according to a patient's personality type (Kahana & Bibring, 1965), personal history, and current life situation. For example, patients with oral or dependent personalities will have a more difficult time with situations that intensify dependent longings, such as dialysis. Narcissistic patients, who experience illness as a threat to self-esteem and an internal image of perfection, may have a particularly difficult time with limb amputation. Weisman (1987) has identified the characteristics of good and bad copers, the pressure points that patients respond to in coping with illness, vulnerabilities to coping, and strategies for coping well. Each new facet of a diabetic's illness will put pressure on some aspect of coping, and it is important to assess a patient's predominant coping style in each clinical situation. For example, someone who copes with experiences of psychologic pain through physical activity will have a difficult time with complications that restrict physical ability, and a person who uses food to cope with distress will have a hard time with dietary restrictions.

The relationship between diabetes and depression is quite complex. As we have seen, there are biologic, environmental, and intrapsychic factors that bear on the relationship. Depression in diabetics is ultimately a product of intricate interrelationships between a patient's central nervous system, neuroendocrine system, psychosocial environment, and inner psychologic world.

Mechanisms Underlying an Association Between Mania and Depression

It is difficult to speculate on potential etiologic links between DM and mania as the evidence for an association between the two remains weak. Nevertheless, as discussed earlier, some investigators have reported an increased prevalence of DM in patients with manic-depressive illness (Lilliker, 1980; van der Velde & Gordon, 1969). The question is then whether the diabetes might exacerbate the manic state, or some aspect of mania might predispose patients toward DM.

Just as there are neuroendocrine and neurotransmitter aberrations in major depression, comparable changes have been postulated in mania. A catecholamine excess (Schildkraut et al., 1983) and a cortisol decrease (Carroll et al., 1976) are the alterations most often suggested to occur. Most authors agree that catecholamine and neuroendocrine changes in mania remain more speculative than those reported for depression (Ettigi & Brown, 1977). This makes it more difficult to propose a mechanism that might underlie an association between mania and DM, and one author has suggested that there is no good reason for such a relationship to exist (Wilkinson, 1981).

It has been hypothesized that lithium carbonate, a common treatment for bipolar disorder, can influence glucose tolerance and might precipitate DM. There have been several case reports of the developmental of DM in patients treated with chronic lithium carbonate therapy (Craig, Abu-Saleh, Smith & Evans, 1977; Crammer, 1982; Johnstone, 1977; Kondeziela, Kaufmann, & Klein, 1985). In addition, van der Velde and Gordon (1969) reported that glucose tolerance increased acutely in 10 bipolar patients treated with lithium and then returned to baseline upon cessation of lithium. No change in mood was observed during that time. It is difficult to assess the clinical implications for patients treated with long-term lithium therapy from this finding. In contrast, Vestergaard and Schou (1987) reported lithium caused no change in fasting blood sugars of 460 psychiatric patients followed over 6 years. It seems unlikely that any relationship that exists between mania and DM is mediated exclusively through lithium carbonate.

Stressful life events have been implicated as a factor in the onset of mania in both young and old patients with bipolar disorder (Ambelas, 1987; Glassner & Haldipur, 1983). This is another potential area of interaction between diabetes and mania. This hypothesis implies that stress might precipitate both mania and DM in genetically vulnerable individuals. Only longitudinal studies that follow diabetic populations for the incidence of mania and bipolar populations for the incidence of DM will be able to begin to sort out this question.

Treatment Issues in Patients With Affective Disorder and DM

The treatment of affective disorders in patients with DM poses special problems. Diabetes is a multisystem disease and can create dilemmas for clinicians in both diagnosis and treatment of coexisting affective disorders.

Depression

The diagnosis of depression in patients with DM can be hard to make because the somatic symptoms of depression may overlap with those of DM. It may be difficult to know whether a patient's complaints of fatigue and lethargy come from depression or uncontrolled diabetes. Many clinicians conclude that depression in diabetics is an appropriate response to a debilitating illness, and therefore miss a treatable affective disorder. In a recent study, Lustman found that depressed diabetics were more likely to complain of diabetic symptoms than were diabetics with elevated HbA_{1c}, values (Lustman et al., 1986). The same investigator found that physicians recognized depression and initiated antidepressant treatment in only one third of depressed diabetics (Lustman & Harper, 1987). Similarly, Wilkinson reported that psychiatric morbidity was identified by physicians in only 28% of a sample of psychiatrically impaired diabetic patients (Wilkinson et al., 1987). This study also found psychiatric illness was most likely to be missed in men, although no explanation was offered for this finding. Depression, it should be remembered, can interfere with diabetic control both behav-

Table 13.5. Potential Complications of Antidepressant use in Diabetics

Polycyclic antidepressants
Anticholinergic effects
Obscure symptoms of hypoglycemia (dry mouth)
Cardiac ischemia (sinus tachycardia)
Confusion
Loss of bowel and bladder tone
Weight gain
Sedation
Orthostatic hypotension (exacerbation of autonomic neuropathy)
Obscure hypoglycemia (block growth hormone response to hypoglycemia)
Hypoglycemia
Hyperglycemia
Cardiac conduction abnormalities
Monoamine oxidase inhibitors
Hypoglycemia
Orthostatic hypotension
Sexual dysfunction
Low-dose psychostimulants
Sinus tachycardia
Elevated blood pressure
Electroconvulsive shock therapy
Hyperglycemia
Hypoglycemia

iorally and endocrinologically and should be treated when identified in diabetics.

In the diagnosis of depression, each item in the DSM-III-R criteria for major depression should be inquired about individually, and prior and family histories of depression should be obtained. Current precipitants and risk factors for depression should also be identified.

Major depression is most commonly treated with a somatic therapy alone or in combination with psychotherapy; the somatic therapy is usually a polycylic antidepressant. Side effects associated with polycyclic antidepressants may make their use difficult in diabetics. Common side effects are sedation, weight gain, orthostatic hypotension and anticholinergic and cardiac conduction effects. Many of these can obviously be problematic for diabetics. The anticholinergic effects can cause sinus tachycardia; this can be dangerous in diabetics with ischemic heart disease. In the elderly, confusion occurs with anticholinergic use. Anticholinergic effects may also interfere with bowel and bladder tone, exacerbating preexisting autonomic neuropathies. Weight gain may make diabetic control more difficult.

Polycyclics also block alpha adrenergic receptors. This may block the growth hormone response to hypoglycemia and mask hypoglycemic episodes in diabetics (Frohman, 1975). Case reports have observed both increased and decreased blood sugars in conjunction with polycyclic use in diabetics (Kronfol et al., 1981; Nelson et al., 1982–83; Thomas et al., 1983; Tollefson & Lesar, 1983; True, Perry, & Burns, 1987). Cardiac conduction abnormalities can occur due to polycyclic mediated decreased conduction through the His-Purkinje system. Sudden death has been associated with use in patients with a corrected QT interval > 440 ms (Cassem, 1987). The potential complications of polycyclic antidepressant use in diabetics are summarized in Table 13.5.

Monamine oxidase inhibitors are another class of antidepressants. They have been associated with hypoglycemia in diabetics (Wickstrom & Pettersson, 1964) and can produce severe orthostatic hypotension and sexual dysfunction. Low-dose psychostimulants are an alternative treatment for depression. These are a particularly safe and effective treatment in the elderly medically ill, including those with diabetes (Woods, Tesar, Murray, & Cassem, 1986). ECT, as discussed earlier, has been associated with both increases and decreases in blood sugar in depressed diabetics (Crammer & Gillies, 1981; Finestone & Weiner, 1984; Normand & Jenike, 1984; Yudofsky & Rosenthal, 1980).

In addition to psychopharmacologic approaches, psychotherapy should be considered in depressed diabetics. Table 13.6 summarizes some of the points to keep in mind when a psychotherapy referral is considered. It is particularly important to try to identify areas in a patient's environment where psychosocial interventions might be helpful, and to identify chronic repetitive patterns of dysfunctional behavior.

Table 13.6. Factors to Consider in Psychotherapy Referral

1. Identifiable precipitant, such as a conflict or loss
2. Precipitant cannot be altered with a simple life change (or patient is unable to make such a change)
3. Chronic sense of hopelessness
4. Patient needs a place to grieve
5. Patient who likes to talk (or does not find talking about inner psychological states frightening or humiliating)
6. Presence of: multiple stresses
   chronic difficulties with relationships
   inability to attend to own feelings
   marital/family problems
7. Patient has failed multiple, adequate antidepressant trials
8. The current situation recreates an earlier psychological trauma
9. Patient is psychologically minded
10. Patient does not have any supportive relationships

Bipolar Disorder

The treatment of depression in bipolar patients is similar to that in unipolar depressives. Lithium carbonate is used for acute manic episodes and maintenance of normal mood. Lithium has effects on renal and thyroid function. It has been associated with the development of interstitial nephritis and nephrogenic diabetes insipidus (Bernstein, 1987), and should be used with great caution in any patients with renal insufficiency. Obviously this will have implications for diabetics. Lithium can also suppress conduction through the sinus node of the heart and should be used with caution in patients with cardiac conduction defects. An alternative treatment to lithium is carbamezapine, known to cause potentially serious hematologic abnormalities which are usually reversed with discontinuation of the treatment. In addition, antipsychotic medications may be needed to control an acute manic episode. Many antipsychotic drugs have anticholinergic effects similar to those discussed for the polycyclic antidepressants. One antipsychotic, loxapine, was reported to cause nonketotic hyperglycemic coma in a nondiabetic woman (Tollefson & Lesar, 1983).

Conclusion

In some ways we have come a long way from Thomas Willis's initial observation of increased depression in diabetics, and in some ways we have not yet traveled far. It appears that diabetes and affective disorders overlap in many ways. It seems increasingly clear that depressive symptoms and major depression occur at high prevalence rates in diabetics, although these rates are within the range reported for other chronic diseases. The evidence for an increased rate of bipolar disorder in diabetics is less convincing.

There are several fascinating neuroendocrine abnormalities common to both diabetes and depression. Thus far it has not been possible to ascertain whether these result from a common underlying abnormality or are merely coincidental. Well-controlled longitudinal studies which use well-specified diagnostic criteria to assess the incidence of diabetes in patients with depression and the incidence of depression in patients with diabetes are needed to address this question. In addition, controlled studies which follow neuroendocrine and neurotransmitter fluctuations in a population of depressed diabetics before and after treatment will help shed some light on the interrelationships between these two systems. An increased understanding of this complex area will help us to better identify and treat depression in our patients. Hopefully, attention to the emotional aspects of medical illness, whether biologic or psychologically based, will help us to treat people, not merely diseases.

References

Ambelas, A. (1987). Life events and mania: a special relationship? *British Journal of Psychiatry, 150*, 235–240.

American Psychiatric Association. (1987). *Diagnostic and Statistical Manual of Mental Disorders* (3rd ed., revised). Washington, DC: American Psychiatric Association.

Arana, G., Baldessarini, R., & Ornsteen, M. (1985). The dexamethasone suppression test in depression for diagnosis and prognosis in psychiatry. *Archives of General Psychiatry, 42*, 1193–1204.

Archer, A., Watkins, P., & Thomas, P. (1983). The natural history of acute painful neuropathy in diabetes mellitus. *Journal of Neurology, Neurosurgery and Psychiatry, 46*, 491–499.

Asfeldt, V. (1972). Hypophyseo-adrenocortical function in diabetes mellitus. *Acta Medica Scandinavia, 191*, 349–354.

Ban, T. (1984). Chronic disease and depression in the geriatric population. *Journal of Clinical Psychiatry, 45*(3), 18–23.

Barglow, P., Hatcher, R., Edidin, D., & Sloan-Rossiter, M. (1984). Stress and metabolic control in diabetes: Psychosomatic evidence and evaluation of methods. *Psychosomatic Medicine, 46*(2), 127–144.

Berkman, L., & Syme, S. (1979). Social network, host resistance, and mortality: A nine year follow-up study of Alameda county residents. *American Journal of Epidemiology, 109*, 186–204.

Bernstein, J. (1987). Psychotropic drug prescribing. In T. Hackett, & N. Cassem (Ed.), *Massachusetts General Hospital Handbook of General Hospital Psychiatry*. Littleton, MA. PSG Publishing Co, Inc.

Bibring, E. (1953). The mechanism of depression. In P. Greenacre (Ed.), *Affective Disorders*. New York: International Universities Press.

Bitar, M., Koulu, M., Rapoport, S., & Linnoila, M. (1986). Diabetes-induced alteration in brain monoamine metabolism in rats. *The Journal of Pharmacology and Experimental Therapeutics, 236*, 432–437.

Blau, R. (1983). Diabetic neuropathic cachexia: Report of a woman with this syndrome and a review of the literature. *Archives of Internal Medicine, 143*, 2011–2012.

Blumer, D., & Heilbronn, M. (1982). Chronic pain as a variant of depressive disease: The pain prone disorder. *Journal of Nervous and Mental Disease, 170*, 381–394.

Bradley, C. (1979). Life events and the control of diabetes mellitus. *Journal of Psychosomatic Research, 23*, 159–162.

Brown, G., Bifulco, A., & Harris, T. (1987). Life events, vulnerability and onset of depression. *British Journal of Psychiatry, 150*, 30–42.

Brown, M., & Greene, D. (1981). Diabetic neuropathy: Pathophysiology and management. In A. Asbury & R. Gilliatt (Ed.), *Peripheral Nerve Disorders—A Practical Approach* (pp. 126–153). London: Butterworths International Medical Reviews.

Cameron, O.G., Kronfol, Z., Greden, J.F., & Carroll, B.J. (1984). Hypothalamic-pituitary-adrenocortical activity in patients with diabetes mellitus. *Archives of General Psychiatry, 41*, 1090–1095.

Carroll, B. (1969). Hypothalamic-pituitary function in depressive illness: Insensitivity to hypoglycemia. *British Medical Journal, 3*(July), 27–28.
Carroll, B.J., Curtis, G.C., & Mendels, J. (1976). Neuroendocrine regulation in depression. *Archives of General Psychiatry, 33*, 1039–1044.
Carroll, B., Feinberg, M., Greden, J., Tarika, J., Albala, A., Haskett, R., James, N., Kronfol, Z., Lohr, N., Steiner, M., de Vigne, J., & Young, E. (1981). A specific laboratory test for the diagnosis of melancholia. *Archives of General Psychiatry, 38*, 15–23.
Cassem, N. (1987). Depression. In T. Hackett & N. Cassem (Ed.), *Massachusetts General Hospital Handbook of General Hospital Psychiatry* Littleton, MA: PSG Publishing Co, Inc.
Cohen, F. (1981). Stress and bodily illness. *Psychiatric Clinics of North America, 4*(2), 269–287.
Cohen, C., Teresi, J., & Holmes, D. (1985). Social networks, stress, and physical health: A longitudinal study of an inner-city elderly population. *Journal of Gerontology, 40*(4), 478–486.
Craig, J., Abu-Saleh, M., Smith, B., & Evans, I. (1977). Diabetes mellitus in patients on lithium. *Lancet, 2*, 1028.
Crammer, J. (1982). Lithium, diabetes, and obesity. *Aggressologie, 23*, 99–101.
Crammer, J., & Gillies, C. (1981). Psychiatric aspects of diabetes mellitus: Diabetes and depression. *British Journal of Psychiatry, 139*, 171–172.
Davis, J., Lewis, S., & Gerich, J. (1977). Peripheral diabetic neuropathy treated with amitriptyline and fluphenazine. *238*, 2291–2292.
Dunbar, F. (1943). *Psychosomatic Diagnosis.* New York: Paul B. Hoeber.
Dunn, S., & Turtle, J. (1981). The myth of the diabetic personality. *Diabetes Care, 4*, 640–646.
Ellenberg, M. (1976). Diabetic neuropathy: Clinical aspects. *Metabolism, 22*, 1627–1655.
Eraker, S.A., Kirscht, J.P., & Becker, M. (1984). Understanding and improving patient compliance. *Annals of Internal Medicine, 100*, 258–268.
Erikson, E. (1963). *Childhood and society.* New York: Norton.
Ettigi, P., & Brown, G. (1977). Psychoneuroendocrinology of affective disorder: An overview. *American Journal of Psychiatry, 134*, 493–501.
Ettigi, P., & Brown, G. (1978). Brain disorders associated with endocrine dysfunction. *Psychiatric Clinics of North America, 1*, 117–136.
Faiman, C., & Moorhouse, J. (1967). Diurnal variations in the levels of glucose and related substances in healthy and diabetic subjects during starvation. *Clinical Science, 32*, 111–126.
Fakhri, O. (1966). Blood sugar after electroplexy. *Lancet, 2*, 587.
Fakhri, O., Fadhli, A., & el Rawi, R. (1980). Effect of electroconvulsive therapy on diabetes mellitus. *Lancet, 2*, 775–777.
Feinmann, C. (1985). Pain relief by antidepressants: Possible modes of action. *Pain, 23*, 1–8.
Finestone, D., & Weiner, R. (1984). Effects of ECT on diabetes mellitus. *Acta Psychiatrica Scandinavia, 70*, 321–326.
Fordyce, W. (1976). *Behavioral methods for control of chronic pain and illness.* St. Louis, MO: Mosby.
France, R., Houpt, J., & Ellinwood, E. (1984). Therapeutic effects of antidepressants in chronic pain. *General Hospital Psychiatry, 6*, 55–63.

Freud, S. (1957). *Studies on Hysteria.* New York: Basic Books.

Frohman, L. (1975). Neurotransmitters as regulators of endocrine function. *Hospital Practice, 10*, 54–67.

Gade, G., Hofeldt, F., & Treece, G. (1980). Diabetic neuropathic cachexia: Beneficial response to combination therapy with amitriptyline and fluphenazine. *243*, 1160–1161.

Geringer, E., Perlmuter, L., Stern, T., & Nathan, D. (1988a). Depression and diabetic neuropathy: A complex relationship. *Journal of Geriatric Psychiatry and Neurology, 1*(1), 11–15.

Geringer, E., Perlmuter, L., Stern, T., & Nathan, D. (1988b). Depression, diabetes, and peripheral neuropathy, manuscript in preparation.

Glassner, B., & Haldipur, C. (1983). Life events and early and late onset of bipolar disorder. *American Journal of Psychiatry, 140*, 215–217.

Gomez-Perez, F., Rull, J., & Dies, H. (1985). Nortriptyline and fluphenazine in the symptomatic treatment of diabetic neuropathy: A double-blind crossover study. *Pain, 23*, 395–400.

Grant, I., Kyle, G., Teichman, A., & Mendels, J. (1974). Recent life events and diabetes in adults. *Psychosomatic Medicine, 36*(2), 121–128.

Greden, W., Sachar, E. Altman, N., & Sassin, J. (1975). Growth hormone responses to hypoglycemia in postmenopausal depressed women. *Archives of General Psychiatry, 32*(January), 31–33.

Heizer, J., Chammas, S., Norland, C., Stillings, W., & Alpers, D. (1984). A study of the association between Crohn's disease and psychiatric illness. *Gastroenterology, 86*, 324–330.

Hendler, N. (1984). Depression caused by chronic pain. *Journal of Clinical Psychiatry, 45*(3), 30–36.

Herzberg, B., Coppen, A., & Marks, V. (1968). Glucose tolerance in depression. *British Journal of Psychiatry, 114*, 627–630.

Hinkle, L., & Wolf, S. (1950). Studies in diabetes mellitus: Changes in glucose, ketone, and water metabolism during stress. *Research Publication of the Association for Research of Nervous and Mental Disease, 29*, 338–358.

Hinkle, L., & Wolf, S. (1952). The effect of stressful life situations on the concentrations of blood glucose in diabetic and non-diabetic humans. *Diabetes, 1*. 383–401.

Hoeper, E., Nycz, G., Cleary, P., Reiger, D., & Goldberg, I. (1979). Estimated prevalence of RDC mental disorder in primary medical care. *International Journal of Mental Health, 8*, 6–15.

Hoogwerf, B. (1985). Amitriptyline treatment of painful diabetic neuropathy: An inadvertent single-patient clinical trial, letter. *Diabetes Care, 8*, 526–527.

Hudson, J.I., Hudson, M.S., Rothschild, A.J., Vignati, L., Schatzberg, A.F., & Melby, J.C. (1984). Abnormal results of dexamethasone suppression tests in nondepressed patients with diabetes mellitus. *Archives of General Psychiatry, 41*, 1086–1089.

Hyman, S. (1988). Recent developments in neurobiology: Part II: Neurotransmitter receptors and psychopharmacology. *Psychosomatics, 29*(3), 254–264.

Jacobson, A.M., & Leibovich, J.B. (1984). Psychological issues in diabetes mellitus. *Psychosomatics, 25*(1), 7–15.

Jenike, M. (1982). ECT and diabetes mellitus. *American Journal of Psychiatry, 139*, 136.

Johnstone, B. (1977). Diabetes mellitus in patients on lithium. *Lancet 2*, 935–936.

Kahana, R., & Bibring, G. (1965). Personality types in medical management. In N. Zinberg (Ed.), *Psychiatry and Medical Practice in a General Hospital* (pp. 108–123). New York: International Universities Press.

Kaplan, G., Roberts, R., Camacho, T., & Coyne, J. (1987). Psychosocial predictors of depression. Prospective evidence from the human population laboratory studies. *American Journal of Epidemiology, 125*, 206–220.

Katon, W. (1984). Depression: Relationship to somatization and medical illness. *Journal of Clinical Psychiatry, 45*, 4–11.

Khurana, R. (1983). Treatment of painful diabetic neuropathy with trazodone [letter] (*Journal of the American Medical Association, 250*, 1392.

Kisch, E. (1986). Stressful events and the onset of non-insulin-dependent diabetes mellitus. *Israel Journal of Medical Sciences, 22*, 466–467.

Kolodney, R. (1971). Sexual dysfunction in diabetic females. *Diabetes, 20*, 557–559.

Kondziela, J., Kaufmann, M., & Klein, M. (1985). Diabetic ketoacidosis associated with lithium: Case report. *Journal of Clinical Psychiatry, 46*, 492–493.

Koranyi, E.K. (1979). Morbidity and rate of undiagnosed physical illnesses in a psychiatric clinic population. *Archives of General Psychiatry, 36*, 414–419.

Kronfol, Z., Greden, J., & Carroll, B. (1981). Psychiatric aspects of diabetes mellitus: Diabetes and depression. *British Journal of Psychiatry, 139*, 172.

Kvinesdal, B., Molin, J., Froland, A., & Gram, L. (1984). Imapramine treatment of painful diabetic neuropathy. *251*, 1727–1730.

Kymiss, P., Shatin, L., & Brown, W. (1979). Relationship between high fasting blood sugar and depression in a mental hygiene clinic population. *Canadian Journal of Psychiatry, 24*, 133–138.

Landis, B., Jovanovic, L., Landis, E., Peterson, C. Groshen, S., Johnson, K., & Miller, N. (1985). Effect of stress reduction on daily glucose range in previously stabilized insulin-dependent diabetic patients, letter. *Diabetes Care, 8*, 624–626.

Leigh, H., & Kramer, S. (1984). The psychiatric manifestations of endocrine disease. *Advances in Internal Medicine, 29*, 413–445.

Lentle, B., & Thomas, J. (1964). Adrenal function and the complications of diabetes mellitus. *Lancet, 2*, 544–549.

Lewinsohn, P., & Amenson, C. (1978). Some relations between pleasant and unpleasant mood-related events and depression. *Journal of Abnormal Psychology, 87*, 644–654.

Lilliker, S.L. (1980). Prevalence of diabetes in a manic-depressive population. *Comprehensive Psychiatry, 21*, 270–275.

Lustman, P.J., Amado, H., & Wetzel, R.D. (1983). Depression in diabetes:A critical appraisal. *Comprehensive Psychiatry, 24*, 65–74.

Lustman, P.J., Griffith, L.S., Clouse, R.E., & Cryer, P.E. (1986a). Psychiatric illness in diabetes mellitus: Relationship to symptoms and glucose control. *Journal of Nervous and Mental Disease, 174*, 736–742.

Lustman, P., & Harper, G. (1987). Nonpsychiatric physicians' identification and treatment of depression in patients with diabetes. *Comprehensive Psychiatry, 28*, 22–27.

Lustman, P., Harper, G., Griffith, L., & Clouse, R. (1986b). Use of the diagnostic interview schedule in patients with diabetes mellitus. *Journal of Nervous and Mental Disease, 174*, 743–746.

MacKenzie, R., & Trulson, M. (1978a). Does insulin act directly on the brain to increase tryptophan levels? *Journal of Neurochemistry, 30*, 1205–1208.

MacKenzie, R., & Trulson, M. (1978b). Effects of insulin and streptozotocin-induced diabetes on brain tryptophan and serotonin metabolism in rats. *Journal of Neurochemistry, 30*, 205–211.

MacKenzie, R., & Trulson, M. (1978c). Regional accumulation of tryptophan and serotonin metabolism following tryptophan loading in diabetic rats. *Journal of Neurochemistry, 31*, 157–160.

Magni, G., De Leo, D., & Schifano, F. (1985). Depression in geriatric and adult medical inpatients. *Journal of Clinical Psychology, 41*, 337–344.

Martin, L. (1981). Impotence in diabetes: An overview. *Psychosomatics, 22*(4), 318–329.

Mason, J. (1968). A review of psychoendocrine research on the pituitary-adrenal cortical system. *Psychosomatic Medicine, 30*, 576–597.

Maudsley, H. (1899). *The pathology of the mind* (3rd ed.). New York: Appleton.

Max, M. Culnane, M., Schafer, S., Gracely, R., Walther, D., Smoller, B., & Dubner, R. (1987). Amitriptyline relieves diabetic neuropathy in patients with normal or depressed mood. *Neurology, 37*, 589–596.

McEwen, B. (1975). The brain as a target organ of endocrine hormones. *Hospital Practice, 10*, 95–104.

McKay, D., Blake, R., Colwill, J., Brent, E., McCauley, J., Umlauf, R., Stearman, G., & Kivlahan, D. (1985). Social supports and stress as predictors of illness. *Journal of Family Practice, 20*, 575–581.

Menninger, W.C. (1935). Psychological factors in the aetiology of diabetes. *The Journal of Nervous and Mental Disease, 81*, 1–13.

Mitas, J., Mosley, C., & Drager, A. (1983). Diabetic neuropathic pain: Control by amitriptyline and fluphenazine in renal insufficiency. *Southern Medical Journal, 76*, 462–467.

Morley, G., Mooradian, A., Levine, A., & Morley, J. (1984). Mechanism of pain in diabetic peripheral neuropathy: Effect of glucose on pain perception in humans. *American Journal of Medicine, 77*, 79–82.

Mueller, P.S., Heninger, G.R., & McDonald, R.K. (1969). Intravenous glucose tolerance test in depression. *Archives of General Psychiatry, 21*, 470–477.

Nathan, D., Singer, D. Godine, J., Hodgson-Harrington, C., & Perlmuter, L. (1986). Retinopathy in older type II diabetics: Association with glucose control. *Diabetes, 35*, 797-801.

Nathan, D., Singer, D. Godine, J., & Perlmuter, L. (1986). Non-insulin-dependent diabetes in older patients: Complications and risk factors. *American Journal of Medicine, 81*, 837–842.

Nelson, W., Orr, W., & Sullivan, C. (1982–83). Use of the dexamethasone suppression test on a combined medicine-psychiatry inpatient unit. *International Journal of Psychiatry in Medicine, 12*, 103–109.

Normand, P., & Jenike, M. (1984). Lowered insulin requirements after ECT. *Psychosomatics, 25*, 418–419.

Nuckolls, K., Cassel, J., & Kaplan, B. (1972). Psychosocial assets, life crisis, and the prognosis of pregnancy. *American Journal of Epidemiology, 95*, 431–441.

O'Neil, M., Lancee, W., & Freeman, S. (1986). Psychosocial factors and depressive disease. *Journal of Nervous and Mental Disease, 174*, 15–23.

Perlmuter, L., Hakami, M., Hodgson-Harrington, C., Ginsberg, J., Katz, J., Singer, D., & Nathan, D. (1984). Decreased cognitive function in aging non-insulin dependent diabetics. *American Journal of Medicine, 77*, 1043–1048.

Poland, R., Rubin, R., Lesser, I., Lane, L., & Hart, P. (1987). Neuroendocrine aspects of primary endogenous depression: Serum concentrations and hypothalamic-pituitary-adrenal cortical activity as determinants of the dexamethasone suppression test response. *Archives of General Psychiatry, 44*, 790–795.

Popkin, M., Callies, A., Lentz, R., Colon, E., & Sutherland, D. (1988). Prevalence of major depression, simple phobia, and other psychiatric disorders in patients with long-standing Type I diabetes mellitus. *Archives of General Psychiatry, 45*, 64–68.

Post, F. (1962). *Significance of affective symptoms in old age: A follow-up study of 100 patients.* New York: Oxford University Press.

Pryce, I. (1964). The relationship between 17-hydroxycorticosteroid excretion and glucose utilization in depressions. *British Journal of Psychiatry, 110*, 90–94.

Pyke, D., & Watkins, P. (1980). Diabetes and ECT. *Lancet, 2*, 980–981.

Rihmer, Z., & Arato, M. (1982). Depression and diabetes mellitus: A study of the relationship between serum cortisol and blood sugar levels in patients with endogenous depression. *Neuropsychobiology, 8*, 315–318.

Robinson, N., & Fuller, J. (1985). Role of life events and difficulties in the onset of diabetes mellitus. *Journal of Psychosomatic Research, 29*, 583–591.

Robinson, R., Lipsey, J., & Price, T. (1985). Post-stroke depression. Diagnosis and management. *Psychosomatics, 26*, 769–778.

Rodin, G. (1983). Psychosocial aspects of diabetes mellitus. *Canadian Journal of Psychiatry, 28*, 219–222.

Rodin, G., & Voshart, K. (1986). Depression in the medically ill: An overview. *American Journal of Psychiatry, 143*, 696–704.

Romano, J., & Turner, J. (1985). Chronic pain and depression: Does the evidence support a relationship? *Psychological Bulletin, 97*, 18–34.

Roy, A., Pickar, D., De Jong, J., Karoum, F., & Linnoila, M. (1988). Norepinephrine and its metabolites in cerebrospinal fluid, plasma, and urine. *Archives of General Psychiatry, 45*, 849–859.

Rubin, R. (1967). Adrenal cortical activity changes in manic-depressive illness. *Archives of General Psychiatry, 17*, 671–679.

Rubin, R., Poland, R., Lesser, I., Winston, R., & Blodgett, A. (1987). Neuroendocrine aspects of primary endogenous depression; Cortisol secretory dynamics in patients and matched controls. *Archives of General Psychiatry, 44*, 328–344.

Ruegg, R., Zisook, S., & Swerdlow, N. (1988). Depression in the aged: An overview. *Psychiatric Clinics of North America, 11*, 83–109.

Sachar, E. (1967). Corticosteroids in depressive illness: A reevaluation of control issues and the literature. *Archives of General Psychiatry, 17*, 544–553.

Sachar, E., Asnis, G., Halbreich, U., Nathan, S., & Halpern, F. (1980). Recent studies in the neuroendocrinology of major depressive disorders. *Psychiatric Clinics of North America, 3*, 313–326.

Sachar, E., Finklestein, J., & Hellman, L. (1971). Growth hormone responses in depressive illness: Response to insulin tolerance test. *Archives of General Psychiatry, 25*, 263–269.

Sachar, E. Hellman, L., Roffwarg, P., Halpern, F., Fukishima, D., & Gallagher, T. (1973). Disrupted 24-hour patterns of cortisol secretion in psychotic depression. *Archives of General Psychiatry, 28*, 19–24.

Sarason, I., Sarason, B., Potter, E., & Antoni, M. (1985). Life events, social support, and illness. *Psychosomatic Medicine, 47*, 156–163.

Schaefer, A., Brown, J., Watson, C., Plemel, D., DeMotts, J., Howard, M., Petrik, N., & Balleweg, B. (1985). Comparison of the validities of the Beck, Zung, and MMPI depression scales. *Journal of Clinical and Consulting Psychiatry, 53*, 415–418.

Schildkraut, J., Schatzberg, A., Mooney, J., & Orsulak, P. (1983). Depressive disorders and the emerging field of psychiatric chemistry. In L. Grinspoon (Ed.), *Psychiatry Update* (pp. 457–471). Washington, DC: American Psychiatric Press.

Schlesser, M., Winokur, G., & Sherman, B.M. (1980). Hypothalamic-pituitary-adrenal axis activity in depressive illness. *Archives of General Psychiatry, 37*, 737–743.

Schulberg, H., Saul, M., McClelland, M., Ganguli, M., Christy, W., & Frank, R. (1985). Assessing depression in primary medical and psychiatric practices. *Archives of General Psychiatry, 42*, 1164–1170.

Seligman, M. (1972). Learned helplessness. *Annual Review of Medicine, 67*, 695–707.

Serio, M., Tarquini, B., Contini, P., Bucolassi, A., & Toccafondi, R. (1968). Plasma cortisol response to insulin and circadian rhythm in diabetic subjects. *Diabetes, 17*, 124–126.

Spring, B., Chiodo, J., & Bowen, D. (1987). Carbohydrates, tryptophan, and behavior: A methodologic review. *Psychological Bulletin, 102*, 234–256.

Surridge, D., Williams Erdahl, D., Lawson, J., Donald, M., Monga, T., Bird, C., & Letemendia, F. (1984). Psychiatric aspects of diabetes mellitus. *British Journal of Psychiatry, 145*, 269–276.

Surwit, R., & Feinglos, M. (1983). The effects of relaxation on glucose tolerance in non-insulin-dependent diabetes. *Diabetes Care, 6*, 176–179.

Thomas, A., Goldney, R., & Phillips, P. (1983). Depression, electroconvulsive therapy and diabetes mellitus. *Australian and New Zealand Journal of Psychiatry, 17*, 289–291.

Tollefson, G., & Lesar, T. (1983). Nonketotic hyperglycemia associated with loxapine and amoxapine: A case report. *Journal of Clinical Psychiatry, 44*, 347–348.

True, B., Perry, P., & Burns, E. (1987). Profound hypoglycemia with the addition of a tricyclic antidepressant to maintenance sulfonylurea therapy. *American Journal of Psychiatry, 144*, 1220–1221.

Trulson, M., & Himmel, C. (1985). Effects of insulin and streptozotocin-induced diabetes on brain norepinephrine metabolism in rats. *Journal of Neurochemistry, 44*, 1873–1876.

Trulson, M., & MacKenzie, R. (1980). Increased tryptophan hydroxylase activity may compensate for decreased brain tryptophan levels in streptozotocin-induced diabetic rats. *The Journal of Pharmacology and Experimental Therapeutics, 212*, 269–273.

Tun, P., Perlmuter, L., Russo, P., & Nathan, D. (1987). Memory self-assessment and performance in aged diabetics and non-diabetics. *Experimental Aging Research, 13*, 151–157.

Turk, D., & Salovey, P. (1984). Chronic pain as a variant of depressive disease: A critical reappraisal. *Journal of Nervous and Mental Disease, 172*, 398–404.

Turkington, R. (1980). Depression masquerading as diabetic neuropathy. *243*, 1147–1150.

van der Velde, C.D., & Gordon, M.W. (1969). Manic-depressive illness, diabetes mellitus, and lithium carbonate. *Archives of General Psychiatry, 21*, 478–485.

Vestergaard, P., & Schou, M. (1987). Does long-term lithium treatment induce diabetes mellitus?: *Neuropsychobiology, 17*, 130–132.

Weisman, A. (1987). Coping with illness. In T. Hackett, & N. Cassem (Ed.), *Massachusetts General Hospital of General Hospital Psychiatry*. Littleton, MA: PSG Publishing Co, Inc.

Weissman, M.M., & Boyd, J.H. (1983). The epidemiology of affective disorders: rates and risk factors. In L. Grinspoon (Ed.), *Psychiatry update* (pp. 406–428). Washington, DC: American Psychiatric Press.

Weissman, M., & Klerman, G. (1977). Sex differences and the epidemiology of depression. *Archives of General Psychiatry, 34*, 98–111.

Wickstrom, L., & Pettersson, K. (1964). Treatment of diabetics with monoamine-oxidase inhibitors. *Lancet, 2*, 995–997.

Wilkinson, D.G. (1981). Psychiatric aspects of diabetes mellitus. *British Journal of Psychiatry, 138*, 1–9.

Wilkinson, G., Borsey, D., Leslie, P., Newton, R., Lind, C., & Ballinger, C. (1987). Psychiatric disorder in patients with insulin-dependent diabetes mellitus attending a general hospital clinic: two stage screening and detection by physicians. *Psychological Medicine, 17*, 515–517.

Willis, T. (1684). *Pharmaceutie rationalis. The works of Thomas Willis* London: Dring Harper and Leigh.

Wing, R., Epstein, L., & Nowalk, M. (1986). Behavioral self-regulation in the treatment of patients with diabetes mellitus. *Psychological Bulletin, 99*, 78–89.

Woods, S., Tesar, G., Murray, G., & Cassem, N. (1986). Psychostimulant treatment of depressive disorders secondary to medical illness. *Journal of Clinical Psychiatry, 47*, 12–16.

Woolf, C., & Wall, P. (1983). Endogenous opiod peptides and pain mechanisms: a complex relationship. *Nature, 306*, 739–1087.

Yudofsky, S., & Rosenthal, N. (1980). ECT in a depressed patient with adult onset diabetes mellitus. *American Journal of Psychiatry, 137*, 100–101.

Author Index

Subject Index